ESSENTIALS OF

MOLECULAR PHARMACOLOGY

Background for Drug Design

ANDREJUS KOROLKOVAS

Doctor in Pharmacy and Biochemistry
Assistant Professor of Pharmaceutical Chemistry
University of São Paulo, São Paulo, Brazil

"The narrow mind seizes upon details;
the large mind grasps the essentials."

John W. Beatty

WILEY-INTERSCIENCE

a Division of John Wiley & Sons, Inc.

NEW YORK · LONDON · SYDNEY · TORONTO

Library of Congress Catalog Card Number: 74–112849

SBN 471   50418   1

Printed in the United States of America

10 9 8 7 6 5 4 3 2 1

This book is dedicated to my wife

R U Z E N A

for her deep affection, unfailing patience,

and unceasing encouragement

PREFACE

The vast progress that came about in the last decades in chemistry and biochemistry as a result of the application of modern theories of chemical structure and the use of refined equipment has produced a real and strong impact on the manner of viewing pharmacology and related sciences, such as pharmacodynamics and pharmaceutical chemistry. The introduction of these new concepts made obsolete the teaching and studying of these sciences as a haphazard accumulation of facts. Countless plausible hypotheses explaining the mechanism of action of many drugs were presented. Several theories on this subject were advanced and properly justified. Some unifying principles were either discovered or proposed. These recent acquisitions have permitted rationalizing the learning and teaching of the biomedical sciences.

This book is an attempt to expound the fundamentals of pharmacology, pharmacodynamics, and pharmaceutical chemistry in the light of not only the modern theories of chemistry and biochemistry—basic sciences—but also of new knowledge discovered in all the related fields. In this introductory text of molecular pharmacology the basic principles of interaction between chemical compounds and biological systems through the most advanced theories on drug action and the mechanisms of drug action are covered in the plane in which all these phenomena are being studied—that is, at the *molecular* or, better still, at the *submolecular* level. This book will also serve as an introduction to the potential new field of *electronic* pharmacology. It provides to interested readers the opportunity to make a more profound study of the items covered. At the end of each chapter a bibliography of recent papers, which have served as sources of information, is given.

This textbook is addressed mainly to students of medicine, veterinary medicine, dentistry, pharmacy, and biochemistry, for whom it can serve both as a text and as a reference source. However in any case it must be necessarily supplemented by traditional textbooks of pharmacology. It is also hoped that students of chemistry and biology will find in it useful information. This basic text will have at least the merit of informing them of the practical applications of chemistry and biology in various fields of the biomedical sciences. Obviously all readers of this textbook are supposed to have a working knowledge of chemistry, physics, biology, and mathematics.

The idea to write this book, a long-cherished desire, was born during the special course on drug design I taught in 1967 at the Universidade de São Paulo and Universidade Federal de Santa Maria, Rio Grande do Sul. The needed stimulus for this undertaking was supplied by appeals not only from my undergraduate students in the regular course of pharmaceutical chemistry but also from those pharmacists, physicians, chemists, biologists, nurses, and other professionals who attended two courses on mechanisms of drug action I organized at the Universidade de São Paulo in 1968.

The first manuscript of this book, which was written in Portuguese, essentially identical to the present text, was completed in December 1968. My work of writing it in Brazil was made easier by the help of many librarians, particularly those from Conjunto das Químicas, Instituto Butantan, Laborterápica-Bristol S.A., Instituto Biológico, Faculdade de Medicina da Universidade de São Paulo, and Escola Paulista de Medicina. To these, I express my gratitude, especially to Sra. Fernanda I. Piochi, head librarian of the library of Conjunto das Químicas da Cidade Universitária da Universidade de São Paulo. Also, my daughter Miriam Mirna was of great help in preparing copies of the manuscript. My colleague Dr. João Fernandes Magalhães read the original copy and gave some profitable suggestions on the arrangement of the matter. Professor Gil Soares Bairão took his valuable time to read the manuscript thoroughly. From both these fellow countrymen I received warm encouragement.

The publication of this book in English was made possible by the keen interest, unceasing stimulation, and invaluable help of Professor Joseph H. Burckhalter, chairman of the Interdepartmental Program in Medicinal Chemistry at the University of Michigan. This is the program with which I have been affiliated since January of this year, owing to a Fulbright Fellowship granted by the Committee on International Exchange of Persons through its Conference Board of Associated Research Councils, whose program officer is Mrs. John D. Leary. Actually the initiative to submit this manuscript for publication was taken by Professor Burckhalter.

My program of studies and research at the University of Michigan gave me the opportunity to bring the original manuscript up to date by adding some comments and references from the most recent research in the field of molecular pharmacology. Some of these papers were brought to my attention by professors, lecturers, and graduate students in medicinal chemistry at this university, especially Bern Hapke and Victor Esteban Marquez-Muskus, who also read critically parts of the manuscript. Mrs. JoAnn Dionne, librarian at the University of Michigan Chemistry–Pharmacy Library, helped me to locate some books and journals.

In the translation of the manuscript from Portuguese to English my former student Eleonora Budniok helped me in two chapters. Most of the language of the final English manuscript was corrected by Professor Joseph H. Burck-halter, Dr. Fortüne Kohen, assistant professor at the University of Michigan, and Mrs. Susan Kruger, a pharmacist graduated from the University of Michigan. However the errors still left are mine. The greatest amount of typing was done by Mrs. Martha P. Harris. The job of proofreading the typed manuscript was again performed with the help of my daughter. To all these dear friends I extend my heartfelt gratitude.

I wish to acknowledge also the assistance of the editors of Wiley-Interscience in preparing the manuscript for publication. And, last but not least, many thanks to the authors who so kindly gave their permission to reproduce portions of their papers and to the editors and publishers who so graciously granted their permission to reprint copyright material.

To all who have contributed to this book in any way, I thank again, this time in Portuguese, "Muito obrigado!"

In spite of the care taken in the preparation of this text, it is certain that mistakes and imperfections still remain, and all criticisms and suggestions toward extirpation of errors or refinement of contents will be welcome.

ANDREJUS KOROLKOVAS

Ann Arbor, Michigan
December 1969

CONTENTS

xi

ESSENTIALS OF
MOLECULAR PHARMACOLOGY

CHAPTER

1

BASIC CONSIDERATIONS

Drug receptor interactions may eventually be visualized as the interaction
of 3-dimensionally defined molecular entities.

Henry G. Mautner

I. INTRODUCTION

"What is man in nature? Nothing before infinity, everything before nothing,
middle term between the nothing and the everything."

In these simple but expressive words, Pascal places man between the
infinitely great and the infinitely small. From this privileged position, since
the time of his appearance on Earth he, incited by innate curiosity and
applying his faculties of intelligence and reasoning, has been trying with
perseverance and even tenacity to penetrate the mysteries of the macrocosm
and extricate the secrets of the microcosm.

Thanks to the very rapid advances of science and technology, admirable
have been his deeds, in one field as well as in another.

In the world of the infinitely great, by using balloons, aerostats, artificial
satellites, and similar engines, he has gathered knowledge concerning the
atmosphere; by resorting to rockets and spaceships, he has collected a
substantial amount of information about outer space and, particularly,

1

about our neighbors the moon and planets; by utilizing the telescope, radar, the radiotelescope, and other instruments, he has obtained data on planets, stars, and galaxies.

In the world of the infinitely small, by availing himself of microscopes with greater and greater powers of resolution, he has succeeded in seeing minuscule beings, such as protozoa, bacteria, rickettsia, and viruses; by using special devices and methods, he has been able to elucidate the structure and chemical constitution of several components of vital unity, including those responsible for the transmission of hereditary characteristics; by employing disintegrators, accelerators, and other instruments that he has been ever improving, he has contrived to detect the elementary particles and determine their mass, electric charge, half-life, and other properties.

This unceasing search for truth has reached all branches of science. This scrutinizing has affected all of them. In consequence in chemistry and biology a real revolution has occurred, not lesser than the one that has taken place in others—particularly in physics. As a result of the influence of new information and of new concepts—which have given origin to bold theories—today efforts are being made to explain the action of chemical compounds on biological systems with increasing specificity. This action is described as it pertains not only to organisms, systems, organs, and tissues but also, and mainly, to cells (*1*), and even to the *molecules* (*2,3*) that constitute the organism, since the fundamental mechanism of action of a certain substance on a living being is usually an interaction of this substance with the biological system at the *molecular level*.

Taking into account a series of factors until recently either unknown or ignored, it is therefore at the *molecular level* and even at the *submolecular level* (*4*)—namely, at the *very intimate of molecules*—that nowadays we seek the whys and hows of interaction between chemical substances used as drugs and the biological effects they cause (*5–7*). As a result of such studies new sciences or branches of already known sciences have sprung up. One of them is *molecular biology* (*8–15*). Others are *molecular biochemistry* (*16*), *molecular biophysics* (*17*), and *molecular pharmacology* (*5–7*).

II. MOLECULAR PHARMACOLOGY

Pharmacology (from the Greek φάρμακον = venom, medicine, drug, and λογια = treatise, dissertation) is the study of drug action and its mechanisms.

A *drug* is a substance of well-defined chemical structure that is used for therapeutical purposes.

Molecular pharmacology is the part of pharmacology that considers molecules as the fundamental functional units. It seeks to explain the pharmacological effects of biologically active compounds at the molecular level; that is, on the basis of molecular interactions and in terms of molecular structures and physicochemical properties. Its aim is to determine and interpret the relationship between chemical structure and biological activity (*5,7,18*).

It is evident that this relationship should be very close, for the chemical substance used as a drug as well as the biological system are, in the last analysis, made up of molecules; these, in turn, of atoms; and these, finally, of fundamental particles. Interaction between a chemical substance and a biological system—or *chemobiodynamic interaction*, as Schueler (*19*) has called it—is the factor responsible for the effect caused by a drug on an organism. Once it is understood what type of interaction occurs between the chemical compound and the molecules of the cells of the organism to which it is administered, it is possible to explain the drug's mechanism of action at the molecular level.

Owing to the paucity of present knowledge, particularly of molecular biochemistry and molecular physiology, attempts to propose such a mechanism of action for most drugs are often disappointing. Usually the explanations that are presented are either incomplete or superficial (*20*). Nevertheless the little that is already known is encouraging researchers to continue their investigations and elaborate new theories to explain further results, which in increasing numbers are being obtained in different areas of knowledge relating to this subject.

REFERENCES

1. G. Deysson, *Actualités Pharmacol.*, **16**, 61 (1963).
2. E. J. Ariëns and A. M. Simonis, *J. Pharm. Pharmacol.*, **16**, 137 (1964).
3. H. G. Mautner, *Pharmacol. Rev.*, **19**, 107 (1967).
4. A. G. Szent-Györgyi, *Introduction to a Submolecular Biology*, Academic, New York, 1960.
5. E. J. Ariëns, Ed., *Molecular Pharmacology*, Vol. I, Academic, New York, 1964.
6. W. C. Holland, R. L. Klein, and A. H. Briggs, *Introduction to Molecular Pharmacology*, Macmillan, New York, 1964.
7. E. J. Ariëns, *Progr. Drug Res.*, **10**, 429 (1966).
8. G. S. Stent, *Molecular Biology of Bacterial Viruses*, Freeman, San Francisco, 1963.
9. G. H. Haggis, D. Michie, A. R. Muir, K. B. Roberts, and P. M. B. Walker, *Introduction to Molecular Biology*, Wiley, New York, 1964.
10. W. Hayes, *The Genetics of Bacteria and Their Viruses: Studies in Basic Genetics and Molecular Biology*, Wiley, New York, 1964.
11. A. L. Lehninger, *Bioenergetics: The Molecular Basis of Biological Energy Transformations*, Benjamin, New York, 1965.
12. R. F. Steiner, *The Chemical Foundations of Molecular Biology*, Van Nostrand, Princeton, N.J., 1965.
13. J. D. Watson, *Molecular Biology of the Gene*, Benjamin, New York, 1965.

14. L. Broglie, Ed., *Wave Mechanics and Molecular Biology*, Addison-Wesley, Reading, Mass., 1966.
15. C. U. M. Smith, *Molecular Biology: A Structural Approach*, Faber and Faber, London, 1968.
16. E. M. Kosower, *Molecular Biochemistry*, McGraw-Hill, New York, 1962.
17. R. B. Setlow and E. C. Pollard, *Molecular Biophysics*, Addison-Wesley, Reading, Mass., 1962.
18. E. J. Ariëns, *Farmaco*, (*Pavia*), *Ed. Sci.*, **23**, 52 (1968).
19. F. W. Schueler, *Chemobiodynamics and Drug Design*, McGraw-Hill, New York, 1960.
20. L. S. Goodman and A. Gilman, Eds., *The Pharmacological Basis of Therapeutics*, 3rd ed., Macmillan, New York, 1965.

2

TYPES OF DRUG ACTION

The structure of a compound affects two properties which are closely interrelated in relation to its biological activity. These two properties are the physical characteristics and the chemical reactivity.

W. A. Sexton

I. THERMODYNAMIC ASPECTS

In order to understand the various and complex chemical and biological mechanisms involved in the action of drugs it is necessary to consider the laws of thermodynamics (*1–3*). These laws rule all processes in which there is liberation or absorption of heat or any other form of energy. Reactions that take place in biological systems are subject to these laws because they are processes that occur with change of energy.

The first law of thermodynamics states that energy cannot be created nor destroyed but only converted from one form into another. This means that the energy consumed in an anabolic process (for example, the binding of a drug to its receptor to form a great molecular complex) should be supplied by a process inverse to the anterior, that is, catabolic, in which there is liberation of energy (as in the case of dissociation of the drug–receptor complex) (*4*).

The second law of thermodynamics imposes some restrictions on the exchange of that energy. It states that conversion of heat into work is accompanied by a change in the temperature of the system. It may be represented by the equation

$$H = G + TS \tag{I}$$

where H is enthalpy, or total energy of the system; G is the Gibbs' free energy—that is, that portion of free energy which a certain system can utilize to perform work; S is entropy, the fraction of total energy that is not available for accomplishment of work—it corresponds to the vibrational energy of atoms and molecules; and T is the absolute temperature.

Since it is not possible to determine the absolute values of any specific system but only their changes, Equation I may be written as

$$\Delta H = \Delta G + T \Delta S \tag{II}$$

where ΔH is the change in enthalpy or change in internal energy, ΔG is the change in Gibbs' free energy, and ΔS is the change in entropy.

Spontaneous reactions, known as *exergonic*, are characterized by decrease in free energy; in these cases ΔG is negative. In *endergonic* reactions, which require increase in free energy, ΔG is positive (4).

In reversible reactions another factor, $\Delta G°$, which is not to be mistaken for ΔG, should be considered. It represents Gibbs' standard free-energy change when all reactants and products are in their normal states or unitary concentrations (1 atmosphere of pressure for pure gases, liquids, and solids; and 1 molal for solutes).

$$\Delta G° = -2.303 RT \log K \tag{III}$$

In the above equation R is the gas constant (1.98 cal/degree/mole), T is the absolute temperature, and K is the reaction equilibrium constant.

In the case of a reaction of the type

$$M + N \longrightarrow P + Q$$

$$\Delta G = \Delta G° + 2.303 RT \log \frac{PQ}{MN} \tag{IV}$$

where $PQ/MN = K$.

In any reaction $\Delta G°$ is always constant, because it is a defined quantity, whereas ΔG may assume any value, depending on the conditions under which the reaction takes place. If reactants and products are in their normal state, $\Delta G = \Delta G°$. In the equilibrium state $\Delta G = 0$, and Equation IV assumes the form of Equation III.

II. THE FERGUSON PRINCIPLE

By observing that in a homologous series certain physical properties—such as solubility in water, vapor pressure, capillary activity, and distribution between immiscible phases—change according a geometric progression, Ferguson (5) concluded that "molar toxic concentrations ... are largely determined by a distribution equilibrium between heterogeneous phases— the external circumambient phase where the concentration is measured and a biophase which is the primary seat of toxic action."

On the basis of this reasoning, from Equation IV he deduced the following:

$$\ln a = \frac{(\bar{G} - \bar{G}_0)}{RT}$$

where a stands for concentration expressed as the thermodynamic activity of a drug in a gas or in a solution, $\bar{G}$ its partial molal free energy in a certain state, $\bar{G}_0$ its partial molal free energy in the normal state, R the gas constant, and T the absolute temperature.

According to Ferguson, it is not necessary to define the nature of biophase nor to measure the concentration of the drug at this site. If equilibrium conditions exist between the drug in the molecular biophase and in exobiophase— that is, in extracellular fluids—the tendency for the drug to escape from each phase is the same, even though the concentrations in the two phases are different (6,7). This tendency is given the name of *thermodynamic activity*. It is equivalent approximately to the degree of saturation of each phase. Therefore thermodynamic activity in the external phase (exobiophase) corresponds to thermodynamic activity in the molecular biophase; in practice it is the first that is measured, since it is not possible to measure the latter.

In the case of volatile drugs their thermodynamic activity is calculated from the expression p_t/p_s, where p_t is the partial pressure of the substance in solution and p_s the saturated vapor pressure of the substance at the experimental temperature. When the drug is nonvolatile, its thermodynamic activity is calculated by employing the ratio S_t/S_0, where S_t is the drug's molar concentration and S_0 its corresponding solubility.

Since both p_s and S_0 are constant, by observing changes in p_t or S_t it is possible to determine, in a relatively simple way, whether drug action is due directly to its physicochemical properties or primarily to its chemical structure.

In the first case the ratio p_t/p_s or S_t/S_0 will be large, usually from 1 to 0.01, because the drug will exert high partial pressure or will be present in high concentration in the external phase, since it is distributed over the whole organism without being firmly attached to any of its cells. The established equilibrium will be between the exobiophase and the molecular biophase.

In the second case the ratio p_t/p_s or S_t/S_0 should be small, usually less than 0.001, since the partial pressure or concentration of the drug in the external phase will be low, because it will be more or less firmly bound to certain receptors in some cells of the organism. The established equilibrium, subject to mass law, will be between drug and receptors on the cell or inside it.

By examining Table 2.1, it is seen that the biological action of the four first substances, the thermodynamic activities of which are comparable, results

TABLE 2.1   Enzymic Inhibition of Succinate Dehydrogenase and Thermodynamic Activity (8)

Compound	Molar Concentration Causing 50% Inhibition of Oxygen Uptake	a
Ethylurethane	0.65	0.117
Phenylurethane	0.003	0.20
Propionitrile	0.48	0.24
Valeronitrile	0.08	0.36
Vanillin	0.011	0.0002

almost certainly from their physicochemical properties. On the other hand, vanillin, with its very low thermodynamic activity, does not fit into the narrow range of the preceding compounds, and it probably acts as a result of its chemical structure (8).

III. STRUCTURE AND ACTIVITY

Based on the mode of pharmacological action, drugs may be divided into two great classes: structurally nonspecific and structurally specific (7–10).

A. Structurally Nonspecific Drugs

Structurally nonspecific drugs are those in which pharmacological action is not directly subordinated to chemical structure, except to the extent that structure affects physicochemical properties (11). Among these properties may be cited adsorption, solubility, pK_a, and oxidation–reduction potential, which influence permeability; and depolarization of the membrane, protein coagulation, and complex formation (12). It is assumed that structurally nonspecific drugs act by physicochemical processes for the following reasons:

1. Their biological action is directly related to thermodynamic activity, which is usually high (8), with values from 1 to 0.01; this means that such drugs act in relatively large doses.

2. Although they vary in chemical structure, they cause similar biological responses.

3. Slight modifications in their chemical structure do not result in pronounced changes in biological action.

Examples of structurally nonspecific drugs are listed in Table 2.2.

TABLE 2.2 Bactericidal Concentration and Thermodynamic Activity of Miscellaneous Compounds (8)

Substance	Bactericidal Concentration (moles/liter)	a
Phenol	0.097	0.11
o-Cresol	0.039	0.17
Ethyl alcohol	4.86	0.32
Octyl alcohol	0.0034	0.88
Propaldehyde	1.08	0.37
Thymol	0.0022	0.38
Acetone	3.89	0.40
Aniline	0.17	0.44
Cyclohexanol	0.18	0.47
Resorcinol	3.09	0.54
Methyl propyl ketone	0.39	0.56
Butyraldehyde	0.39	0.76

B. Structurally Specific Drugs

Structurally specific drugs are those whose biological action results essentially from their chemical structure, which should adapt itself to the three-dimensional structure of receptors in the organism by forming a complex with them (9,11,13). Hence in these drugs chemical reactivity, shape, size, stereochemical arrangement of the molecule, and distribution of functional groups, as well as resonance, inductive effects, electronic distribution, and possible binding with receptors, besides other factors, will play decisive roles.

Several considerations suggest that the pharmacological effect produced by these drugs results from complexation with a chemically reactive minuscule area of certain body cells whose topography and functional groups are usually complementary to those of the drugs:

1. Their biological action does not depend solely on thermodynamic activity, which is usually low (less than 0.001); this means that structurally specific drugs are effective in lesser concentration than the structurally nonspecific ones (7).

2. They have some structural characteristics in common, and the fundamental structure present in all of them, by orienting functional groups into a

similar spatial direction, is responsible for the analogous biological response they cause.

3. Slight modifications in their chemical structure may result in substantial changes in pharmacological activity, so that substances thus obtained may have actions ranging from antagonistic to similar to that of the parent compound.

To distinguish structurally nonspecific drugs from those that are structurally specific it is not enough to consider only one or two of several points of differentiation, some of which have been mentioned. *All* of them should be considered. Frequently certain drugs that have no structural similarity nevertheless exhibit similar pharmacological effects, which are not appreciably altered by slight structural variations within each chemical category. For instance, diuretics present a broad variety of chemical structure (*14–20*)—methylxanthinic, sulfamido, organomercurial, benzothiadiazino, spiro-lactonic, etc.—and their diuretic action is not much affected by slight structural modifications of the molecule of each group (*21,22*). Yet, contrary to what at first seems to be the case, diuretics are structurally *specific*. Actually they produce *analogous* pharmacological response—but by interfering with *different* biochemical processes. This phenomenon is not uncommon. Many other drugs are known to cause similar effects through different mechanisms (*6*). This consideration supports the efforts of those who seek to understand at the molecular level the various ways of producing not only diuresis but several other pharmacological effects by different types of drugs.

REFERENCES

1. G. J. Van Wylen and R. E. Sonntag, *Fundamentals of Classical Thermodynamics*, Wiley, New York, 1965.
2. R. Wurmser and R. Banerjee, "Equilibrium and Thermodynamic Considerations," in M. Florkin and E. H. Stotz, Eds., *Comprehensive Biochemistry*, Vol. XII, Elsevier, Amsterdam, 1964, pp. 18–61.
3. T. L. Hill, *Thermodynamics for Chemists and Biologists*, Addison-Wesley, Reading, Mass., 1968.
4. W. C. Holland, R. L. Klein, and A. H. Briggs, *Introduction to Molecular Pharmacology*, Macmillan, New York, 1964.
5. J. Ferguson, *Proc. Roy. Soc. (London)*, Ser. B, **127**, 387 (1939).
6. F. N. Fastier, *Ann. Rev. Pharmacol.*, **4**, 51 (1964).
7. T. C. Daniels and E. C. Jorgensen, "Physicochemical Properties in Relation to Biologic Action," in C. O. Wilson, O. Gisvold, and R. F. Doerge, Eds., *Textbook of Organic Medicinal and Pharmaceutical Chemistry*, 5th ed., Lippincott, Philadelphia, 1966, pp. 4–62.

8. W. A. Sexton, *Chemical Constitution and Biological Activity*, 3rd ed., Spon, London, 1963.
9. A. H. Beckett, *Progr. Drug Res.*, **1**, 455 (1959).
10. J. J. Lewis, *An Introduction to Pharmacology*, 3rd ed., Williams and Wilkins, Baltimore, 1964.
11. R. B. Barlow, *Introduction to Chemical Pharmacology*, 2nd ed., Methuen, London, 1964.
12. A. Sekera, *Actualités Pharmacol.*, **14**, 197 (1961).
13. T. Z. Csáky, *Introduction to General Pharmacology*, Appleton-Century-Crofts, New York, 1969.
14. T. H. Maren, *Physiol. Rev.*, **47**, 595 (1967).
15. N. Bank, *Ann. Rev. Med.*, **19**, 103 (1968).
16. A. N. Brest, R. Seller, G. Onesti, O. Ramirez, C. Swartz, and J. H. Moyer, *Am. J. Cardiol.*, **22**, 168 (1968).
17. E. J. Cafruny, *Pharmacol. Rev.*, **20**, 89 (1968).
18. E. J. Cafruny, *Ann. Rev. Pharmacol.*, **8**, 131 (1968).
19. H.-J. Hess, *Ann. Rep. Med. Chem.*, **3**, 62 (1968).
20. W. M. Kirkendall and J. H. Stein, *Am. J. Cardiol.*, **22**, 162 (1968).
21. R. W. Berliner and J. Orloff, *Pharmacol. Rev.*, **8**, 137 (1956).
22. K. H. Beyer and J. E. Baer, *Pharmacol. Rev.*, **13**, 517 (1961).

INFLUENCE OF PHYSICO-CHEMICAL PROPERTIES

The physico-chemical properties of a drug molecule are determinative as far as its ability to induce a particular biological effect is concerned. This implies that there is a relationship between the physico-chemical properties of the drug and its biological activity.

E. J. Ariëns

I. FACTORS RELATED TO BIOLOGICAL ACTIVITY

The complexity of biological systems and the series of phenomena that occur from the time the proper dosage of the drug is introduced into the organism until its final interaction with a specific receptor or organized tissues in which the desired stimulus is started can be represented schematically as shown in Figure 3.1. Hence in the transport processes of drugs, in their concentration at a certain site, and in their metabolism and interaction with biological systems three groups of factors should be considered (*1–8*):

1. The physicochemical properties: solubility, partition coefficients, degree of ionization, surface-tension activity.
2. The chemical structure: resonance, inductive effects, isosterism,

13

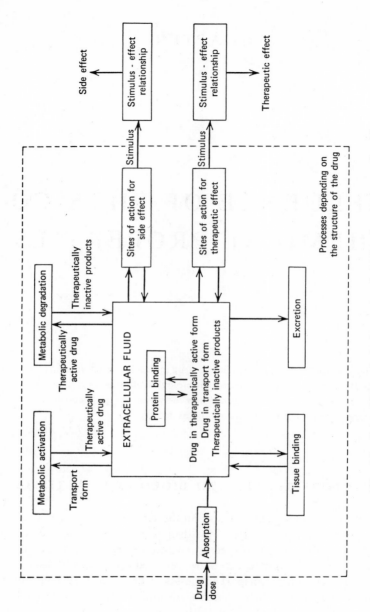

Fig. 3.1. Some of the principal processes that take place in drug action (*1*).

14

oxidation–reduction potentials, types of chemical bonds, chelation, electronic distribution, light absorption.

3. The spatial conformation: dimensional factors, interatomic distances between functional groups, stereochemistry.

II. SOLUBILITY

The term *solubility* refers to solubilities in different media and varies between two extremes: polar solvents, such as water, and nonpolar solvents, such as lipids. The name *hydrophilia*, or *lipophobia*, refers to solubility in water—and *lipophilia*, or *hydrophobia*, to that in lipids. The relationship between both is schematically represented in Figure 3.2.

Solubility is particularly relevant in homologous series, as shown in Figure 3.3. For instance, the antibacterial activities of certain normal primary alcohols, cresols, and alkyl phenols; the estrogenic activity of alkyl 4,4′-stilbenediols; and the anesthetic activity of esters of *p*-aminobenzoic acid are directly related to their liposolubility (7).

Solubility can play a fundamental role in the biological action of some drugs. For instance, in a series of isatin-β-thiosemicarbazone derivatives it was found that the antiviral activity is directly proportional to the solubility of those compounds in chloroform (Table 3.1).

Closely related to solubility is drug absorption, which is of primary importance, because the intensity of a drug's biological action will depend on the degree of absorption. Absorption processes can be active or passive. Transport across the membrane takes place through one of the following modes: direct passage, movement across membrane pores, and pinocytosis (10). For details the reader is referred to Chapter 10, Section V.

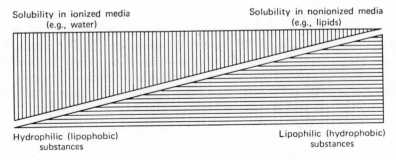

Fig. 3.2. Relationship between hydrophiles and lipophiles (4).

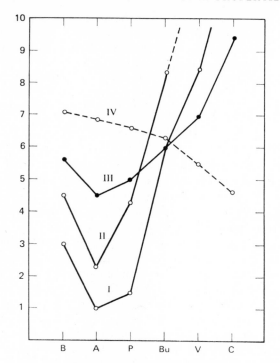

Fig. 3.3. Influence of some physicochemical properties on biological activity (7). Acids: B = Benzoic, A = phenylacetic, P = β-phenylpropionic, Bu = γ-phenylbutyric, V = δ-phenylvaleric, C = ε-phenylcaproic. I. Solubility (concentration l/m × 10^{-1}). II. Distribution coefficient (cottonseed oil–water). III. Bactericidal activity (concentration l/m × 10^{-3}). IV. Surface tension (dynes/cm × 10^{-1}).

Drugs whose chemical structures are similar to those of normal cellular metabolites can cross cellular membranes through an active absorption process. A number of lipid-insoluble substances penetrate by a passive diffusion process, although, owing to the constant motion of the cells, which confers to living tissue a character of a "stirred system," the term *passive* seems to be inadequate (*11,12*). Passive diffusion depends on the size of the pores, the molecular volume of the drugs dissolved in water, and the differences in concentrations of fluids separated by cellular membranes.

Since most drugs are not structurally similar to actively transported normal cellular metabolites, the rate of their passage across cellular membranes, which are of lipid and protein nature, will be greatly determined by their liposolubility. Compounds that are very soluble in lipids will cross membrane barriers rapidly. The contrary will happen with drugs of low solubility. Details can be found elsewhere (*13,14*).

TABLE 3.1 Correlation between Liposolubility and Anti-viral Activity of Isatin-β-thiosemicarbazone Derivatives (9)

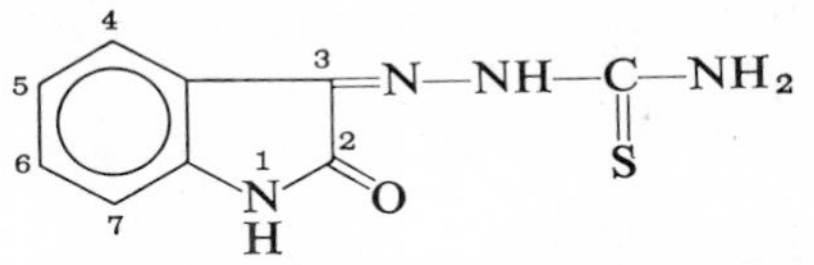

Substituent	Solubility in Chloroform	Relative Antiviral Activity
7-Carboxy	0	0
5-Methoxy	3	0.03
4-Methyl	8	3.4
4-Chloro	10	8.6
6-Fluoro	16	39.8
7-Chloro	29	85
None	32	100

Reprinted with permission from the Williams and Wilkins Company.

III. PARTITION COEFFICIENTS

The biological activity of several groups of compounds can be correlated with their partition coefficients in polar and nonpolar solvents (15,16). Overton (17) and Meyer (18) were the pioneers in these studies. They resorted to partition coefficients first to explain the activity of certain narcotics and, later, of general anesthetics. According to these authors, such compounds, because of their greater affinity for lipids (as they showed from their distribution coefficients in water–oil mixtures), fix primarily to nervous system cells, rich in lipids, and thus they owe their biological action to this phenomenon.

A better correlation was found with the oil–gas partition coefficient. By measuring the minimal alveolar concentration of several anesthetics necessary to produce a standard analgetic effect, Eger and co-workers (19) concluded that anesthetics of high liposolubility are efficient in low alveolar concentrations. According to those authors, anesthesia is induced when anesthetics reach relative saturation in some lipid structure situated in the brain. In recent studies (20,21) Eger and collaborators found good correlation between minimal alveolar concentrations and the solubilities of some general anesthetics in olive oil, but relatively poor correlation with hydrate dissociation pressure at 0°C (Figure 3.4). However, they admitted that the difference in

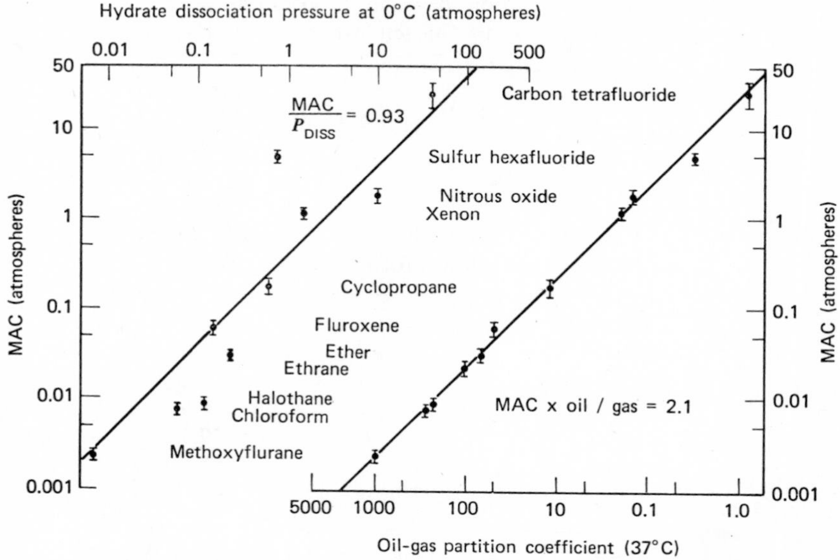

Fig. 3.4. Comparison of the correlations of minimal alveolar concentration (MAC) with hydrate dissociation pressure (left graph, upper scale) and lipid solubility (right graph, lower scale). If the data followed the correlation MAC/hydrate dissociation pressure equals a constant or MAC × oil–gas partition coefficient equals a constant, then the data should be along the 45° angle slopes as indicated. The data obtained in the experiment show that the correlation between MAC and liposolubility is far better than the one between MAC and hydrate dissociation pressure (20).

the correlations is not enough to invalidate hydrate theories (20), which will be discussed further.

The results obtained by Eger and co-workers are in agreement with the Ferguson principle, according to which, as it was seen in Chapter 2, the potency of structurally nonspecific drugs depends on the relative saturation of the biophase, that is, of some cellular compartment.

The aforementioned correlations do not explain, however, the mechanism of action of general anesthetics. They only point out the relevance of partition coefficients in predicting the biological action of these drugs.

On the basis of the fact that xenon produces narcosis, Wulf and Featherstone (22) advanced the hypothesis that anesthetic activity results from the molecular size of the compounds utilized. They showed that anesthetic activity is related to molecular volume b, which appears in the van der Waals equation

$$\left(P + \frac{a}{V^2}\right)(V - b) = RT$$

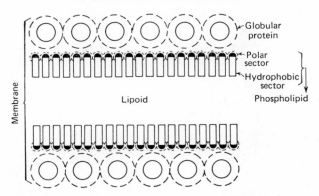

Fig. 3.5.   Danielli–Davson model of membrane structure (*23*).

The molecular volume b should be greater than that of those substances—such as water, oxygen, and nitrogen—that could normally occupy the lateral space between the lipid and the protein layers of the cellular membrane (Figures 3.5 and 3.6).

Actually the values of b for such substances are, respectively: water, 3.05; oxygen, 3.18; and nitrogen, 3.91. With a greater b value (nitrous oxide, 4.4; xenon, 5.1; ethylene, 5.7; cyclopropane, 7.5; chloroform, 10.2; ethyl ether, 13.4), when occupying the space between the lipid layers normally occupied by water, oxygen, and nitrogen, general anesthetics would cause alteration in the cellular structure and subsequent depression of function, resulting in anesthesia.

A more recent and suggestive theory of the mode of action of general anesthetics is that of Pauling (*25,26*). According to this author, the important phase of the central nervous system in anesthesia is not the lipid one, as assumed in former theories, but the aqueous one. Considering that certain

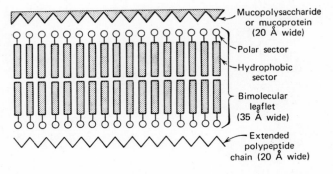

Fig. 3.6.   Schematic representation of the unit membrane hypothesis of Robertson (*24*).

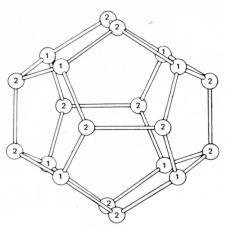

Fig. 3.7. Microcrystalline hydrate (1 = hydrogen; 2 = oxygen).

compounds, such as chloroform and xenon, form *in vitro* microcrystalline hydrates, Pauling postulated that similar crystals, made up by water molecules and called *clathrates*, would be formed in the encephalic fluid and stabilized by general anesthetics bound by the van der Waals forces to side chains of proteins and other solutes. These microcrystalline hydrates (Figure 3.7) would alter the conduction of electrical impulses necessary for the maintenance of wakefulness; in consequence narcosis or anesthesia would occur. However, in a recent paper Erlander (27) presented evidence to contradict the clathrate theory. Nevertheless it is interesting to combine Wulf and Featherstone's theory with Pauling's. By building up molecular models, both of microcrystalline hydrates and of general anesthetics, it is seen that the latter ones can be easily enclosed inside the former ones.

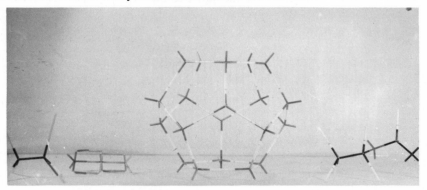

Comparative sizes of microcrystalline hydrate (second from right) and some general anesthetics (halothane, nitrous oxide, and ethyl ether).

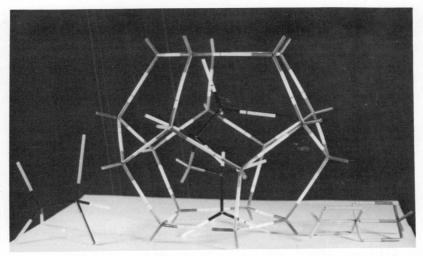

Microcrystalline hydrate containing ethyl ether in its interior. Halothane (to the left) and nitrous oxide (to the right) are outside. Both these general anesthetics can be perfectly enclosed inside the microcrystalline hydrate.

Miller (*28*) advanced a hypothesis analogous to the clathrate theory. Like Pauling, he assumes that increasing the amount of water in a more organized state in the nervous system results in a decrease in its activity. Miller's theory differs from Pauling's, however, in requiring the presence not of clathrates but of *icebergs*, microcrystals of smaller size, which would encompass the molecules of the general anesthetics. Details of the theories of the structure of water (*29–35*) and anesthesia (*36–41*) can be found in the cited references.

A. Influence of Inductive and Resonance Effects

Until the last decade no attempt was made to establish quantitatively structure–activity relationships, since this area was considered to be too complicated. Lately, however, several authors have attempted to express the degree of pharmacological action of drugs by mathematical equations (*42*). For instance, with the purpose of correlating chemical structure with the physical properties and biological activity of drugs, Hansch (*11,12,43–45*) has been studying two complex processes:

1. Movement of the drug from the point of application in the biological system to the sites of action.

2. Occurrence of a rate-limiting chemical or physical reaction in receptor sites.

Both these processes are often distant (in time and space) from the observed biological response, because the drug, before producing an effect, must cross a series of compartments made up essentially of aqueous or organic phases.

Owing to the success of Overton and Meyer and their disciples in correlating biological activity with partition coefficients, Hansch has employed a model analogous to the one used by those authors.

Hansch starts from a chemical substance of known biological action and compares its activity with that of compounds of analogous structure, differing from it only in substituent groups. He determines the distribution coefficients of the parent compound and its derivatives between water, a polar solvent, and normal octanol, a nonpolar solvent (46,47). The difference between the respective logarithms of the distribution coefficients is called π:

$$\pi_{\text{COOH}} = \log P_{\text{COOH}} - \log P_{\text{H}}$$

In the equation above π, the hydrophobicity constant, is the measure of contribution of the substituent to solubility in a series of partitions; P_{COOH} is the partition coefficient of the carboxylic derivative; P_{H} is the partition coefficient of the parent compound. If π has a positive value, it means that the substituent group increases the solubility of the compound in nonpolar solvents. If it has a negative value, the substituent group will increase the solubility of the compound in polar solvents.

Furthermore in his studies Hansch takes into consideration Hammett's equation (48), which relates the chemical structure both to equilibrium constants and to rate constants. Two parameters enter in this equation: σ, characteristic only of the substituent—it represents the ability of the group to attract or repel electrons through a combination of inductive and resonance effects; ρ, characteristic of the reaction considered—it measures the sensitivity of this type of reaction to substitution in the parent compound (49).

Hammett's equation is expressed by the formula

$$\log \left(\frac{k}{k_0} \right) = \rho \sigma$$

where k and k_0 refer to the rate constants for reaction of the derivative and the parent compound, respectively; such constants can be substituted by the equilibrium constants, K and K_0; in this case the equation takes the form

$$\log \left(\frac{K}{K_0} \right) = \rho \sigma$$

The value of σ can be obtained almost directly (49) by measuring the effect of the substituent in the ionization constant of the parent compound, because

$$\sigma = \log \left(\frac{K_{\text{COOH}}}{K_{\text{H}}} \right)$$

in which K_{COOH} and K_{H} are the ionization constants of the substituted and nonsubstituted compounds, respectively. If a substituent presents a positive

σ-value, it means that it attracts electrons; if it has a negative σ-value, it means that it donates electrons.

By using the parameters π, σ, and ρ and not taking into account steric factors, which were assumed to be constant, Hansch and his co-workers derived the following equation (50):

$$\log\left(\frac{1}{C}\right) = -k\pi^2 + k'\pi + \sigma\rho + k''$$

where C is the drug concentration necessary to produce the biological effects, and k, k', k'' are constants for the system being studied, determined through regression analysis of the equations corresponding to the derivative bio- logically tested in the series.

This equation, with slight adaptations in some cases, was applied to various groups of drugs—chloramphenicol derivatives (50), penicillins (51–53), barbiturates (54,55), sulfonamides (56), a series of monoamine oxidase inhibitors (57,58), antihistaminics (58), β-haloalkylamines (59), analgetics of the imidazoline series (60), and several antibacterial agents (61,62). Correla- tions obtained between the observed and calculated activities were good, about 0.8 to 0.9, in most cases. Examples are shown in Tables 3.2 and 3.3.

Besides the immediate interest to molecular pharmacology, the work of Hansch and colleagues toward relating the biological action to numerical constants—although on a semiempirical basis—constitutes a potentially

TABLE 3.2 Observed and Calculated Concentrations of Nonbarbiturates That Cause Hypnosis (55)

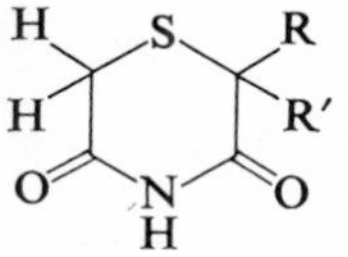

Substituents		log 1/C	
R	R'	Observed	Calculated
Methyl	Methyl	2.40	2.429
Ethyl	Ethyl	2.97	2.854
Propyl	Propyl	2.78	2.842
Butyl	Butyl	2.40	2.390
Ethyl	Butyl	3.02	2.842
Ethyl	Phenyl	2.67	2.883

Reprinted by permission of the American Chemical Society.

TABLE 3.3   Comparison of $\log K$ with $\Sigma\pi$ Where K is the *n*-Octanol–Water Partition Coefficient of the Penicillin Free Acid and $\Sigma\pi$ is the Partition-Coefficient Function of the Penicillin Side Chain (*53*)

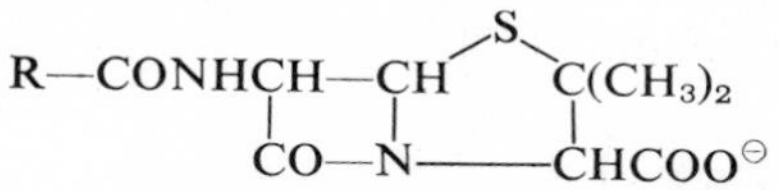

$$R\text{—CONHCH—CH} \overset{\displaystyle S}{} C(CH_3)_2$$
$$\text{CO—N———CHCOO}^{\ominus}$$

R	$\log K$	Calculated $\Sigma\pi$	Estimated $\Sigma\pi$
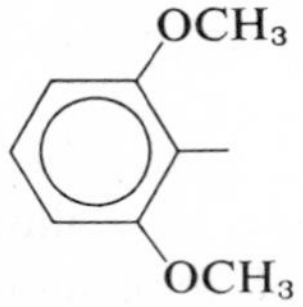 (2,6-dimethoxyphenyl with OCH$_3$ groups)	1.22	1.47	1.25
$C_6H_5CH_2$—	1.83	2.69	2.03
$C_6H_5\underset{\overset{\vert}{OH}}{CH}$—	1.40	0.89	1.48
$C_6H_5OCH_2$—	2.09	2.11	2.36
$C_6H_5\underset{\overset{\vert}{CH_3}}{OCH}$—	2.28	2.61	2.60
$C_6H_5\overset{\overset{CH_3}{\vert}}{\underset{\underset{CH_3}{\vert}}{OC}}$—	2.76	3.11	3.21
$C_6H_5\underset{\overset{\vert}{C_2H_5}}{OCH}$—	2.65	3.11	3.07

valuable contribution to the rational design of new drugs and to the elucidation of the roles played by hydrophobic, electronic, and steric factors in the interaction of drugs with receptors.

B. Influence of Polarizability

In a series of studies on the mechanism of action of antibiotics on microorganisms, Garrett and co-workers (*61*) found that data from a kinetic analysis of bacterial growth gave significant structure-activity correlations. This technique of analysis was called *microbial kinetics*. They suggested that several parameters, including molecular size and binding constants peculiar to substituents, should be taken into account in the prediction of substituents effects on biological activities.

Cammarata (63), arguing that in the case of chloramphenicol derivatives the equation derived by Hansch gives a good, but not necessarily significant, correlation ($r = 0.824$), modified Hansch's equation in the study of such compounds by resorting to microbial kinetics. He not only introduced the electronic polarizability f, which is also a measure of volume, but also divided Hammett's constant σ into its inductive and resonance parameters, σ_I and σ_R, respectively, and derived the following equation:

$$\log A = a\pi^2 + b\pi + c\sigma_I + d\sigma_R + f$$

where A is biological activity.

By using this new equation, he obtained correlations of about 0.99, or very close to unity. Although the interest in physicochemical parameters in drug design is growing, both the equation derived by Hansch and the modification of it introduced by Cammarata present some limitations and cannot be applied to all groups of drugs.

C. Utilization of Quantitative Models

Besides the linear free-energy relationship that attributes the biological activity of a molecule to contributions from various free-energy-related physicochemical parameters of the substituents, several empirical mathematical models are also being employed in the study of structure-activity relationships. In these quantitative models the observed biological activity is expressed as a function of parameters ascribed to each substituent group and/or parent portion of the molecule (42,64). These studies were started by Bruice and collaborators (65), have been developed by Free and Wilson (66), and are being pursued by Purcell and co-workers (64,67–70), Kopecký, Boček, and colleagues (71–74), and Ban and Fujita (75). Their empirical method is based on an additive mathematical model in which it is assumed that a certain substituent in a specific position contributes additively and constantly to the biological activity of a molecule in a series of chemically related compounds.

Among the equations used in such studies, the following one presented a statistically significant correlation of data for both *para-* (71) and *meta-* disubstituted benzenes (72):

$$BA = b_x + b_y + e_x e_y$$

where BA is the biological activity and the indices x and y refer to the contribution of a substituent in the positions X and Y, respectively.

Results of a successful application of the Free and Wilson's approach are shown in Table 3.4.

However, it is evident that not all biological activities can be described by this additive empirical model (64).

TABLE 3.4   Free and Wilson's Approach Applied to Some Tetracyclines (63)

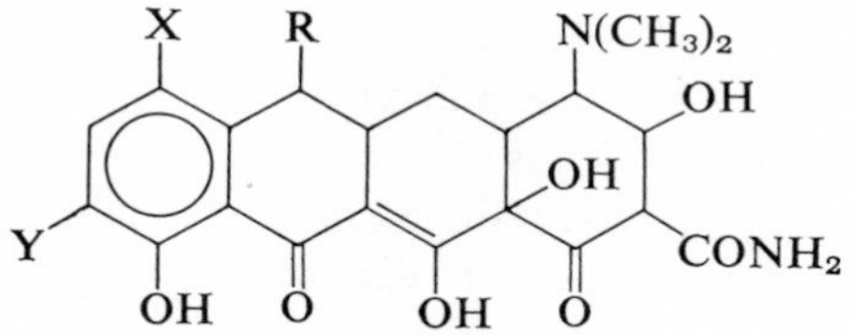

Substituents			In vitro Activity Against Staphylococcus aureus Relative to Tetracycline	
R	X	Y	Observed	Calculated
H	Cl	NH_2	525	443
H	Br	NH_2	320	343
H	NO_2	NH_2	275	333
CH_3	NO_2	NH_2	160	146
CH_3	Br	NH_2	140	156
CH_3	Br	CH_3CONH	75	51
H	NO_2	NO_2	60	-8
H	Cl	NO_2	21	102
H	Br	NO_2	15	2
CH_3	NO_2	CH_3CONH	15	41

Reprinted by permission of the American Chemical Society.

D. Use of Molar Attraction Constants

With the purpose of determining the relative degree of drug–receptor interaction in a series of structurally related compounds, Ostrenga (76) used the molar attraction constants, expressed by the equation

$$F = (EV)^{\frac{1}{2}}$$

where E is the potential energy and V is the molar volume. This equation is deduced from the solubility parameter δ:

$$\delta = \frac{(EV)^{\frac{1}{2}}}{V} = \frac{F}{V}$$

which appears in an equation that relates the enthalpy of two chemical species that interact in terms not of free energy and entropy but of other physical parameters: molar volume V, mole fraction X, volume fraction ϕ, and the solubility parameter δ:

$$\Delta H \simeq (V_1 X_1 + V_2 X_2)\phi_1\phi_2(\delta_1 - \delta_2)^2$$

By applying this constant to six different classes of compounds Ostrenga found a high degree of correlation between chemical structure and biological activity: in one case, of 0.965. He therefore concluded that F is related to Hansch's π, which is conceivable since the partition phenomena and the physical interactions are dependent on chemical structure. Table 3.5 shows the results obtained with penicillin derivatives. However, this method has also limited applicability (76).

TABLE 3.5 Effective Concentration for the Activity of Penicillin Derivatives on *Staphylococcus aureus* in Mice (76)

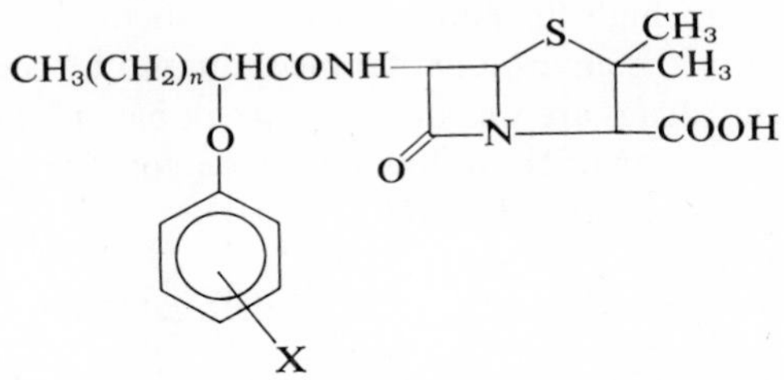

Function	F	Log $(1/C)$ Observed	Calculated	Δ Log $(1/C)$
H	1061	5.86	5.75	0.11
4-Cl	1239	5.79	5.43	0.36
4-OCH$_3$	1253	5.69	5.40	0.29
α-Et ($n = 1$)	1194	5.54	5.51	0.03
4-NO$_2$	1256	5.53	5.40	0.13
2-Cl	1239	5.40	5.43	0.03
2,5-Cl$_2$	1417	5.24	5.11	0.13
α-Pr ($n = 2$)	1327	5.03	5.27	0.24
3,5-(CH$_3$)$_2$	1305	5.03	5.31	0.28
α-Bu ($n = 3$)	1460	5.01	5.03	0.02
2,4-Cl$_2$	1417	4.97	5.11	0.14
2,4-Br$_2$	1557	4.87	4.86	0.01
2,3,6-Cl$_3$	1595	4.72	4.79	0.07
4-Cyclohexyl	1762	4.70	4.49	0.21
4-*tert*-Bu	1518	4.67	4.93	0.26
3,4,5-(CH$_3$)$_3$	1427	4.65	5.09	0.44
4-*tert*-Amyl, α-Et	1784	4.57	4.45	0.12
Cl$_5$	1951	4.25	4.15	0.10

Although numerous attempts to correlate biological activity with several physicochemical and empirical parameters have been reported, their ultimate value in drug design, even when correlations are statistically significant, remains to be tested.

IV. DEGREE OF IONIZATION

The partially lipidic nature of cellular membranes (such as the ones that enwrap the stomach, small intestine, mucosa, nervous tissue) facilitates the passage of drugs with high liposolubility across them. This liposolubility is affected by the pH of the environmental medium and by the degree of dissociation pK_a. Usually drugs are weak acids or weak bases. The degree of dissociation pK_a is calculated from the following Henderson–Hasselbach equations:

In the case of acids: $RCOOH \rightarrow RCOO^{\ominus} + H^{\oplus}$

$$pK_a = pH + \log \frac{[\text{undissociated acid}]}{[\text{ionized acid}]}$$

$$= pH + \log \frac{[RCOOH]}{[RCOO^{\ominus}][H^{\oplus}]}$$

In the case of bases: $R\overset{\oplus}{N}H_3 \rightarrow RNH_2 + H^{\oplus}$

$$pK_a = pH + \log \frac{[\text{ionized base}]}{[\text{undissociated base}]}$$

$$= pH + \log \frac{[R\overset{\oplus}{N}H_3]}{[RNH_2]}$$

Weak acids have a high pK_a; weak bases, a low pK_a. Data on the pK_a of many organic acids (77) and bases (78) are available. The biological activity of certain acids and bases is directly related to their degree of ionization. Whereas some (e.g., phenols, carboxylic acids) act in the molecular form, others (e.g., quaternary ammonium salts, acetylcholine) act in an ionized form (7). In these cases the pH plays an important role, as can be seen in Figure 3.8.

Thiopental, secobarbital, and barbital, although having comparable pK_a values (7.6, 7.9, and 7.8, respectively), present very different chloroform–water partition coefficients (> 100, 23.3, and 0.7, respectively) and for this reason are absorbed at very different rates: the first one is absorbed very rapidly; the second one, less rapidly; and the last one, very slowly (79). For details about membranes see Chapter 10, Section V.

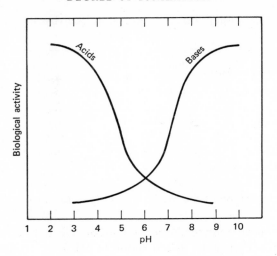

Fig. 3.8.   Biological activity of acids and bases as a function of pH (*7*).

A. Relevance of pK$_a$ in Biological Action

Some compounds, such as quaternary ammonium salts and sulfonic acids, because they are completely ionized and, for this very reason, poorly soluble in lipids, are not well absorbed at the pH of the gastrointestinal tract. As a consequence these compounds remain for a long time in contact with pathological agents localized in the gastrointestinal tract. The action of certain antiprotozoan agents, such as pyrvinium pamoate, which acts against *Enterobius vermicularis* and other parasitic worms, and of the so-called intestinal sulfonamides, which act against some bacterial infections, is due to the above-mentioned fact.

There is therefore an optimal pK$_a$ for each group of drugs. Bell and Roblin (*80*) postulated that the optimal pK$_a$ for sulfonamides would range from 6.0 to 7.5; that is, the maximal activity of a sulfonamide is reached when about 50% of its molecules are in the ionized form and about 50% in the molecular form, since the anion alone is active, but only the neutral molecule is able to cross the cellular membrane (Table 3.6).

However, Cammarata and Allen (*82*) disprove Bell and Roblin's conclusions. They cite several examples of sulfonamides that, although having a pK$_a$ outside the limit prescribed by those authors, are very active. This is especially so in the case of those which contain substituents at N^1 having a negative inductive effect ($-I$) and which are potentially able to manifest high activity *in vitro*, provided they can cross the bacterial cellular wall. By

TABLE 3.6 Relationship between Biological Activity and pK_a of Certain Sulfonamides (81)

Sulfonamide	Minimal Effective Concentration ($M \times 10^{-6}$)	pK_a	Percentage of Ionization at pH 7
Sulfanilamide	2500	10.5	0.03
Sulfapyridine	20	8.5	3.4
Sulfathiazole	4	6.8	61.6
Sulfadiazine	4	6.4	80.0

Reprinted by permission of the McGraw-Hill Book Company.

making a graphical representation of the bacteriostatic concentration for many different sulfonamides as a function of pH, they obtained a parabolic curve (Figure 3.9).

Foernzler and Martin (83), by applying molecular-orbital calculations to 50 different sulfonamides, tried to relate bacteriostatic activity not only with pK_a, as Bell and Roblin (80) had already done with the same sulfonamides, but also with the electronic charge on the ionizing nitrogen N^1 atom, having observed that the bacteriostatic activity increases with increase in the formal charge on N^1. Details on the mode of action of sulfonamides are found elsewhere (84–87).

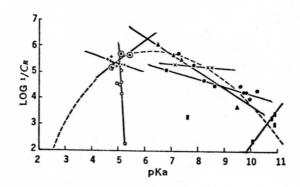

Fig. 3.9. Bacteriostatic activity of sulfanilamides as a function of pK_a (82). Key: $\bigcirc$ = 2-sulfanilamido (substituted) thiadiazoles; + = *meta-* and/or *para*-substituted N^1-benzoylsulfanilamides; $\bigcirc$ = *ortho*-substituted N^1-benzoylsulfanilamides; $\blacktriangle$ = 2-sulfanilamido (substituted) pyrimidines; × = 2-sulfanilamido (substituted) pyridines; $\bullet$ = N^1-(substituted) phenylsulfanilamides; $\blacksquare$ = N^1-(substituted) methylsulfanilamides. (Reproduced by permission of the copyright owner.)

B. Role of Ionization in the Activity of Drugs

When the biological activity of a drug is due to ions, this activity will increase with increase in the degree of ionization. However, if it results from undissociated molecules, increase in the degree of ionization of the active compounds will cause a decrease in activity. Besides, there are some drugs that exert their activities as free radicals (88,89).

Ionization affects other physicochemical properties. The increase in ionization increases a drug's water solubility and decreases its liposolubility and, consequently, its adsorption and passage across lipid barriers and membranes, and its concentration in tissues rich in lipids (4).

In general drugs cross cellular membranes in undissociated forms as intact molecules and act in dissociated forms, as ions (Figure 3.10).

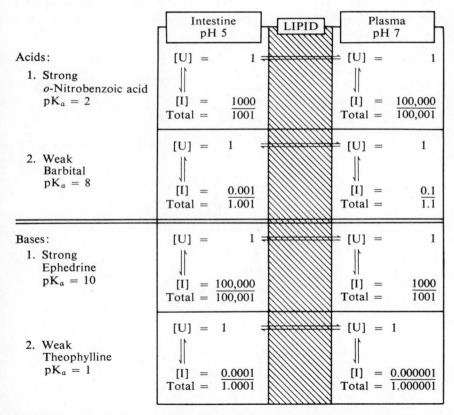

Fig. 3.10. Theoretical distribution between the gastrointestinal tract and the plasma of organic acids and bases of various approximate pK_a values. [U] and [I] represent concentrations of the un-ionized and ionized forms, respectively.

This happens because the passage of ions across the cellular membrane is prevented by two factors:

1. The cellular membrane is made up of layers of electrically charged macromolecules (lipids, proteins, and mucopolysaccharides—Figure 3.11), which attract or repel the ions (90).

2. The hydration of ions increases their volumes, rendering difficult their diffusion through pores.

It is known that the biological action of amino acridines increases with the degree of ionization (Table 3.7). Very likely drugs of this type act at the external part of the cell, since they cannot cross cellular membranes.

By considering that a number of drugs act in the form of ions, Stearn and Stearn (92) assumed that the bacteriostatic action of derivatives of acridine and of triphenylmethane, as well as of other basic dyes, should result

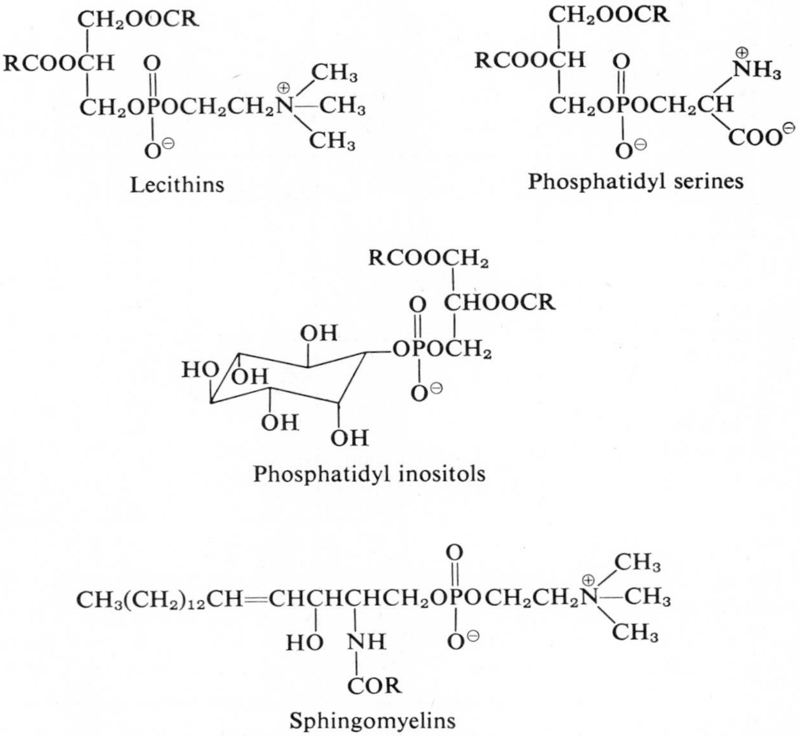

Fig. 3.11.   Formulas of some common lipids that make up the cellular membrane.

TABLE 3.7 Ionization and Bacteriostatic Effects of Amino Acridines (*91*)

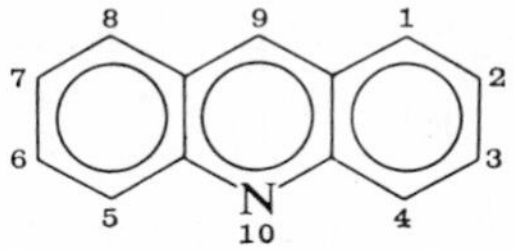

Acridine	Minimal Bacteriostatic Concentration (*Streptococcus pyogenus*)	Percentage of Ionization (pH $= 7.3$ at $37°C$)
9-NH$_2$	1/160,000	100
3,9-di-NH$_2$	1/160,000	100
3,6-di-NH$_2$	1/160,000	99
4,9-di-NH$_2$	1/ 80,000	98
3-NH$_2$	1/ 80,000	73
2,7-di-NH$_2$	1/ 20,000	3
2-NH$_2$	1/ 10,000	2
1-NH$_2$	1/ 10,000	2
4-NH$_2$	1/ 5,000	<1

from a reaction of their respective cations with essential anions of bacterial cells:

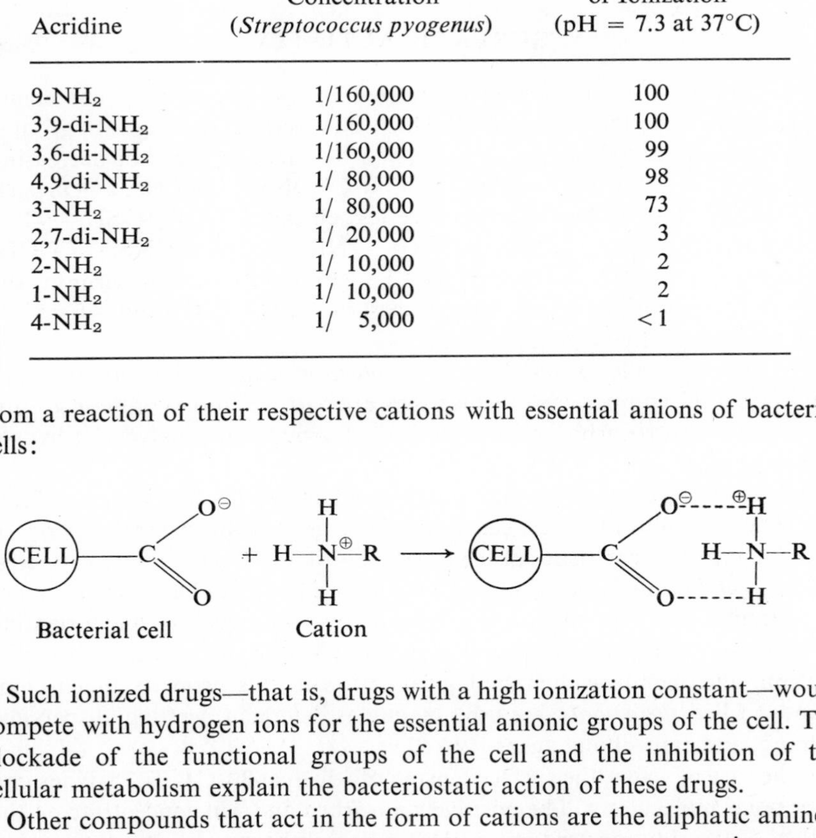

Bacterial cell   Cation

Such ionized drugs—that is, drugs with a high ionization constant—would compete with hydrogen ions for the essential anionic groups of the cell. The blockade of the functional groups of the cell and the inhibition of the cellular metabolism explain the bacteriostatic action of these drugs.

Other compounds that act in the form of cations are the aliphatic amines, diamines, amidines, guanidines, biguanidines, quaternary ammonium compounds, and pyridinium salts (*7*).

On the other hand, in contrast to what happens with invert soaps (which act in the form of cations), ordinary soaps exert their antibacterial action in the form of anions, competing for hydroxyl ions in a cationic group of an essential enzyme. Nevertheless their activity is very weak, because the living cells present a predominantly anionic nature. This is what happens with

$$Cl^{\ominus} \left[R^1—\overset{\overset{\displaystyle R^2}{\displaystyle |}}{\underset{\underset{\displaystyle R^3}{\displaystyle |}}{N^{\oplus}}}—R^4 \right] \qquad RCOO^{\ominus}\ Na^{\oplus}$$

bacteria, the isoelectric point of which is approximately 4, so that in pH 7 they manifest an anionic character.

V. SURFACE ACTIVITY

Some chemical groups are characterized by the property of conferring water solubility on the molecules to which they belong. Among such groups, called *hydrophilic, lipophobic,* or *polar,* can be cited, in order of decreasing efficiency, the following: $—OSO_2ONa$, $—COONa$, $—SO_2Na$, $—OSO_2H$, and $—SO_2H$. The following groups are less efficient: $—OH$, $—SH$, $—O—$, $=CO$, $—CHO$, $—NO_2$, $—NH_2$, $—NHR$, $—NR_2$, $—CN$, $—CNS$, $—COOH$, $—COOR$, $—OPO_3H_2$, $—OS_2O_2H$, $—Cl$, $—Br$, and $—I$. Furthermore the presence of unsaturated bonds, such as exist in $—CH=CH—$ and $—C\equiv C—$, helps to promote hydrophilicity (*93*).

Other groups, called *lipophilic, hydrophobic,* or *nonpolar,* increase the liposolubility of the compounds of which they are part. Examples of these groups are aliphatic hydrocarbon chains, aryl alkyl groups, and polycyclic hydrocarbon groups.

Compounds carrying hydrophilic and lipophilic groups, and provided there is a proper equilibrium between both these groups, have the property of modifying the characteristics of the interface—that is, the boundary surface—between two liquids, or a liquid and a solid, or a liquid and a gas. Some types of molecules decrease the surface tension by concentrating and orienting themselves in a definite arrangement in the interface or on the surface of a solution, and they owe their biological action to this property. Such compounds, called *surfactants,* are used mainly as detergent, wetting, dispersing, foaming, and emulsifying agents (*94–97*).

In the case of water, the surface tension of which at 20°C is 72.75 dynes/cm, fewer polar molecules will be positively adsorbed and will concentrate on the surface of the solution; the more polar ones will be negatively adsorbed, so the solute will disperse itself within the solution.

In the case of a mixture of liquids the nonpolar (hydrocarbon) part of the molecule will orient itself toward the nonpolar liquid, whereas the polar groups (such as $—NO_2$, $—NH_2$, $—OH$, $—COOH$) will be attracted toward the polar liquid. In this orientation van der Waals forces, hydrogen bonds, and ionic dipoles play a role.

Surfactant agents present two distinct regions of lipophilic and hydrophilic character. For this reason they are called *amphiphilic*, or *amphiphils* (from the Greek ἄνφι = both, and φιλος = friend). Their greater or lesser hydrophilicity and lipophilicity depends on the degree of polarity of the groups present. Taking this factor into consideration, they can be classified into four categories (*94,95*):

1. *Nonionic.* They are not ionizable and contain weakly hydrophilic and lipophilic groups, which render them soluble or water dispersible (*98*); examples: polyoxyethylene ethers and polyol esters of fatty acids (polysorbates, or Tweens).

2. *Cationic.* The lipophilic group is located on the cation; examples: quaternary ammonium salts and aliphatic amines of high molecular weight.

3. *Anionic.* The lipophilic group is in that part of the molecule which, when it is ionized, acquires a negative charge; examples: ordinary soaps, salts of bile acids, alkyl sulfates and sulfonates, sulfate and phosphate esters.

4. *Amphoteric.* Also called *ampholytic*, or *ampholytes*, these compounds contain, besides the lipophilic group, one cationic hydrophilic group and at least one anionic hydrophilic group; examples: Derifats and Miranols.

In diluted concentrations the surfactant agents act as inorganic electrolytes, from electric and osmotic points of view; in high concentrations they can associate themselves by forming polymers that impart a colloidal nature to the solution. Such a process, however, is reversible.

The concentration in which the polymerization of surfactant agents occurs is known as critical micelle concentration (CMC). It varies from one compound to another, but in a homologous series it can be represented by the following expression (*99*):

$$\log{(\text{CMC})} = A - \beta N$$

where A is a constant characteristic of the homologous series and depends on the molecular structure; β, a constant that is equal to $\log 2$ for most anionic and cationic surfactants and $\log 3$ for amphoteric surfactants (*100*); and N, the length of the alkyl chain. The term βN should be constant for all compounds that carry a normal alkyl chain. For determining CMC several methods are used, including nuclear magnetic resonance (*101*).

Surfactant agents deeply affect cellular-membrane permeability, whether by disintegrating or lysing it (this happens with those of high activity, by denaturation of proteins of which the membrane is a part) or by simply enwrapping it with a layer and in this way interfering with the absorption of other compounds (this occurs with compounds of low activity).

Because they disorganize cellular membranes and cause hemolysis, besides being easily adsorbed by proteins, surfactant agents are not, in general, applied internally but only topically, as skin disinfectants or sterilizers of instruments. This is the case for cationic surfactants. Nonionic surfactants are largely employed in pharmaceutical forms for oral (sometimes even parenteral) use as solubilizing agents of water-insoluble or slightly soluble drugs.

The physicochemical properties of some nonionic detergents were reviewed by Elworthy and Macfarlane (102), and their interaction with water was studied by Corkill and Goodman (103).

REFERENCES

1. E. J. Ariëns, *Progr. Drug Res.*, **10**, 429 (1966).
2. E. J. Ariëns, *Farmaco*, *(Pavia)*, Ed. *Sci.*, **23**, 52 (1968).
3. B. B. Brodie and C. A. M. Hogben, *J. Pharm. Pharmacol.*, **9**, 345 (1957).
4. A. Sekera, *Actualités Pharmacol.*, **14**, 197 (1961).
5. K. J. Brunings, Ed., *Modern Concepts in the Relationship Between Structure and Pharmacological Activity*, Pergamon, Oxford, 1963.
6. D. R. H. Gourley, "Factors Modifying Drug Action in the Body," in W. F. M. Fulton, Ed., *Modern Trends in Pharmacology and Therapeutics*, Vol. I, Appleton-Century-Crafts, New York, 1967, pp. 1–40.
7. T. C. Daniels and E. C. Jorgensen, "Physicochemical Properties in Relation to Biologic Action," in C. O. Wilson, O. Gisvold, and R. F. Doerge, Eds., *Textbook of Organic Medicinal and Pharmaceutical Chemistry*, 5th ed., Lippincott, Philadelphia, 1966, pp. 4–62.
8. A. Cammarata and A. N. Martin, "Physical Properties and Biological Activity," in A. Burger, Ed., *Medicinal Chemistry*, 3rd ed., Interscience, New York, 1970, pp. 118–163.
9. P. W. Sadler, *Pharmacol. Rev.*, **15**, 407 (1963).
10. A. C. Brown, "Passive and Active Transport," in T. C. Ruch and H. D. Patton, Eds., *Physiology and Biophysics*, 19th ed., Saunders, Philadelphia, 1965, pp. 820–842.
11. C. Hansch, *Farmaco*, *(Pavia)*, Ed. *Sci.*, **23**, 293 (1968).
12. A. Leo, C. Hansch, and C. Church, *J. Med. Chem.*, **12**, 766 (1969).
13. L. S. Schanker, *Ann. Rev. Pharmacol.*, **1**, 29 (1961).
14. L. S. Schanker, *Advan. Drug Res.*, **1**, 71 (1964).
15. D. J. Lamb and L. E. Harris, *J. Am. Pharm. Assoc.*, **49**, 583 (1960).
16. K. Kakemi, T. Arita, S. Kitazawa et al., *Chem. Pharm. Bull.*, **15**, 1705, 1819, 1828 (1967).
17. E. Overton, *Vierteljahrsschr. Naturforsch. Ges. Zürich*, **44**, 88 (1899).
18. H. Meyer, *Arch. Exptl. Pathol. Pharmakol.*, **42**, 109 (1899); *ibid.*, **46**, 338 (1901).
19. E. I. Eger, II, B. Brandstater, L. J. Saidman, M. J. Regan, J. W. Severinghaus, and E. S. Munson, *Anesthesiology*, **26**, 771 (1965).
20. E. I. Eger, II, C. Lundgren, S. L. Miller, and W. C. Stevens, *Anesthesiology*, **30**, 129 (1969).

21. E. I. Eger, II, and R. O. Shargel, *Anesthesiology*, **30**, 136 (1969).
22. R. J. Wulf and R. M. Featherstone, *Anesthesiology*, **18**, 97 (1957).
23. J. F. Danielli and H. A. Davson, *J. Cell. Comp. Physiol.*, **5**, 495 (1935).
24. J. D. Robertson, "Unit Membranes: A Review with Recent New Studies of Experimental Alterations and a New Subunit Structure in Synaptic Membranes," in M. Locke, Ed., *Cellular Membranes in Development*, Academic, New York, 1964, pp. 1–81.
25. L. Pauling, *Science*, **134**, 15 (1961).
26. J. F. Catchpool, "The Pauling Theory of General Anesthesia," in A. Rich and N. Davidson, Eds., *Structural Chemistry and Molecular Biology*, Freeman, San Francisco, 1968, pp. 343–355.
27. S. R. Erlander, *J. Macromol. Sci.-Chem.*, A2, 595 (1968).
28. S. L. Miller, *Proc. Natl. Acad. Sci. U.S.*, **47**, 1515 (1961).
29. H. S. Frank and W.-Y. Wen, *Discussions Faraday Soc.*, **24**, 133 (1957).
30. G. Némethy and H. A. Scheraga, *J. Chem. Phys.*, **36**, 3382, 3401 (1962).
31. G. Némethy and H. A. Scheraga, *J. Phys. Chem.*, **66**, 1773 (1962); *ibid.*, **67**, 2888 (1963).
32. J. L. Kavanau, *Water and Solute-Water Interactions*, Holden-Day, San Franscisco, 1964.
33. W. Luck, *Fortschr. Chem. Forsch.*, **4**, 653 (1964).
34. M. J. Sparnaay, *J. Colloid Interface Sci.*, **22**, 23 (1966).
35. H. J. C. Berendsen, "Water Structure," in A. Cole, Ed., *Theoretical and Experimental Biophysics*, Vol. I, Dekker, New York, 1967, pp. 1–76.
36. L. J. Mullins, *Chem. Rev.*, **54**, 289 (1954).
37. L. D. Vandam, *Ann. Rev. Pharmacol.*, **6**, 379 (1966).
38. B. P. Schoenborn and R. M. Featherstone, *Advan. Pharmacol.*, **5**, 1 (1967).
39. E. R. Larsen, R. A. Van Dyke, and M. B. Chenoweth, "Mechanisms of Narcosis," in A. Burger, Ed., *Drugs Affecting the Central Nervous System*, Dekker, New York, 1968, pp. 1–24.
40. Pharmacology Society Symposium, "The Molecular Pharmacology of Anesthesia," *Federation Proc.*, **27**, 870–913 (1968).
41. A. Cherkin, *Ann. Rev. Pharmacol.*, **9**, 259 (1969).
42. W. P. Purcell, J. A. Singer, K. Sundaram, and G. L. Parks, "Quantitative Structure–Activity Relationships and Molecular Orbitals in Medicinal Chemistry," in A. Burger, Ed., *Medicinal Chemistry*, 3rd ed., Interscience, New York, 1970, pp. 164–192.
43. C. Hansch, *Ann. Rep. Med. Chem.*, **2**, 347 (1967); *ibid.*, **3**, 348 (1968).
44. C. Hansch, "The Use of Substituent Constants in Structure–Activity Studies," in E. J. Ariëns, Ed., *Physico-Chemical Aspects of Drug Action*, Pergamon, Oxford, 1968, pp. 141–167.
45. C. Hansch, *Accounts Chem. Res.*, **2**, 232 (1969).
46. C. Hansch and T. Fujita, *J. Am. Chem. Soc.*, **86**, 1616 (1964).
47. C. Hansch, J. E. Quinlan, and G. L. Lawrence, *J. Org. Chem.*, **33**, 347 (1968).
48. L. P. Hammett, *Physical Organic Chemistry*, McGraw-Hill, New York, 1940.
49. E. S. Gould, *Mechanism and Structure in Organic Chemistry*, Holt, Rinehart and Winston, New York, 1959.

50. C. Hansch, R. M. Muir, T. Fujita, P. P. Maloney, F. Geiger, and M. Streich, *J. Am. Chem. Soc.*, **85**, 2817 (1963).

51. C. Hansch and A. R. Steward, *J. Med. Chem.*, **7**, 691 (1964).

52. C. Hansch and E. W. Deutsch, *J. Med. Chem.*, **8**, 705 (1965).

53. A. E. Bird and A. C. Marshall, *Biochem. Pharmacol.*, **16**, 2275 (1967).

54. C. Hansch and S. M. Anderson, *J. Med. Chem.*, **10**, 745 (1967).

55. C. Hansch, A. R. Steward, S. M. Anderson, and D. Bentley, *J. Med. Chem.*, **11**, 1 (1968).

56. T. Fujita and C. Hansch, *J. Med. Chem.*, **10**, 991 (1967).

57. R. W. Fuller, M. M. Marsh, and J. Mills, *J. Med. Chem.*, **11**, 397 (1968).

58. E. Kutter and C. Hansch, *J. Med. Chem.*, **12**, 647 (1969).

59. C. Hansch and E. J. Lien, *Biochem. Pharmacol.*, **17**, 709 (1968).

60. W. B. Neely, H. C. White, and A. Rudzik, *J. Pharm. Sci.*, **57**, 1176 (1968).

61. E. R. Garrett, O. K. Wright, G. H. Miller, and K. L. Smith, *J. Med. Chem.*, **9**, 203 (1966).

62. C. Hansch, E. Kutter, and A. Leo, *J. Med. Chem.*, **12**, 746 (1969).

63. A. Cammarata, *J. Med. Chem.*, **10**, 525 (1967); *ibid.*, **11**, 1111 (1968); *ibid.*, **12**, 314 (1969).

64. J. A. Singer and W. P. Purcell, *J. Med. Chem.*, **10**, 1000 (1967).

65. T. C. Bruice, N. Kharasch, and R. J. Winzler, *Arch. Biochem. Biophys.*, **62**, 305 (1956).

66. S. M. Free, Jr., and J. W. Wilson, *J. Med. Chem.*, **7**, 395 (1964).

67. W. P. Purcell, *Biochim. Biophys. Acta*, **105**, 201 (1965).

68. W. R. Smithfield and W. P. Purcell, *J. Pharm. Sci.*, **56**, 577 (1967).

69. W. P. Purcell and J. M. Clayton, *J. Med. Chem.*, **11**, 199 (1968).

70. W. P. Purcell and J. M. Clayton, *Ann. Rep. Med. Chem.*, **4**, 314 (1969).

71. K. Boček, J. Kopecký, M. Krivucová, and D. Vlachová, *Experientia*, **20**, 667 (1964).

72. J. Kopecký, K. Boček, and D. Vlachová, *Nature*, **207**, 981 (1965).

73. K. Boček, J. Kopecký, and M. Krivucová, *Experientia*, **23**, 1038 (1967).

74. R. Zahradník, K. Boček, and J. Kopecký, "Empirical Equations for Correlating Biological Efficiency of Organic Compounds," in E. J. Ariëns, Ed., *Physico-Chemical Aspects of Drug Action*, Pergamon, Oxford, 1968, pp. 127–139.

75. T. Ban and T. Fujita, *J. Med. Chem.*, **12**, 353 (1969).

76. J. A. Ostrenga, *J. Med. Chem.*, **12**, 349 (1969).

77. G. Kortüm, W. Vogel, and K. Andrussow, *Dissociation Constants of Organic Acids in Aqueous Solution*, Butterworths, London, 1961.

78. D. D. Perrin, *Dissociation Constants of Organic Bases in Aqueous Solution*, Butterworths, London, 1965.

79. C. A. M. Hogben, L. S. Schanker, D. J. Tocco, and B. B. Brodie, *J. Pharmacol. Exptl. Therap.*, **120**, 540 (1957).

80. P. H. Bell and R. O. Roblin, Jr., *J. Am. Chem. Soc.*, **64**, 2905 (1942).

81. F. W. Schueler, *Chemobiodynamics and Drug Design*, McGraw-Hill, New York, 1960.

82. A. Cammarata and R. C. Allen, *J. Pharm. Sci.*, **56**, 640 (1967).

83. E. C. Foernzler and A. N. Martin, *J. Pharm. Sci.*, **56**, 608 (1967).

84. J. K. Seydel, *Mol. Pharmacol.*, **2**, 259 (1966).
85. J. K. Seydel, "Molecular Basis for the Action of Chemotherapeutic Drugs, Structure–Activity Studies on Sulfonamides," in E. J. Ariëns, Ed., *Physico-Chemical Aspects of Drug Action,* Pergamon, Oxford, 1968, pp. 169–180.
86. J. K. Seydel, *J. Pharm. Sci.*, **57**, 1455 (1968).
87. T. Struller, *Antibiot. Chemother.*, (*Basel*), **14**, 179 (1968).
88. M. S. Blois, Jr., H. W. Brown, R. M. Lemmon, R. O. Lindblom, and M. Weissbluth, Eds., *Free Radicals in Biological Systems*, Academic, New York, 1961.
89. T. N. Tozer, L. D. Tuck, and J. C. Craig, *J. Med. Chem.*, **12**, 294 (1969).
90. A. W. Cuthbert, *Pharmacol. Rev.*, **19**, 59 (1967).
91. A. Albert, *Selective Toxicity*, 4th ed., Methuen, London, 1968.
92. A. E. Stearn and E. W. Stearn, *J. Bacteriol.*, **9**, 491 (1924).
93. D. Hummel, *Identification and Analysis of Surface-Active Agents*, Interscience, New York, 1962.
94. A. M. Schwartz and J. W. Perry, *Surface Active Agents*, Interscience, New York, 1949.
95. A. M. Schwartz, J. W. Perry, and J. Berch, *Surface Active Agents and Detergents*, Vol. II, Interscience, New York, 1958.
96. J. L. Moilliet, B. Collie, and W. Black, *Surface Activity*, 2nd ed., Van Nostrand, Princeton, N.J., 1961.
97. International Congress on Surface Active Substances, *Chemistry, Physics, and Application of Surface Active Substances*, 3 vols., Gordon and Breach, New York, 1967.
98. M. J. Schick, Ed., *Nonionic Surfactants*, Dekker, New York, 1967.
99. H. B. Klevens, *J. Am. Oil Chemists' Soc.*, **30**, 74 (1953).
100. A. H. Beckett and R. J. Woodward, *J. Pharm. Pharmacol.*, **15**, 422 (1963).
101. J. F. Yan and M. B. Palmer, *J. Colloid Interface Sci.*, **30**, 177 (1969).
102. P. H. Elworthy and C. B. Macfarlane, *J. Pharm. Pharmacol.*, **17**, 65, 129 (1965).
103. J. M. Corkill and J. F. Goodman, *Advanc. Colloid Interface Sci.*, **2**, 297 (1969).

PHARMACOLOGICAL EFFECTS OF SPECIFIC MOIETIES

The molecular modification of a promising "lead" compound is still a major line of approach to new drugs. Structural variations bring about new physical properties and alter the reactivity of a molecule, which in turn may cause changes in distribution in cells and tissues, in access to active sites of enzymes and receptors, in reaction rates at such sites, and in excretion patterns. Even an apparently very minor change in chemical structure may thus uncover biological effects that have been dormant or overshadowed by side effects in the parent material.

Alfred Burger

I. CHEMICAL STRUCTURE AND BIOLOGICAL ACTION

In the preceding chapters it was shown that the biological action of structurally specific drugs depends directly on their size, shape, and electronic distribution, as recent reviews point out (*1–3*).

With the purpose of correlating pharmacological activity with chemical constitution, Burger (4) compiled in an extensive table biological activities associated with specific structural entities. In addition, he listed a series of biological activities associated with special ring systems (Table 4.1).

TABLE 4.1   Biological Activities Associated with Special Ring Systems (4)

Ring System	Drug Prototypes	Biological Activities
Indole and condensed systems	Ergotamine	Sympatholytic
	Lysergic acid diethylamide	Psychotomimetic
	Serotonin	Pressor
	Reserpine	Hypotensive, ataractic
Isoquinoline	Emetine	Emetic, amebicidal
	Papaverine	Vasodilator
	Morphine	Analgetic, euphoric
	Tubocurarine	Curariform
Phenothiazine	Phenothiazine	Anthelmintic
	Phenopropazine	Antiparkinsonism
	Promethazine	Antihistaminic
	Chlorpromazine	Antiemetic, ataractic
Pyrazolone	Antipyrine	Antineuralgic, analgetic
Pyrimidines and condensed systems	Pyrimethamine	Antimalarial
Purines, pteridines	Caffeine, theophylline	Analeptic, diuretic
	Pteroylglutamic acid	Vitamin
	Amethopterin	Antileukemic
	6-Mercaptopurine, fluorouracil	Tumor inhibitory
Quinolines and condensed systems	Primaquine	Antimalarial
	Cinchophen	Antiarthritic
	Surfen	Trypanocidal

Although the presence of a specific moiety does not necessarily mean that the molecule will possess a particular biological activity, since this activity depends on the molecule as a whole (5), the chemical groupings present in, or introduced into, a drug are important for two reasons:

1. They may be essential for the manifestation of a particular biological action, owing to their chemical reactivity or spatial arrangement.

2. They may modify the intensity of a certain biological action, as a consequence of characteristic effects exerted by them.

For maximal biological activity, however, the chemical reactivity must be within a definite range. On one hand, too reactive groupings—those that react easily with various cell constituents—may prevent the drug's reaching the site in which it must act. On the other hand, relatively unreactive moieties may render negligible the biological activity of the parent drug. Therefore biological activity demands optimal chemical reactivity and optimal physicochemical properties (5). By resorting only to structural modifications in parent compounds, several researches were accomplished with the purpose of obtaining new drugs (6–13).

Using chemical and biological criteria relating to the structure of drugs, Ariëns (12,13) distinguishes between *chemofunctional* moieties (those that contribute to the binding of drug to receptor through various forces) and *biofunctional* moieties (those responsible for biological activity). Since *chemofunctional* moieties are discussed in Chapter 7, the present chapter is concerned mainly with biofunctional moieties. Various effects displayed by different groupings are studied, especially those directly involved in pharmacological activity as well as those that increase or diminish it.

In biofunctional moieties distinction must be made between *essential* and *nonessential* parts. The first ones demand high structural specificity, because they as active parts will interact with receptors to produce pharmacological action. It is evident, therefore, that these parts cannot undergo great modification in their chemical structures. However, the last ones—namely, nonessential parts—are not involved in drug–receptor complexation, so that great variability in their chemical structures is permissible.

Ariëns (12) classifies biofunctional moieties as (a) carrier moieties, (b) vulnerable moieties, (c) critical and noncritical moieties, (d) bioisosteric groups, and (e) haptophoric and pharmacophoric groups.

II. CARRIER MOIETIES

Most substances introduced into an organism undergo metabolic processes in which their structures may be deeply altered. This modification may activate or deactivate a drug (6,8). In order to make the compound's pharmacologically active part reach the site in which it must act it is often necessary to supply it with an appropriate carrier group, through proper application of the principle of drug latentiation. This subject is being thoroughly studied by some authors (6,8,12–14). What is stated next about this topic is a summary of the excellent and exhaustive reviews of these researchers, especially that of Harper (8).

Drug latentiation consists essentially in converting, through chemical modification, a biologically active compound to an inactive carrier form that, after enzymic attack, will release the active drug. *Drug latentiation* must not be confused with two related terms: (a) *structural formulation*—modification of a biologically active compound at a point not essential to its complexation with the receptor; (b) *pharmaceutical formulation*—technical processes through which, without altering the chemical structure of the drug, it is obtained in an easily dispensable form by modification of its physical properties, by physical combination with some inert material, or by adjustment of physical properties of the medium in which it is administered (*8*).

A classical example of drug latentiation is Prontosil rubrum. Although it contains sulfanilamide, the well-known antibacterial agent, it is inactive, *in vitro*, as result of the carrier-group effect; but *in vivo*, through the enzymic action of azoreductase, it releases sulfanilamide, the active part:

Prontosil rubrum
(inactive)

Sulfanilamide
(active)

According to their physiological function, carrier groups may be (*12*) *restricting*, *selecting*, *fixed*, or *disposable*.

Among *restricting* groups are the bulky groups, which prevent passage of the drug through cell membranes; the ionized groups, which reduce or prevent penetration of the drug through the lipid barriers; and the strongly lipophilic groups, which tend to cause the drug to accumulate in compartments with pronounced lipophilic nature. An example is succinylsulfathiazole; as a consequence of its anionic carrier part, it is poorly absorbed, and its action is restricted to the intestine (*13*).

Selecting groups are those that can assist in the choice of specific pathways in the distribution of drug. This applies to, for instance, amino acids (*15*), sugars, steroids, and purine derivatives, which are actively transported and for this reason frequently utilized, particularly as carriers of alkylating agents. Uracil mustard, used as a carcinostatic agent, has low toxicity because of its high affinity for cell nuclei due to the carrier group uracil.

The name *fixed* is given to groups that may be fixed to the rest of the drug

Uracil mustard

molecule so firmly that they release the active part only after induction of effect. The just mentioned example illustrates this: uracil is a *fixed selecting* carrier group.

Disposable groups are those that, after playing their role as carriers, are rejected, liberating the active part by a process of bioactivation. This is the case for Prontosil rubrum, already mentioned.

Carrier groups have been introduced with the following objectives in mind from a pharmacological point of view (*6,8*):

1. To modify the duration of drug action.
2. Provided the interconversion could be localized in a particular target cell or tissue, to achieve (a) direct exclusive attack in the target cell with the active compound (particularly in the case of compounds with systemic toxicity) and (b) differentiation between the various possible effects of a compound, thus attaining greater clinical specificity.
3. To overcome difficulties encountered during pharmaceutical formulation.
4. To modify drug transport and distribution in the body.
5. To reduce the toxicity of certain compounds.

Owing to a lack of knowledge of chemical structures of the enzymes responsible for activating or inactivating certain classes of drugs, latentiation is as a rule undertaken empirically. Nevertheless some interesting results have been obtained. It is evident that the nature of the carrier group will affect not only absorption and distribution of the inactive form that is transported but also the rate of release of the active drug through enzymic attack. Some possible forms of transport are listed in Table 4.2.

Steric factors, as result of their role in drug transport, should be taken into account. It is often necessary to increase or diminish the volume of a carrier group, to prevent or to ease its rotation around a linkage, to make its structure flat or nonflat. For instance, the simple introduction of a properly placed double bond in a compound of type I, so that it may assume structure II, converts it from nonplanar to planar, owing to the possibility of conjugation of the π-electron cloud of the aromatic ring with the π-electron cloud of the double bond of the heterocyclic ring (III). This does not occur in the parent compound, in which the saturated heterocyclic ring can rotate freely around the bond linking it to the aromatic ring. Nevertheless introduction of a

TABLE 4.2   Schematic Representation of Some
Active Drugs and Their Possible Forms of Transport
(6)

Active Drug	Inactive Form of Transport[a]
R—OH	R—O—C(=O)—X
R—SH	R—S—C(=O)—X
R—COOH	R—C(=O)—O—X
R—N(R')—H	R—N(R')—C(=O)—X
R—OH	R—phosphate
R—SH	R—phosphate

[a] X stands for the greater portion of the carrier molecule.

Reproduced by permission of the American
Chemical Society.

methyl group in the *ortho* position of the phenyl ring makes the unsaturated
compound (II) nonplanar (IV) (8).

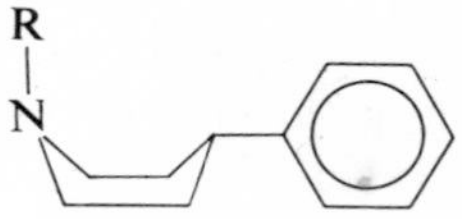

I
Nonplanar

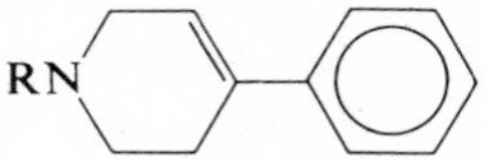

II
Planar

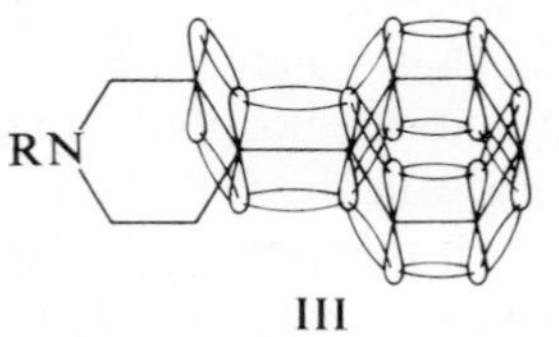

III
Planar

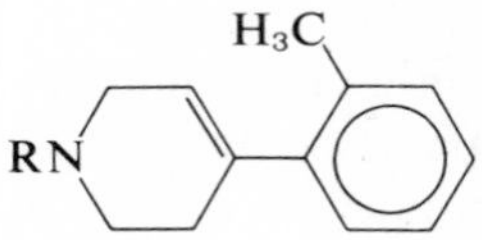

IV
Nonplanar

A. Prolongation or Shortening of Action

Usually it is desirable for a drug to have prolonged action. For example, in the case of antibiotics it is often necessary to achieve and maintain high blood levels of these chemotherapeutic agents. With hormones, efforts are made to avoid frequent administration, particularly in slow treatments. The means used to prolong the action of drugs are several:

1. Esterification, mainly of steroids (such as androgens, estrogens, progestogens, glucocorticoids, mineral corticoids) and certain antibiotics (oleandomycin, erythromycin).

2. Complex formation (zinc–protamine–insulin, vitamin B_{12}–zinc–tannic acid, amphetamine tannate).

3. Salt formation (penicillin salts, such as procaine penicillin, benzylpenicillin potassium).

4. Conversion of unsaturated to saturated compounds (prednisone and prednisolone, in the place of cortisone and cortisol).

On the other hand, one wishes at times to shorten instead of prolonging the duration of action of a drug. This can often be accomplished by replacing a stable chemical group by a labile one. Thus substitution of Cl of chlorpropamide by CH_3 (besides the replacement, at the end of the side chain, of C_3H_7 by C_4H_9) results in tolbutamide. Since CH_3 is labile, this group is soon oxidized to COOH, giving an inactive product. As a consequence tolbutamide's half-life is only 5.7 hours, whereas chlorpropamide's is 33 hours (12).

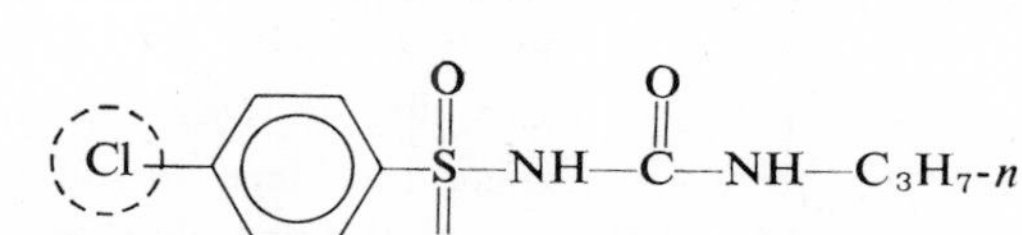

$$H_3C-\bigcirc-\overset{\overset{O}{\|}}{\underset{\underset{O}{\|}}{S}}-NH-\overset{\overset{O}{\|}}{C}-NH-C_4H_9\text{-}n$$

labile moiety

Tolbutamide
(short acting)
quickly degradated

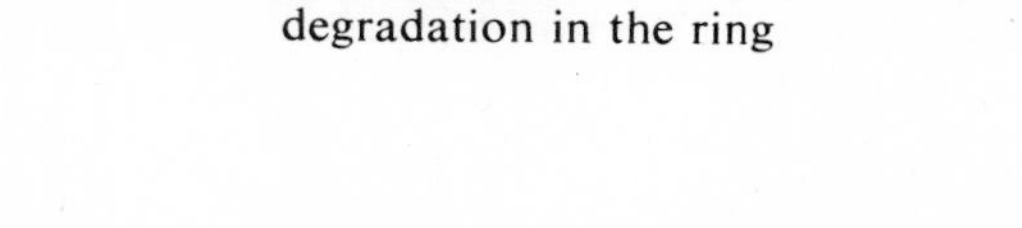

$$Cl-\bigcirc-\overset{\overset{O}{\|}}{\underset{\underset{O}{\|}}{S}}-NH-\overset{\overset{O}{\|}}{C}-NH-C_3H_7\text{-}n$$

stable moiety

Chlorpropamide
(long acting)
resistant against oxidative
degradation in the ring

B. Drug Localization

In the case of compounds with high systemic toxicity but beneficial therapeutic effect in diseased cells, the problem is to add to these drugs a carrier that will transport them to those cells and as a result of enzymic action release them near the receptor site where they will exert their effect *in situ* (8). Several examples of compounds with latent activity may be cited:

1. Cytostatic or anticancer agents, such as cyclophosphamide, and melphalan, in which the carriers are, respectively, cyclophosphamide ester and phenylalanine:

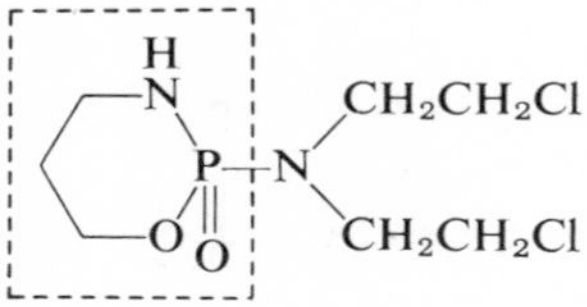

Cyclophosphamide 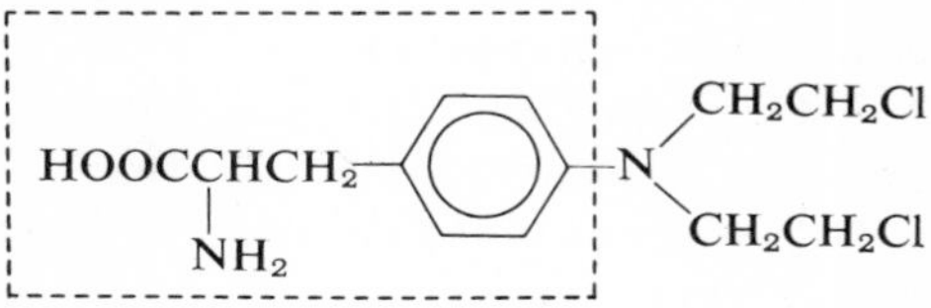   Melphalan

2. Chelating agents, such as an 8-hydroxyquinoline derivative, in which the carrier is glucuronic acid:

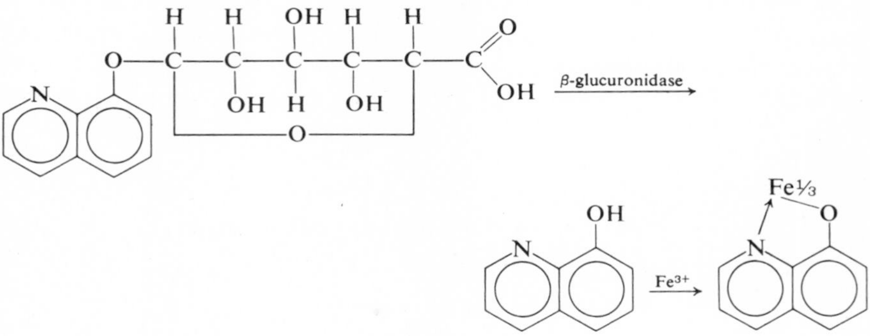

C. Transport Regulation

There are a number of recent examples of drug latentiation in which increased efficiency of the active moiety has been brought about through regulation of transport and penetration of the drug within the body. One is the condensation of the tuberculostatic isoniazid or certain thiosemicarbazones with starch or other polysaccharides that have been oxidized by periodate. The same approach has been used in the preparation of iron–dextran complexes, molecular complexes of sennosides, peptide–vitamin B_{12} complex, and

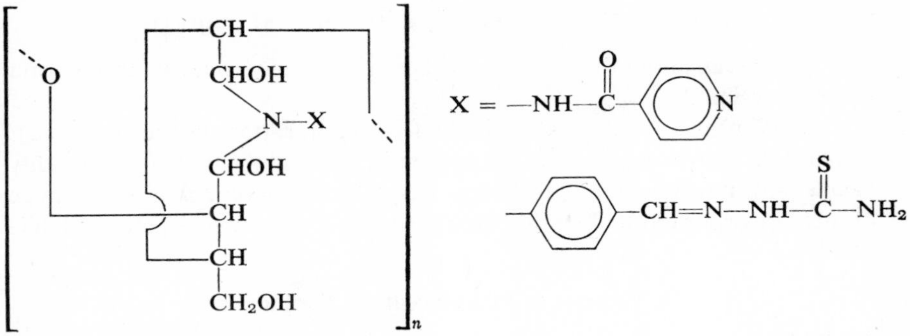

Antitubercular
complexes

TABLE 4.3 Sulfonamides Used in Intestinal Infections (*12*)

Formula[a]	Compound
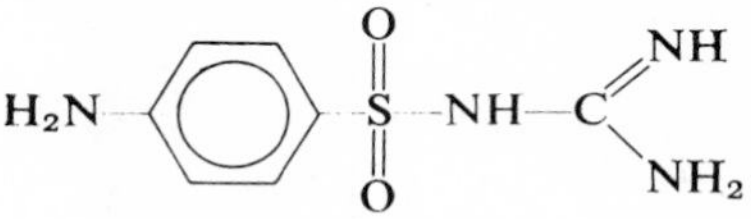	Sulfaguanidine
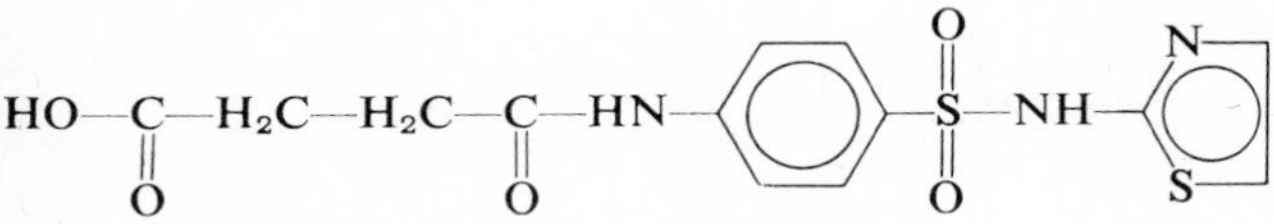	Succinylsulfathiazole
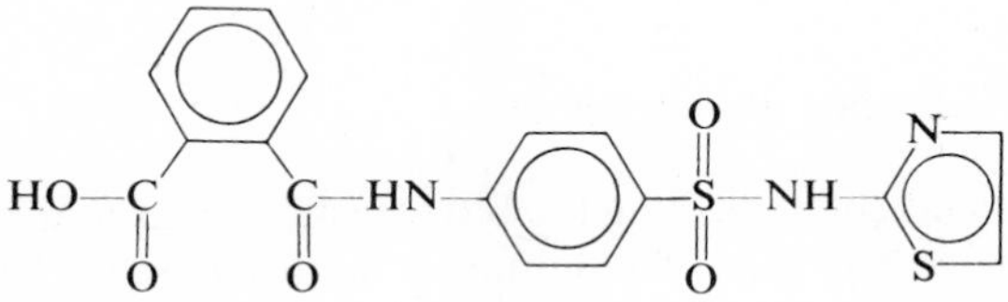	Phthalylsulfathiazole
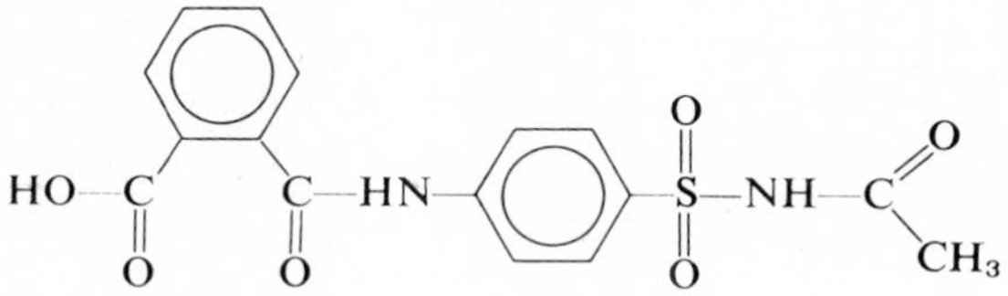	Phthalylsulfacetamide
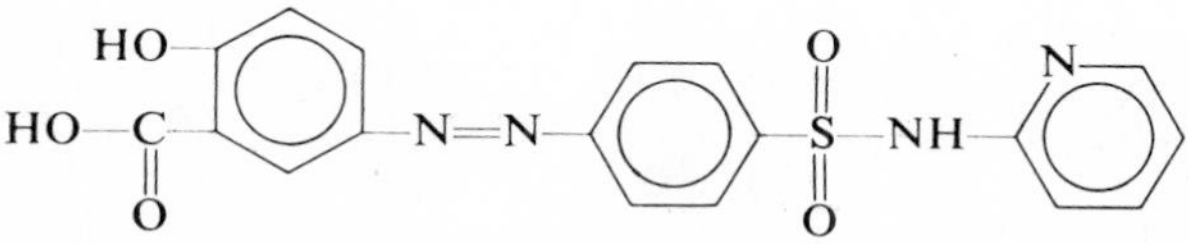	Salazosulfapyridine

[a] Strongly hydrophilic transport forms.

salts of various antibiotics, such as streptomycin, neomycin, viomycin, and streptothrycin.

Various means are utilized to regulate drug transport in the body (*12*): increase or decrease of volume, alteration of hydrophilicity or liposolubility (Table 4.3), introduction or removal of cationic or anionic moieties, change of pH, incorporation of hydrocarbon and other suitable stable or labile moieties.

D. Adjunct to Pharmaceutical Formulation

Structural modifications of known drugs have been used as adjuncts to pharmaceutical formulation, as a means of achieving drug latentiation (*8*).

After the discovery that ethyl mercaptan is antitubercular *in vitro*, researches were conducted with the aim of obtaining a derivative without the disadvantages of the parent compound: foul smell, low boiling point, and inflammability. As a result of these investigations, diethyl dithiolisophthalate was developed, in which the thiol groups are masked.

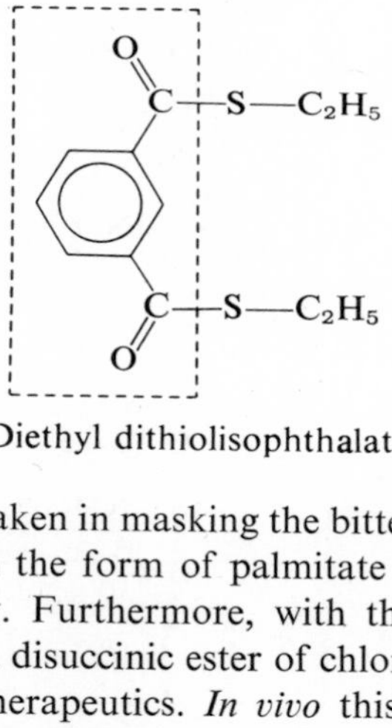

Diethyl dithiolisophthalate

A similar measure was taken in masking the bitter taste of chloramphenicol (*16*); it was found that in the form of palmitate it is tasteless but, *in vivo*, releases the active moiety. Furthermore, with the purpose of obtaining a water-soluble compound a disuccinic ester of chloramphenicol was prepared, and it is being used in therapeutics. *In vivo* this derivative is hydrolyzed, yielding first the monosuccinate and then the parent compound, free chloramphenicol.

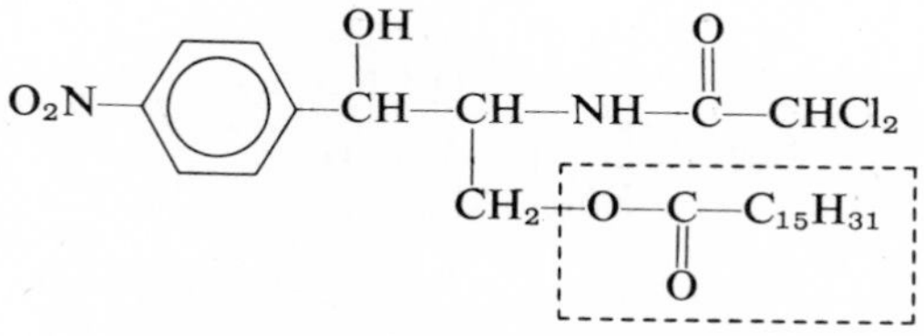

Chloramphenicol palmitate

Triacetin acts through a similar means. This fungistatic owes its activity to acetic acid, which is released slowly through hydrolysis not only by esterases present on human skin but also by fungi that parasitize the skin. Here glycerol plays simply the role of a carrier:

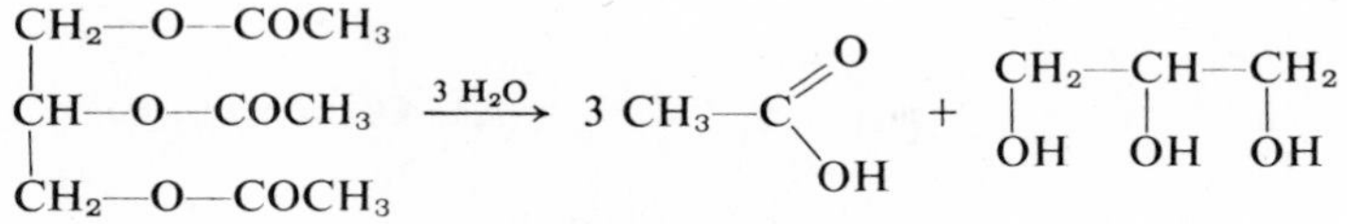

$$
\begin{array}{l}
CH_2\!-\!O\!-\!COCH_3 \\
CH\!-\!O\!-\!COCH_3 \\
CH_2\!-\!O\!-\!COCH_3
\end{array}
\xrightarrow{\;3\,H_2O\;}
3\ CH_3\!-\!C\!\!\underset{OH}{\overset{O}{\diagdown}}
\ +\
\begin{array}{ccc}
CH_2 & CH & CH_2 \\
OH & OH & OH
\end{array}
$$

Formaldehyde is an effective preservative. However, because of its unpleasant odor and irritant action, it cannot be used in cosmetics. To overcome these undesirable properties dimethylol urea and monomethylol dimethylhydantoin were prepared; under slightly acidic conditions both compounds release formaldehyde in sufficient amount to exert a preservative action.

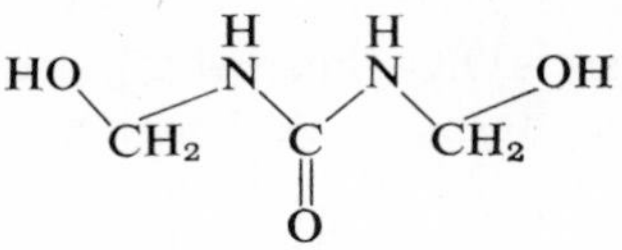

Dimethylol urea 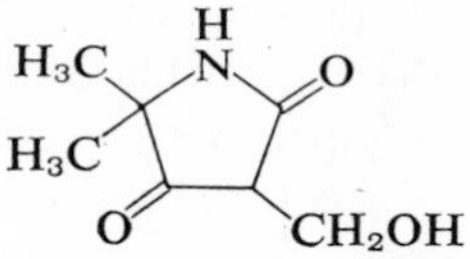   Monomethylol dimethylhydantoin

E. Lessening of Toxicity and Side Effects

Several examples can be listed of drugs obtained through the supply of suitable carrier moieties to biologically active compounds which are too toxic or which have serious side effects.

The simple sulfonation of β-naphthylamine, which is carcinogenic, converts it into an innocuous product (*12*):

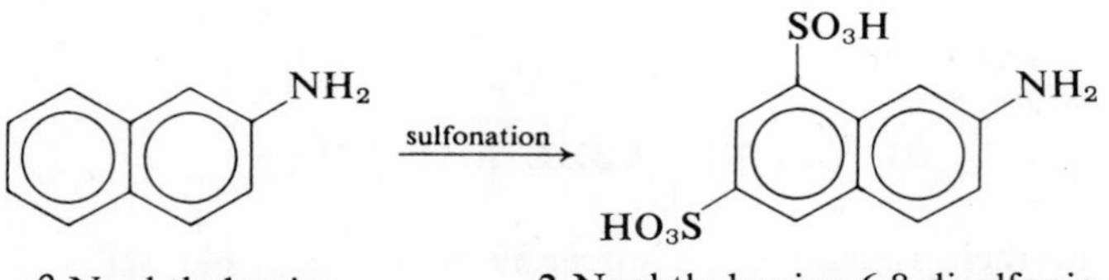

β-Naphthylamine   2-Naphthylamine-6,8-disulfonic acid
(highly carcinogenic)   (noncarcinogenic)

Chloral hydrate, although a very effective hypnotic, is restricted in use because, besides its unpleasant odor and taste, it produces gastrointestinal

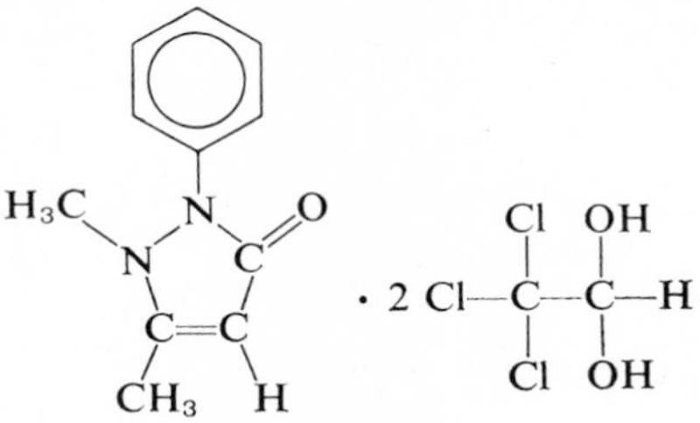

Dichloralphenazone

irritation. Dichloralphenazone, a product of the complexation of two molecules of chloral hydrate, has none of those disadvantages.

Para-aminosalicylic acid (PAS), used as tuberculostatic, presents the inconvenience of being irritant to the gastrointestinal tract. Its *p*-tolyl ester is not only of low toxicity but also tasteless. It produces the same intensity of action as equivalent doses of sodium PAS (*12*).

Sometimes the presence of a vulnerable moiety is sufficient for low toxicity. This occurs with the pesticide GS 13005, which is O,O-dimethyl-S-[2-methoxy-1,3,4-thiadiazol-5-(4H)onyl-(4)methyl]-dithiophosphate. Although it is highly toxic to insects, this organic phosphate is less toxic to mammals and plants, because, in contrast to insects, mammals and plants can degrade it readily by cleaving the substituted thiadiazole ring and thus inactivating the compound (*13*).

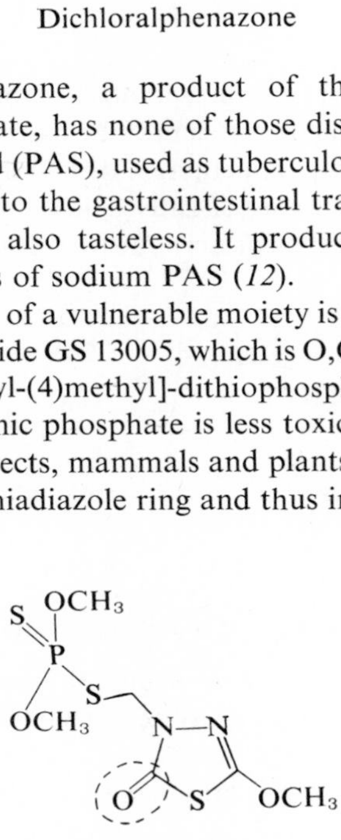

GS 13005

III. VULNERABLE MOIETIES

Because of their resistance or susceptibility to enzymic action, certain moieties present or introduced into drugs can either prolong or reduce their time of action, depending on whether they lead to activation or inactivation of the drugs. These moieties include ester links, certain peptide linkages in polypeptides, and alkyl chains with terminal OH or NH_2 groups (Table 4.4).

In order to stabilize a vulnerable moiety medicinal chemists often resort to

TABLE 4.4 Elimination and Stabilization of Vulnerable Moieties (*13*)

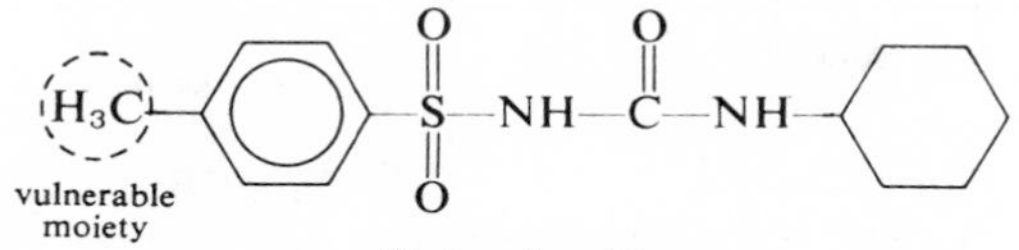

Tolcyclamide

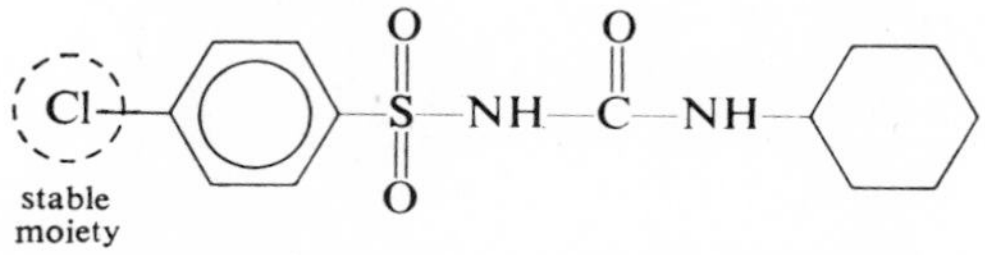

1-(*p*-Chlorobenzenesulfonyl)-3-cyclohexylurea

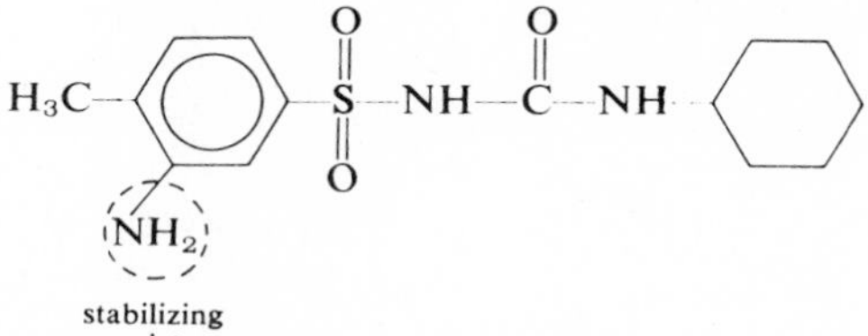

Metahexamide

the steric effect of alkyl groups. Thus the simple introduction of a methyl in close proximity to the ester link of acetylcholine results in compounds with far greater resistance to hydrolysis by acetylcholinesterase (Table 4.5).

Another example is found in procaine derivatives—that is, in esters of *p*-aminobenzoic acid (Table 4.6).

By introducing into lidocaine a vulnerable group, such as —CO—O—, between the aromatic ring and one of the methyl groups attached to that ring, tolycaine is obtained, which has a far shorter action than lidocaine (*12*):

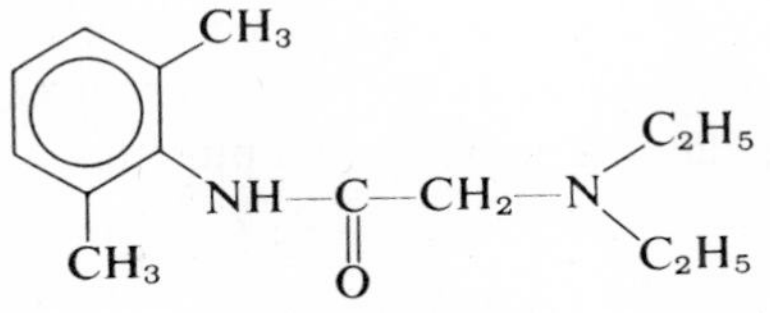

Lidocaine

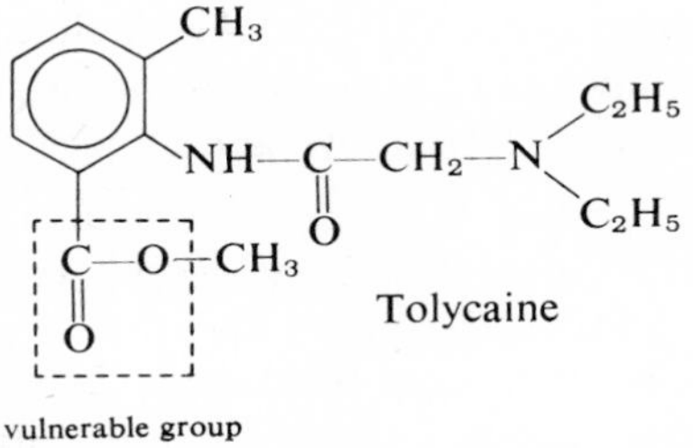

Tolycaine

vulnerable group

Long Acting

Short Acting

TABLE 4.5   Stabilization of the Vulnerable Group in Acetylcholine by Suitable Substitution (8)

Formula	Compound	Rate of Hydrolysis by Acetylcholinesterase
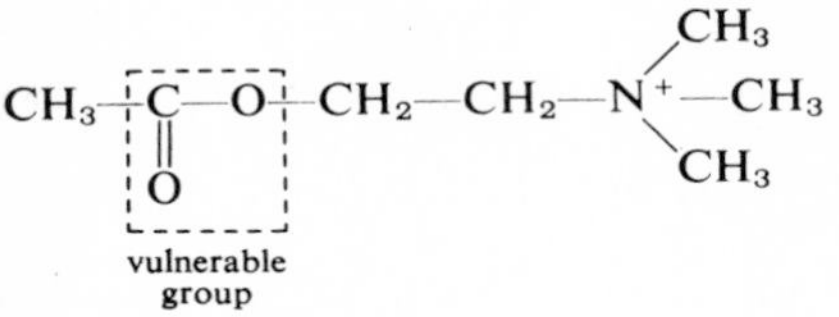 vulnerable group	Acetylcholine	100
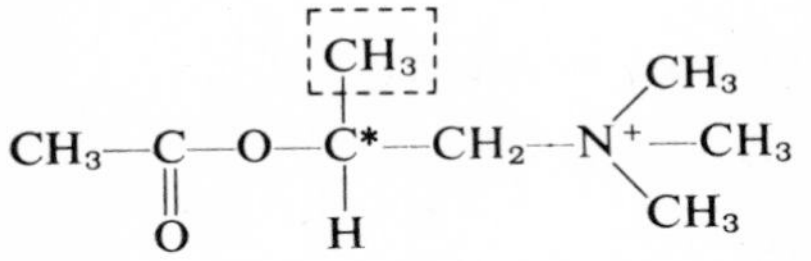	L-(+)-Acetyl-β-methylcholine	54.5
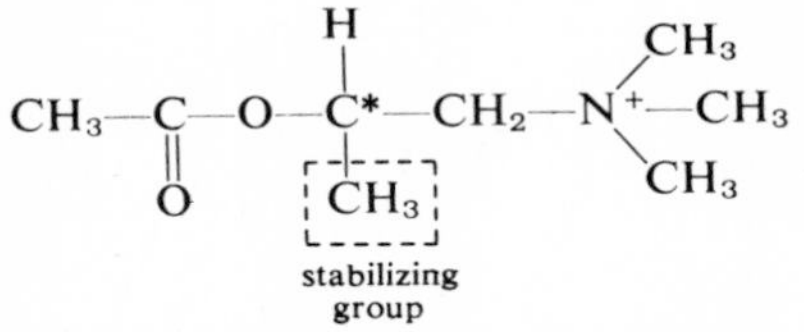 stabilizing group	D-(−)-Acetyl-β-methylcholine	Inhibition of hydrolysis

IV. CRITICAL AND NONCRITICAL MOIETIES

Critical moieties are the groups involved in drug–receptor complexation and are therefore essential to pharmacological action. *Noncritical* moieties are the groups that do not interact with the receptor; consequently they are susceptible to relatively wide structural variation. This offers the possibility of modifying the physicochemical characteristics of drugs and hence their distribution in the body. For example, in anticholinergic esters the acidic group is essential, but the choline moiety is not, since it can be eliminated without causing disappearance of anticholinergic activity. In a recent review Ariëns (17) lists several examples of essential and nonessential moieties.

V. BIOISOSTERIC GROUPS

Isosteric and bioisosteric groups have great application in molecular pharmacology, especially in the design of new drugs through the method of variation, or molecular modification (9,11,15,18–20).

TABLE 4.6 Stabilization of Vulnerable Groups by Suitable Substitution (14)

Structure	R	R′	R″	Rate of Hydrolysis in Human Serum
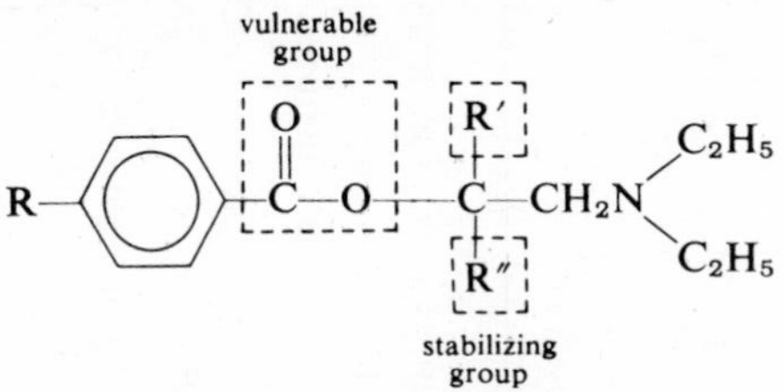	—NH_2	—H	—H	500
	—NH_2	—H	—CH_3	15
	—NH_2	—CH_3	—CH_3	0
	—F	—H	—H	3000

Reprinted by permission of the Williams and Wilkins Company.

In 1919 Langmuir (*21*) defined as *isosteres* those compounds or groups of atoms that have the same number and arrangement of electrons; for example, N_2 and CO, N_2O and CO_2, N_3^- and NCO^-. Isosteres are characterized by similar physical properties.

By introducing the hydride displacement law in 1925, Grimm (*22*) widened the concept of isosterism. Addition of a hydrogen atom with its lone electron to another atom results in what was conventionally called *pseudoatom*. Both the pseudoatom and the atom having one more electron than the atom from which the pseudoatom was derived have some analogous physical properties.

Later on Erlenmeyer (*23*) redefined isosteres as "atoms, ions or molecules in which the peripheral layers of electrons can be considered to be identical" (Table 4.7).

TABLE 4.7   An Expanded Table of Isosteres (*24*)

Grimm's Hydride Displacement

Total electrons	6	7	8	9	10	11
	C	N	O	F	Ne	Na^+
		CH	NH	OH	FH	—
			CH_2	NH_2	OH_2	FH_2^+
				CH_3	NH_3	OH_3^+
					CH_4	NH_4^+

Atoms and Groups of Atoms with the Same Number of Peripheral Electrons

Peripheral electrons	4	5	6	7	8
	N^+	P	S	Cl	ClH
	P^+	As	Se	Br	BrH
	S^+	Sb	Te	I	IH
	As^+	—	PH	SH	SH_2
	Sb^+	—	—	PH_2	PH_3

At the present time groups with similar steric and electronic configurations are also considered isosteres in spite of the number of electrons involved. Such is the case with the following groups:

carboxylate —COO—	ketone —CO—	chlorine —Cl
sulfonamido —SO_2NR—	sulfone —SO_2—	trifluoromethyl —CF_3

For instance, antihistaminic agents have the following general structure:

$$R-X-CH_2-CH_2-N \overset{\displaystyle R'}{\underset{\displaystyle R'}{}}$$

in which X can be any of these isosteric groups: O, NH, or CH_2. Another example is cholinergic blocking agents, which have the same general formula shown above, but X can be one of the following groups: —COO—, —CONH—, —COS—.

Considering the vast application of the concept of isosterism in molecular pharmacology, Friedman (25) has introduced the term *bioisosteres* as meaning "compounds which fit the broadest definition for isosteres, and have the same type of biological activity," even antagonistic.

In its broadest sense, therefore, the term *isosteres* may be applied to groups that merely bear resemblance in their external electronic shells or more restrictedly to groups with similar localization of regions of high or low electron density in molecules of similar size and shape (20). According to this criterion there are at least two types of isosteres:

1. *Classical isosteres*: those encompassed by Erlenmeyer's definition; that is, those represented in the hydride-displacement law, the elements of every group of the periodic table, and annular equivalents such as —CH=CH— and —S— (Table 4.8).

TABLE 4.8   Classical Isosteres (20)

Monovalents	Bivalents	Trivalents	Tetra-substituted Atoms	Annular Equivalents
F, OH, NH_2, CH_3	—O—	—N=	=C=	—CH=CH—
Cl, SH, PH_2	—S—	—P=	$=N^+=$	—S—
Br	—Se—	—As=	$=P^+=$	—O—
I	—Te—	—Sb=	$=As^+=$	—NH—
		—CH=	$=Sb^+=$	

2. *Nonclassical isosteres*: those that, substituted in a certain molecule, give origin to a compound whose steric arrangement and electronic configuration are similar to those of the parent compound; examples of pairs of these isosteres are H and F, —CO— and —SO_2—, —SO_2NH_2 and —$PO(OH)NH_2$ (Table 4.9).

TABLE 4.9   Nonclassical Isosteres (20)

—CO—	—COOH	—SO_2NH_2	H	Annular structures	$-O-\overset{\displaystyle O}{\overset{\displaystyle \|}{C}}-$	—OH
—SO_2—	—SO_3H	—$PO(OH)NH_2$	F	Open structures	$-\overset{\displaystyle O}{\overset{\displaystyle \|}{C}}-O-$	—NH_2

Although it is not possible to achieve pure isosterism (*10*), the principles of isosterism and bioisosterism are extensively employed to modify the structure of biologically active compounds. This substitution yields not only products whose action is identical to that of compounds taken as models but antagonists as well. Several examples may be cited of natural product equivalents, parametabolites, paravitamins, parahormones, and mimetics, as well as their specific antagonists, antimetabolites, antivitamins, antihormones, and lytics developed by applying the concept of isosterism (*7,9,10,12,17,19, 20,24*):

1. Aminopyrine and its isostere exert more or less the same antipyretic activity:

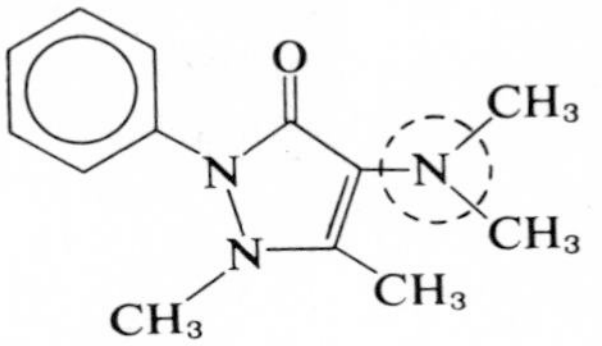

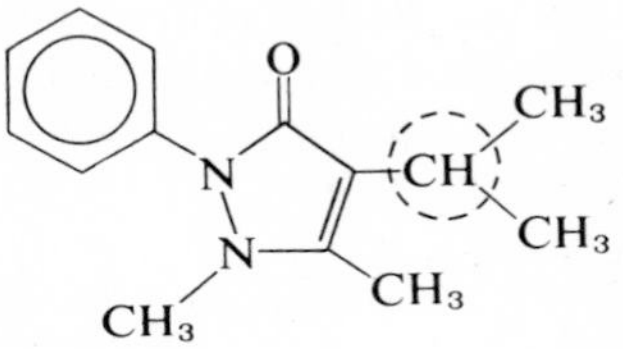

2. Acetylcholine and carbachol have similar muscarinic action:

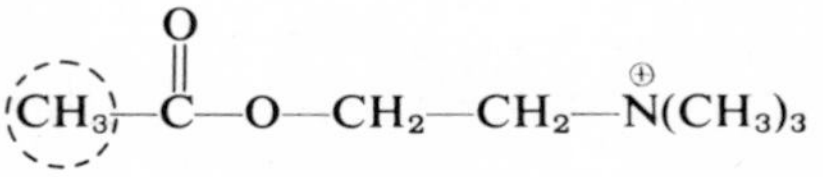

Acetylcholine 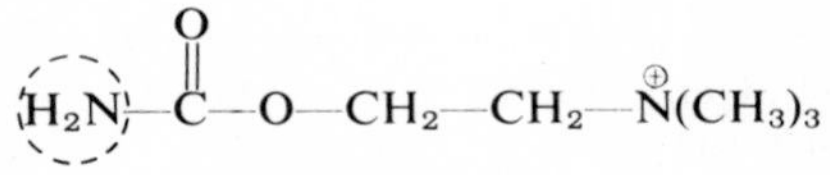　　　　　　　　　　Carbachol

3. 2-Thenylalanine is a biological antagonist of phenylalanine:

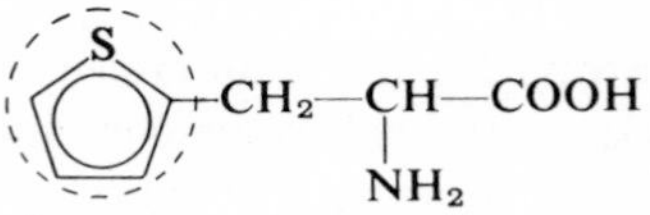

2-Thenylalanine 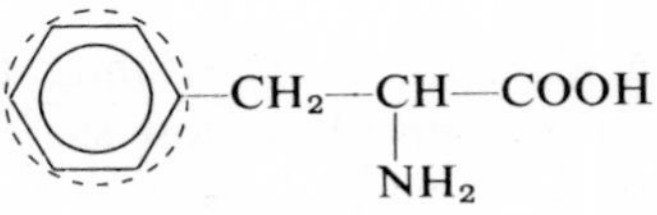　　　　　　　　　　Phenylalanine

4. 5-Bromouracil is an antagonist of thymine:

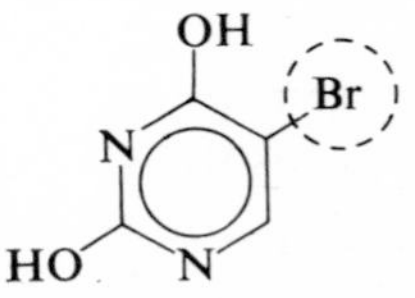

5-Bromouracil 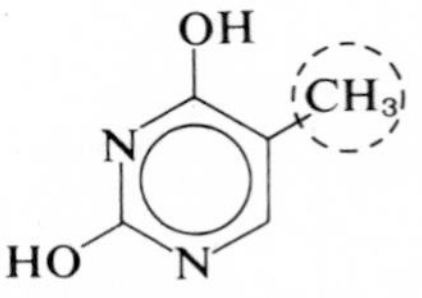　　　　　　　　　　Thymine

It should be recalled that the replacement of certain groups or atoms of natural metabolites by so-called deceptor groups (5), some of which are listed in Table 4.10, generally, but not always, results in competitive antagonists

TABLE 4.10   Deceptor Groups (5)

Normal Atom or Group	Deceptor Atoms or Groups	Examples of Competitive Metabolites
—H	—F	Fluorocitric acid; 5-Fluorouracil
	—Br	5-Bromouracil
	—CH$_3$	—CHOHCH$_3$ (terminal) in pantothenic acid
—OH	—NH$_2$	Aminopterin
—NH$_2$	—OH	Oxythiamine
	—NHNH$_2$	β-Phenylethylhydrazine
—CH$_3$	—Cl	2-Chloronaphthoquinone
	—C$_2$H$_5$	Ethionine
—S—	—O—	In methionine
	—CH$_2$CH$_2$—	In biotin
	—CH=CH—	Pyrithiamine
	—NH—	Thiamine analog
—COOH	—SO$_2$NH$_2$	Sulfanilamide
	—SO$_3$H	In nicotinic acid
	—COCH$_3$	β-Acetylpyridine
—COR	—PO(OR)$_2$	Antagonists of acetylcholinesterase
	—CONR$_2$	Carbamylcholine
—CO—	—CH$_2$—	Deoxypyridoxal

(4,26). These, once incorporated into biochemical processes, can lead to what is called *lethal synthesis* (27); that is, they cause finally the death of the microorganism that has used them instead of metabolites.

VI. HAPTOPHORIC AND PHARMACOPHORIC GROUPS

Haptophoric groups are groups that assist in binding drug to receptor. *Pharmacophoric* groups are those responsible for biological action. Thus diphenylmethyl and dicyclic moieties are haptophoric groups present in various drugs (Table 4.11).

Variety of actions that some drugs exert results from the presence of pharmacophoric and haptophoric groups able to complexate by different mechanisms with different types of receptors. This occurs with some sulfonic derivatives that can elicit various activities (Table 4.12).

TABLE 4.11 Prevalence of Diphenylmethyl and Related Dicyclogroups as Haptophoric Moieties in Drugs (12)

Formula	Compound	Formula	Compound
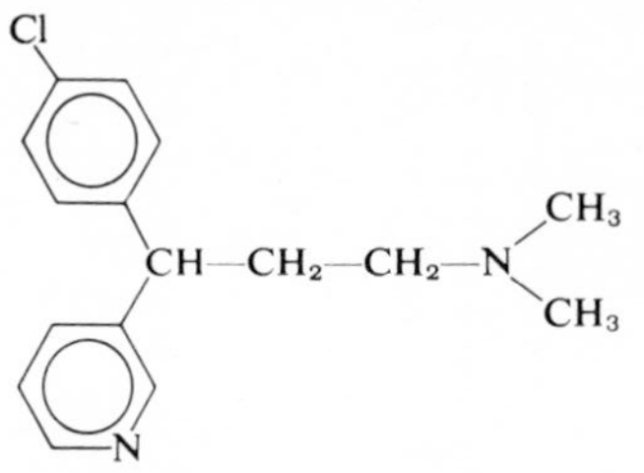	Chlorpheniramine (antihistaminic)	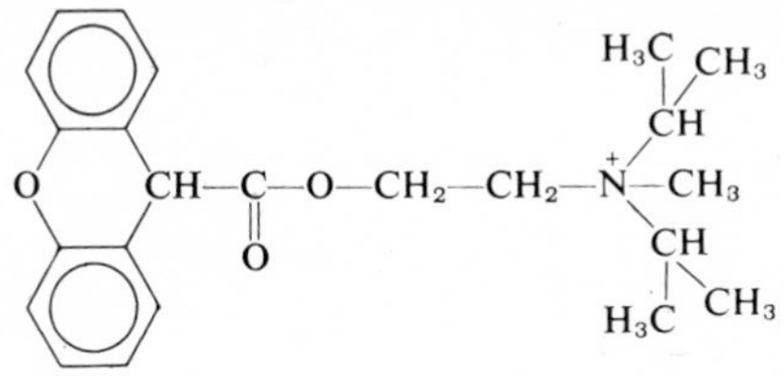	Propantheline (anticholinergic)
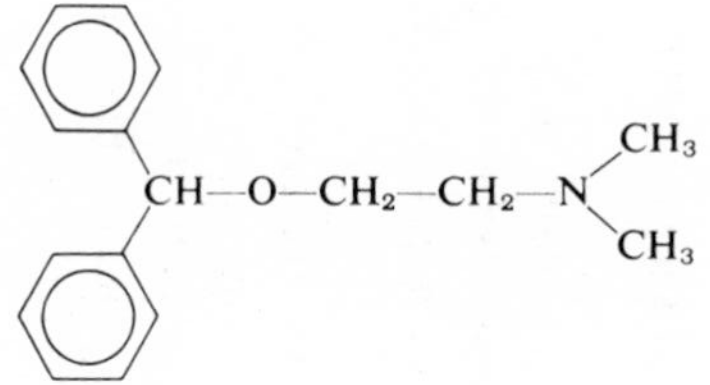	Diphenhydramine (antihistaminic)	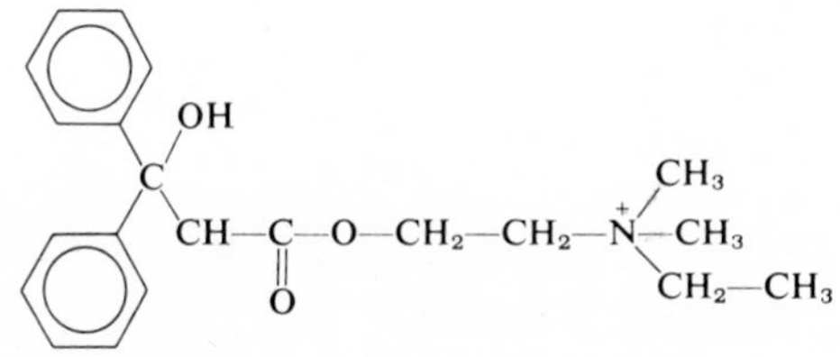	Lachesine (anticholinergic)
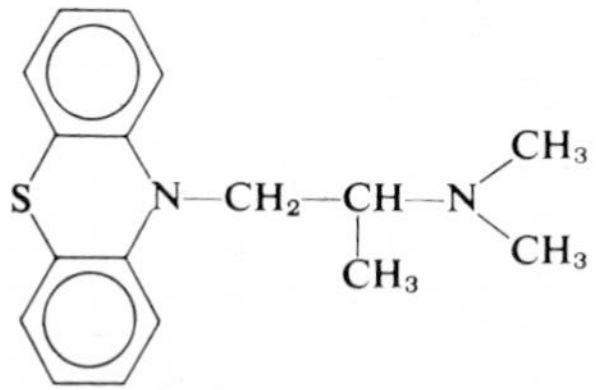	Promethazine (antihistaminic)	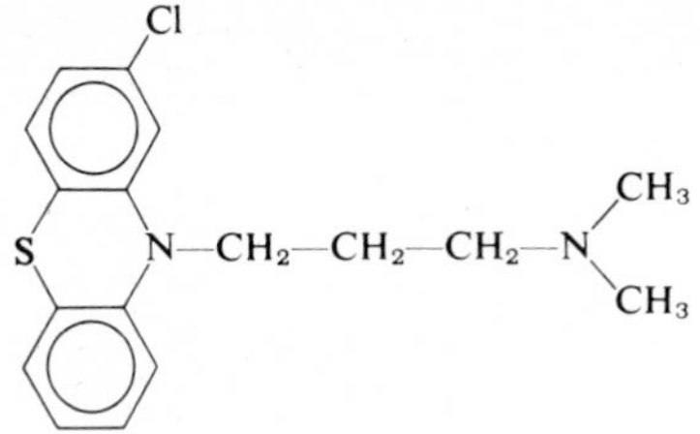	Chlorpromazine (tranquilizer)
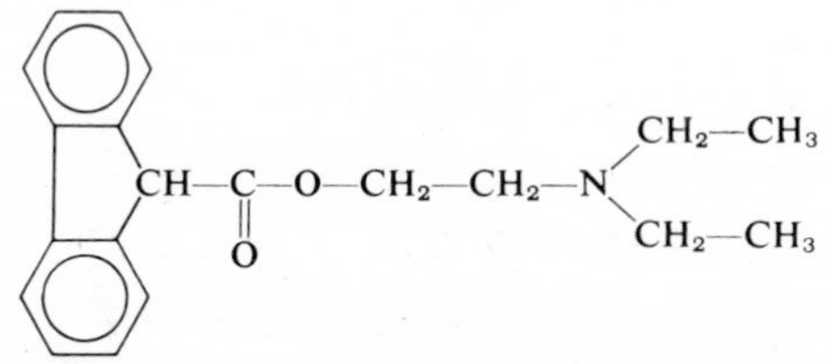	Pavatrine ® (spasmolytic, anticholinergic)	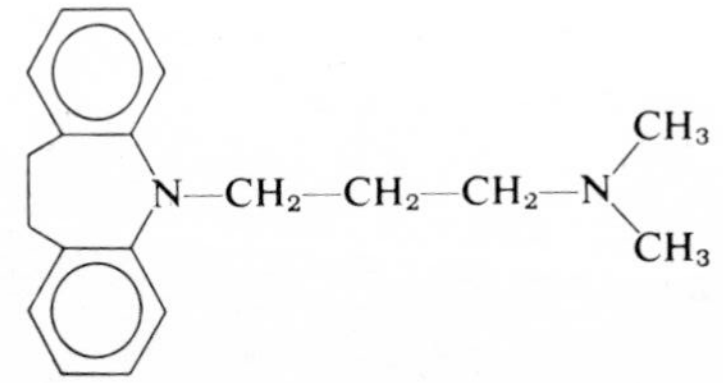	Imipramine (antidepressant)

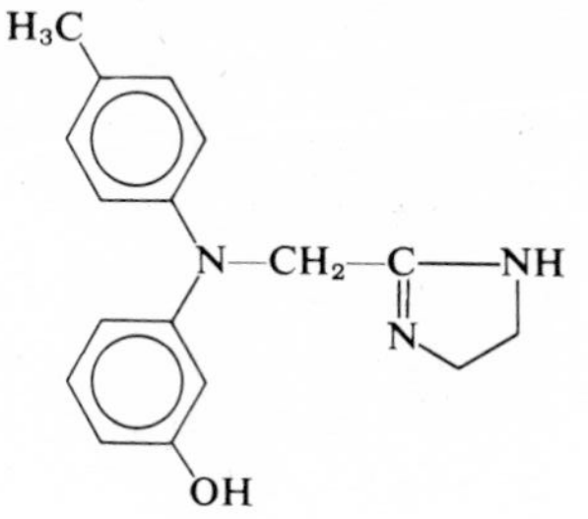

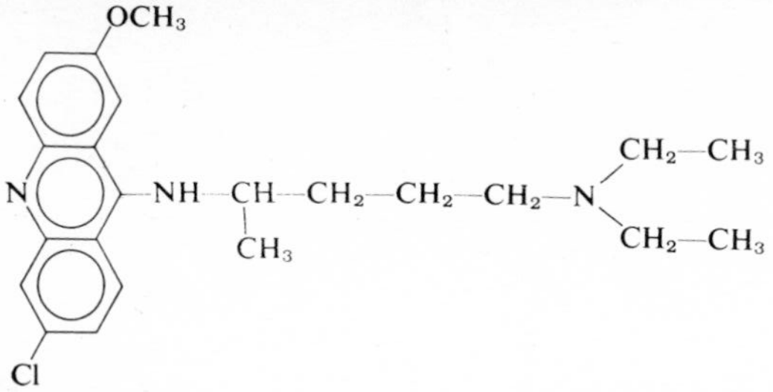

Quinacrine (antimalarial)

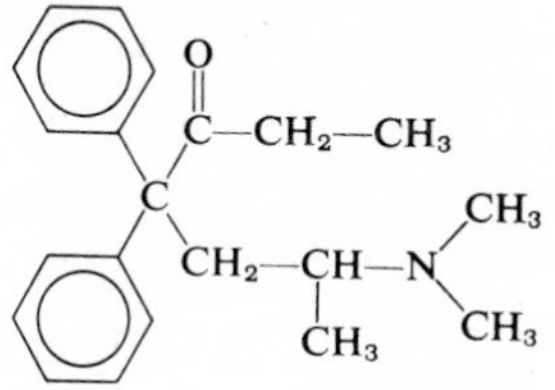

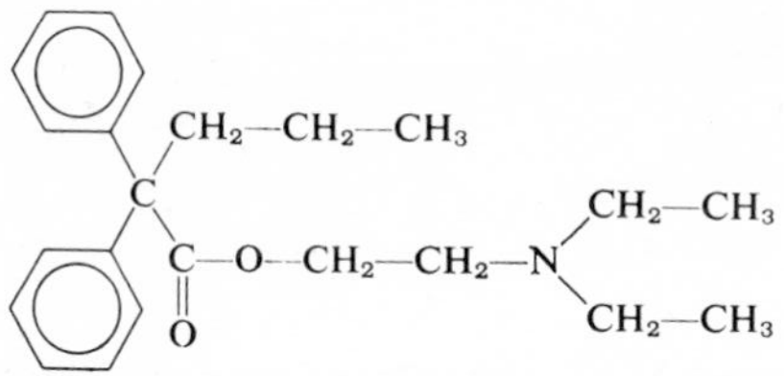

SKF 525A (multipotent enzyme inhibitor)

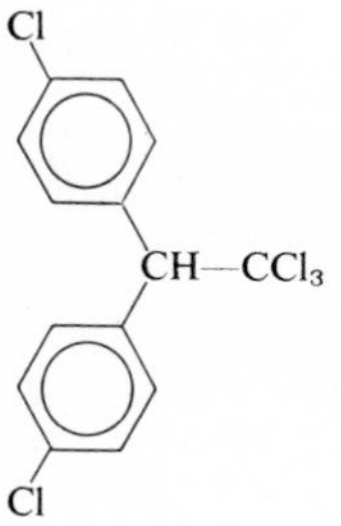

DDT (insecticide)

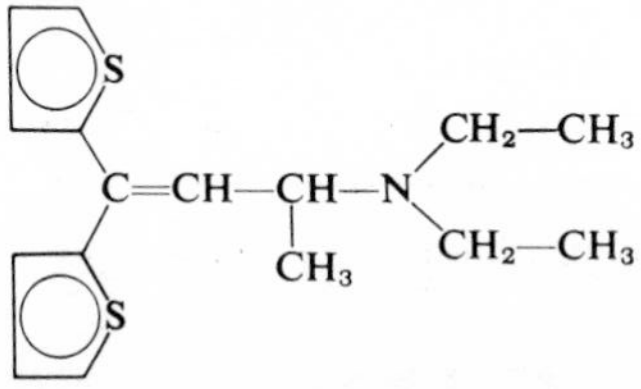

PR 186 (anticoagulant)

Phentolamine (sympatholytic)

Methadone (analgetic)

Thiambutene (analgetic)

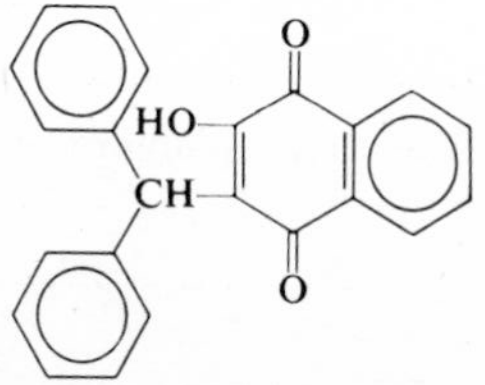

TABLE 4.12 Biological Action of Related Sulfonylureas (I), Sulfonamides (II), and Sulfones (III, IV) (12)

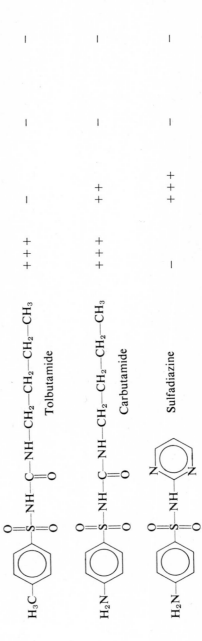

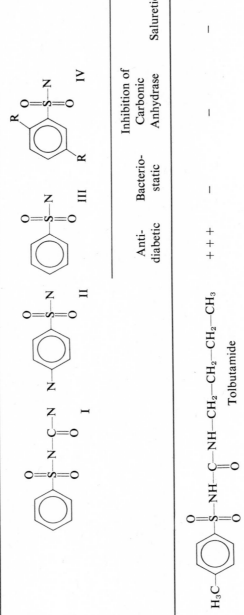

	Anti-diabetic	Bacterio-static	Inhibition of Carbonic Anhydrase	Saluretic
Tolbutamide	+ + +	–	–	–
Carbutamide	+ + +	+ +	–	–
Sulfadiazine	–	+ + +	–	–

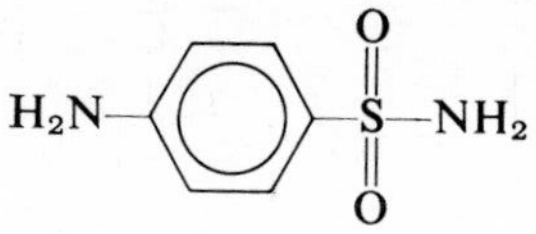 Sulfanilamide	−	++	++	−
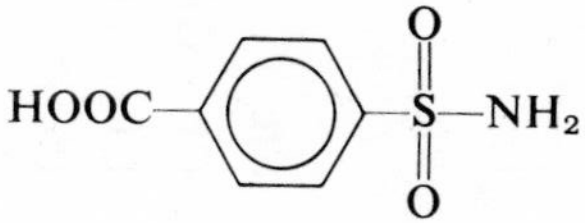 Carzenide	−	−	+++	−
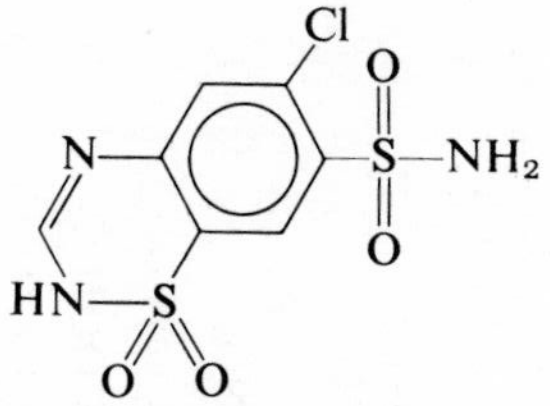 Chlorothiazide	−	−	++	+++ / +

63

VII. ELECTRONIC EFFECTS OF SPECIFIC GROUPS

Basic studies of organic chemistry, expanded in specialized literature (*28–35*), have demonstrated that certain chemical groups produce two important electronic effects: inductive and conjugative.

A. Inductive Effects

Inductive (or *electrostatic*) effects result from electronic shifts along simple bonds owing to the attraction exerted by certain groups because of their electronegativity (Table 4.13). Thus, as shown in Table 4.14, groups that

TABLE 4.13   Electronegativity of Some Chemical Elements (*36*)

		H 2.1						
	B 2.0			C 2.5		N 3.0	O 3.5	F 4.0
Si 1.8		P 2.1		S 2.5		Cl 3.0		
	As 2.0		Se 2.4		Br 2.8			
Sb 1.8		Te 2.1		I 2.5				
	2.0			2.5		3.0	3.5	4.0

Reprinted by permission of Cornell University Press.

TABLE 4.14   Inductive Effects of Some Chemical Groups (*28*)

− *I* Groups			+ *I* Groups
—NH₃⁺	—CHO	—OR	—CH₃

—NR₃⁺	—C=O
	  |
	  R
		—SH	—CH₂R

—NO₂	—F	—SR	—CHR₂
—C≡N	—Cl	—CH=CH₂	—CR₃

—COOH	—Br	—CR=CR₂	—C—O⁻
			  ‖
			  O

—COOR	—OH	—C≡C—H	

Reprinted by permission of Holt, Rinehart and Winston, Inc.

attract electrons more strongly than hydrogen display negative inductive effects $(-I)$, whereas those that attract electrons less strongly than hydrogen manifest positive inductive effects $(+I)$. Similar effects exerted through space between dipoles or charges of the substituent group and the reaction center are called *field effects* (29,30). Groups that manifest a $-I$ effect are called electron acceptors; those that show a $+I$ effect, electron donors (29).

Thus alkyl groups, which exert an effect toward donating or repelling electrons, have a positive inductive effect. This fact is borne out by comparing the dissociation constants of formic and acetic acids: the mere replacement of H by CH_3 reduces the dissociation constant by a factor of 10 (31):

$$H-COOH \qquad K = 1.76 \times 10^{-4}$$

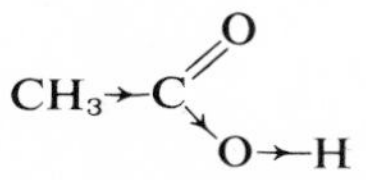

$$K = 1.76 \times 10^{-5}$$

Alkyl groups can manifest, besides inductive effects, the phenomenon of hyperconjugation as a consequence of the possibility of σ-electrons of the C—H bond interacting with the π-electrons of the neighboring bond. The phenomenon of hyperconjugation is a very important, although particular, case of σ-π conjugation and can explain, at least partially, differences in heats of hydrogenation (28). Examples of hyperconjugation are found in the following molecules:

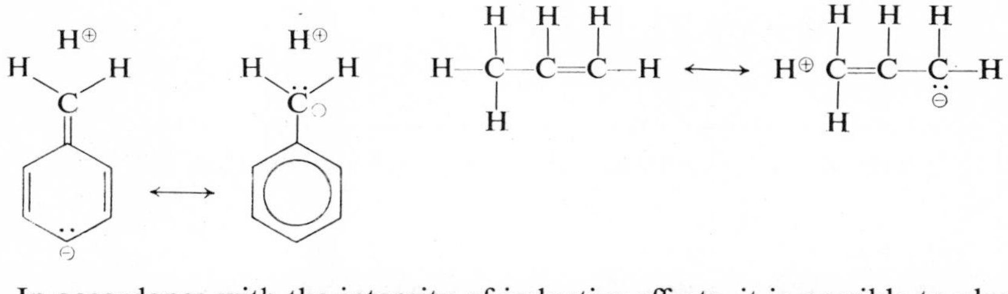

In accordance with the intensity of inductive effects, it is possible to place certain groups in decreasing order of the $-I$ effect or in increasing order of the $+I$ effect (31):

$$F > Cl > Br > I > OCH_3 > C_6H_5 \qquad -I \text{ effect}$$

$$CH_3 < C_2H_5 < CH(CH_3)_2 < n\text{-}C_3H_7 < C(CH_3)_3 \quad +I \text{ effect}$$

B. Conjugative Effects

Conjugative (or *resonance*) effects result from the delocalization and high mobility of π-electrons and are manifested in compounds with conjugated double bonds. Groups that increase the electronic density in conjugated systems have $+R$ character; those that decrease such density, $-R$ character (Table 4.15). Usually each of the $+R$ groups is attached to the remainder of the molecule by an atom having one or more unshared pairs of electrons (28).

TABLE 4.15   Resonance Effect of Some Chemical Groups (28)

$+R, -I$ Groups	$-R, -I$ Groups	$+R, +I$ Groups
—F	—NO₂	—O⊖
—Cl	—C≡N	—S⊖
—Br	—CHO	—CH₃
—I	—C=O	
—OH	R	
—OR	—COOH	—CR₃
—O—C—R ‖ O	—COOR	
—SH	—CONH₂	
—SR	O ‖ —S—R ‖ O	
—NH₂		
—NR₂		
—NH—C—R ‖ O	—CF₃	

Reprinted by permission of Holt, Rinehart and Winston, Inc.

VIII. EFFECTS OF HALOGENATION

There are many nonpharmacological reasons for synthesizing halogenated compounds analogous to others already known (37):

1. Some are easily obtained as starting materials in organic syntheses.

2. Halogens are often used as blocking or directing groups during the synthesis of aromatic compounds, and, once these have been prepared, halogens are not removed because of economic considerations.

3. Sometimes certain manufacturers, whose sole purpose is to market products similar to those of their competitors, halogenate drugs simply to circumvent manufacturing patents.

Such commercial and economic reasons are not those that lead medicinal chemists concerned with the design and preparation of new drugs to introduce halogens in molecules of biologically active compounds. Their purpose in resorting to halogenation, a common practice, is to obtain structurally analogous compounds with modified biological activity. Effects produced by this replacement may be the following (5):

1. Purely physical, as, for example, in the case of general anesthetics and antiseptics, whose biological activity is related to physical properties, such as liposolubility, surface tension, and vapor pressure.

2. Direct result of chemical reactivity of the halogen, as in alkylating agents and acylating agents.

3. Combination of physical and chemical effects, as in halogen-substituted p-aminobenzoic acids.

Interest in this type of molecular modification therefore stems from the steric and electronic effects of halogens, whose atomic volume is substantially greater than that of hydrogen (Table 4.16). Furthermore all C–halogen bonds except C—F are weaker than C—H (Table 4.17).

TABLE 4.16 Atomic Radii of Hydrogen and Halogens (38)

Atom	Atomic Radius (Å)
Hydrogen	0.29
Fluorine	0.64
Chlorine	0.99
Bromine	1.14
Iodine	1.33

TABLE 4.17 Characteristics of Carbon–Halogen Bonds (38)

Bond[a]	Interatomic Distance (Å)	Bond Strength (kcal/mole)
C—H	1.14	93
C—F	1.45	114
C—Cl	1.74	72
C—Br	1.90	59
C—I	2.12	45

[a] In aliphatic series.

For the manifestation of conjugative effect a uniform electronic system should be established among the molecule's component groups, with over-lapping of electronic clouds; as a consequence a necessary condition for conjugation is that the axes of π-electron clouds (and of p-electrons) be parallel (*31*). This occurs in the system —CH=CH—CH=CH—, which behaves not as an agglomerate of double bonds but as a uniform system that transmits atomic interaction as a result of the overlapping of π-orbitals, axes of which are disposed parallel (*39*).

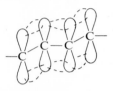

The contrary occurs in 2-quinuclidone. Although it has an amide group with expected amide properties, the rigid bicyclic system forces the axes of the p-electron clouds of nitrogen to stay perpendicular (and not parallel as in the case of true amides) to the axes of the electron clouds of the carbonyl group. Conjugation not being possible, 2-quinuclidone behaves less like an amide and more like an amine and a ketone.

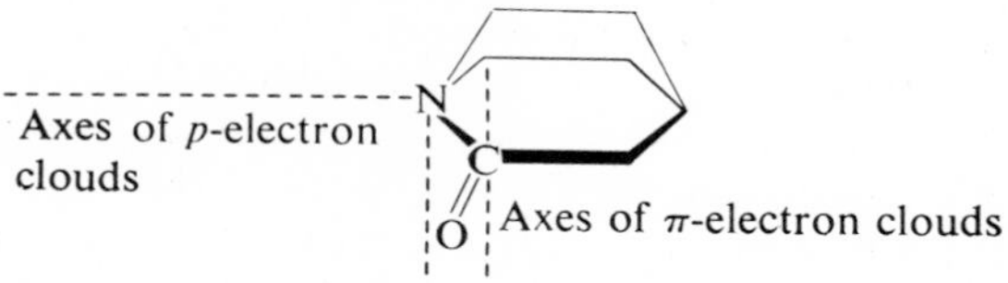

Axes of p-electron clouds

Axes of π-electron clouds

The electronic effects exerted by halogens are of two types: inductive $-I$, owing to their avidity for electrons, and conjugative $+R$, owing to their high electron density as a consequence of having three pairs of unshared electrons.

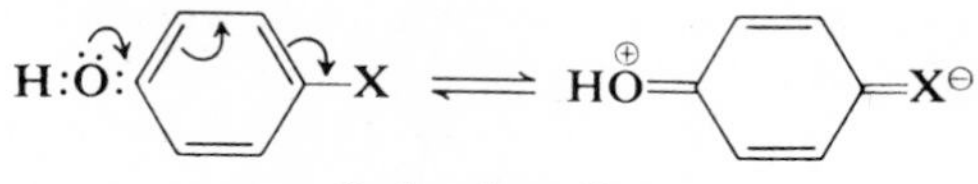

Inductive effect

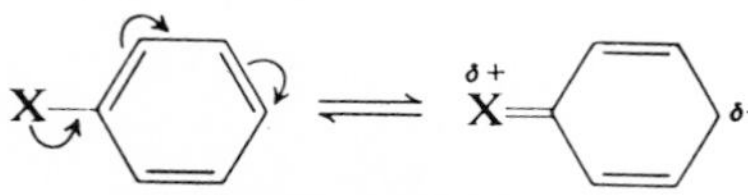

Conjugative effect

In some cases, such as when inductive and conjugative effects are equal and opposite in sign, they cancel each other. In other cases, however, the inductive effect prevails over the conjugative one or vice versa, depending on the position of the halogens and on the moiety to which they are bound (5).

Therefore halogens can exert three main effects: steric effects, electronic effects, and obstructive halogenation. Several anesthetics and other drugs have been prepared with the aim of taking advantage of these effects of halogenation (4,37,38). This section merely mentions *labile halogens*, whose presence characterizes compounds such as nitrogen mustards and adrenergic blocking agents. These covalently bonded halogens are released spontaneously in the form of halide ions from the compound of which they are part, as shown in Chapter 7, Section II. Another type not covered in detail are the chloramines, whose antiseptic action is due to hypochlorous acid, which results from hydrolysis:

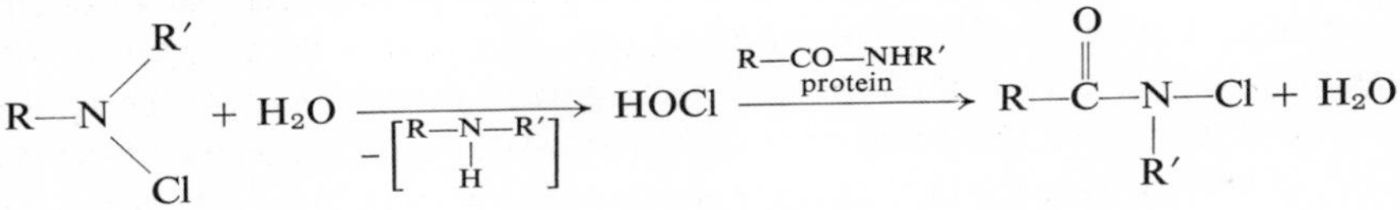

A. Steric Effects

In many halogenated compounds the action of the halogen results from its steric effect. For example, it was shown that 9-α-halogen substitution in cortisol and cortisone increases activity in the following order: $H < F < Cl < Br < I$ (37).

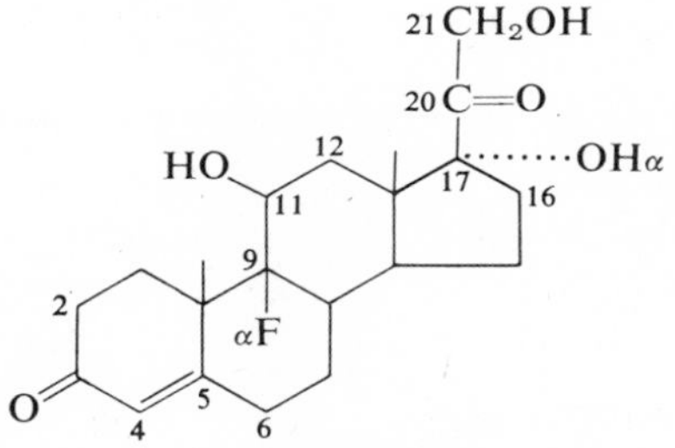

Fludrocortisone

In the case of thyroxine the bulky atoms of iodine prevent the free rotation around the ether bond and maintain the planes of aromatic rings in a perpendicular position to each other (37):

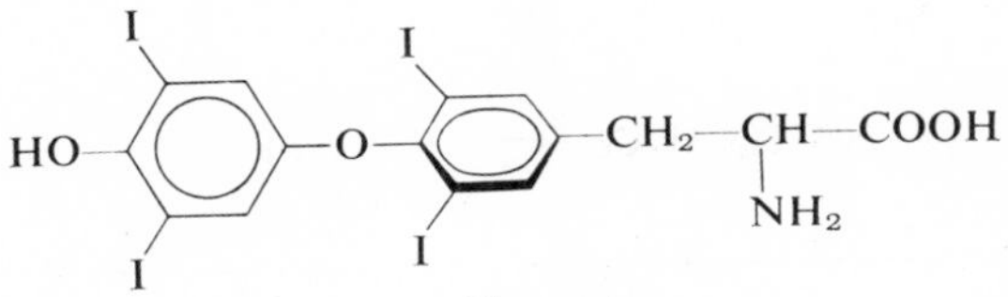

Thyroxine

Another example is found in bretylium. Substitution of bromine by other halogens and groups, such as CH_3 or NO_2, does not alter its activity. From this fact it follows that the function of the halogen is merely steric (37):

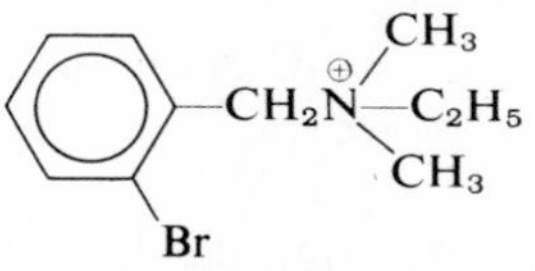

Bretylium

B. Electronic Effects

Several examples of electronic effects on the biological activity of a certain compound can be found in the aromatic series, probably because electronic effects are easily transmitted through conjugated systems. Alkylating agents may have decreased the percentage of hydrolysis as a result of the inductive effect of halogen, with a consequent reduction in the biological activity of the resulting compound (Table 4.18).

TABLE 4.18   Electronic Effects on the Activity of Alkylating Agents (37)

Compound	Hydrolysis (%)	Biological Activity
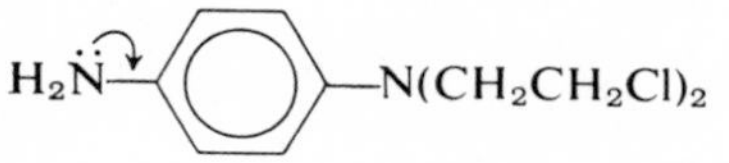	100	+
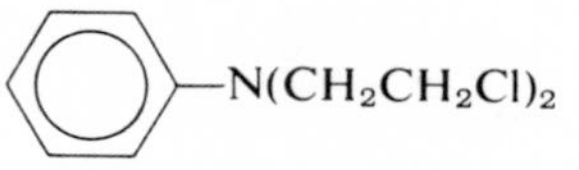	20	+
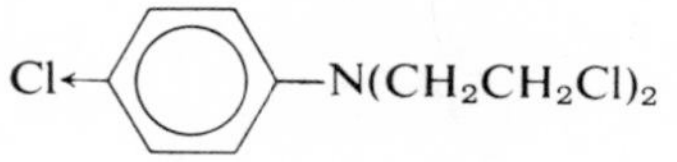	9	−
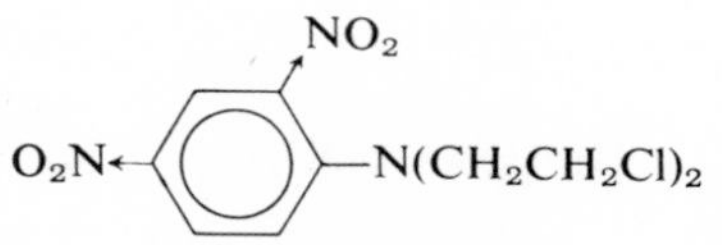	< 1	−

Reprinted by permission of the Williams and Wilkins Company.

The pharmacological activity of several bacteriostatic and fungicidal substances is enhanced by the introduction of one or more halogens. The same enhancement occurs in the local anesthetics, as in the case of procaine derivatives. The greater activity is perhaps related not only to electronic effects but to steric effects as well (Table 4.19).

TABLE 4.19 Relative Rates of Hydrolysis
of Some Procaine Derivatives (37)

Compound	Relative Rate of Hydrolysis
Procaine	1.00
2-Chloroprocaine	4.63
2-Bromoprocaine	2.44
3,5-Dichloroprocaine	0.26

In some instances halogens present in certain drugs can be replaced by other groups that exert negative inductive effects. This happens in the case of chloramphenicol, whose antimicrobial activity is directly related to the electronegativity of the *para* substituent of the aromatic ring and to the molar volume and the electronegativity of the acyl substituent of the dichloroacetamide chain (41).

C. Obstructive Halogenation

In the process of detoxication aromatic rings are hydroxylated and afterward conjugated with glucuronic acid:

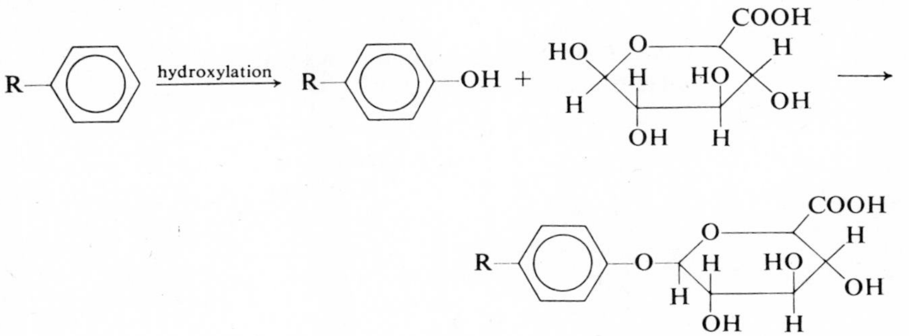

The presence of a halogen in the *para* position of aromatic rings of some drugs prevents this process. Anticonvulsant agents that are derived from phenobarbital and contain chlorine bound to the *para* position of the phenyl have more persistent action than the parent compound. This is a good example of obstructive halogenation, because it is known that phenobarbital is hydroxylated in this position (26,37).

Replacement of the methyl group by chlorine in tolbutamide increases its half-life from 5.7 to 33 hours (12). This prolongation of action is also ascribed to obstructive halogenation.

D. Special Effects Due to Fluorine Introduction

Fluorine is the most electronegative of halogens. For this reason the strength of trifluoroacetic acid is similar to that of more dissociated mineral acids. Furthermore, since its atomic radius is nearly equal to that of hydrogen, fluorine differs from hydrogen less than other halogens. This explains the ease with which the molecules of fluorinated antimetabolites can replace those of normal metabolites in the organism at the molecular level. Such is not the case with chlorinated, brominated, and iodinated compounds. Also, the p-electrons of halogens other than fluorine, as a result of their promotion to vacant d-orbitals, can enter into resonance with the π-electrons of electron-donating chemical groups, as illustrated by halogenated o-phenols and p-phenols, and o-anilines and p-anilines:

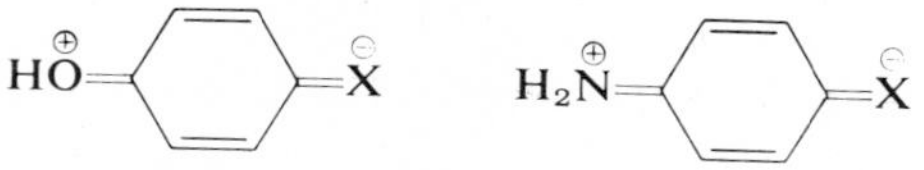

Fluorine does not possess this property, because it has no d-orbitals, since its electronic configuration is $1s^2 2s^2 2p_x^2 2p_y^2 2p_z$. For this reason p-fluorophenol is slightly less acidic than phenol itself, whereas other p-halogenated phenols are much more acidic in increasing order of the atomic number of the halogen considered (Table 4.20).

TABLE 4.20   Dissociation   Constants   of
p-Halogenated Phenols (38)

Compound	Dissociation Constant $K_a \times 10^{-10}$
Phenol	0.32
p-Fluorophenol	0.26
p-Chlorophenol	1.32
p-Bromophenol	1.55
p-Iodophenol	2.19

It must be recalled that the C—F bond is stronger than the C—H, C—Cl, C—Br, and C—I bonds (Table 4.17). The CF_3 moiety, so much used in drugs (38,42), has a high negative inductive effect and also exerts an influence through hyperconjugation:

$$F \xleftarrow{} \overset{F}{\underset{F}{C}}{-} \longleftrightarrow F{-}\overset{F\oplus}{\underset{F}{C}}{=} \longleftrightarrow F\oplus \ \overset{F}{\underset{F}{C}}{=} \longleftrightarrow F{-}\overset{F}{\underset{F\oplus}{C}}{=}$$

The electronic properties of the C—F bond have a direct influence on its biochemical properties, among which the most prominent is its great stability to metabolic processes (37,38). Thus, although the compound $ClCH_2CH_2$-$SCH_2CH_2SCH_2CH_2Cl$ is a very potent vesicant poison, the corresponding fluorinated derivative, due to the stability of fluorine atoms, is entirely innocuous (38). Furthermore, although the CF_3 group is not attacked, the remainder of the molecule can undergo degradation (37).

The small volume of the fluorine atom does not interfere with the interaction of the drug of which it is part with the respective cellular receptor. This is the reason that some biochemical systems accept fluoroacetic acid in place of acetic acid (43). This fraudulent incorporation leads to lethal synthesis, caused also by 5-fluorouracil and 5-fluoronicotinic acid (27).

In short, the stability of the C—F bond, the small volume of the fluorine atom, and its highly electronegative character have made appealing the introduction of this halogen into pharmacodynamic and chemotherapeutic agents. For instance, therapeutics have recently been enriched by many fluorinated drugs (37,38): anesthetics (38,42,44,45); antimetabolites; diuretics and saluretics (44); convulsant, anticonvulsant, and muscle-relaxant agents;

$$FCH_2(CH_2)_7\underset{\underset{CH_3}{|}}{CH}(CH_2)_8COOH$$

Fluorotuberculostearic acid (analogous to tuberculostearic acid and active against *Mycobacterium tuberculosis in vitro*)

Trifluoromethylphenol
(vermifuge)

o-, m-, or p-fluoroalanine (antimetabolite of phenylalanine and bacteriostatic)

psychotherapeutic and antiemetic agents (44); steroids; neuroleptics, anti-histaminics, and analgetics; vermifuges, antibacterials, antivirals, and anti-fungics; as well as various other drugs (44).

IX. EFFECTS OF ALKYL GROUPS

By exerting effects on the physical properties—such as solubility, diffusi-bility, or surface tension—of an organic substance, alkyl groups substantially influence biological activity (5). Examples of drugs where this was the accomplished objective are certain antiseptics, phenolic fungicides and bactericides, and several anesthetics.

For instance, the methyl group exerts mainly two types of effect (46): steric and electronic. Steric effects are of two sorts:

1. Those manifested in aqueous solution, involving solubility, covalent hydration, and chelation (Table 4.21).

TABLE 4.21 Increased Solubility in Water Caused by Insertion of Methyl Groups (46, 47)

Drug	R′	R″	pK$_a$	Ionization at pH 5.2 (%)	Solubility at pH 5.2 (g-mole/l at 37°C)
Sulfadiazine	H	H	6.5	3.9	0.0005
Sulfamerazine	H	CH$_3$	7.1	1.4	0.0013
Sulfamethazine	CH$_3$	CH$_3$	7.4	0.7	0.024

2. Those that require a complementary surface in order to be manifested; that is, on receptors and enzymes.

Electronic effects, owing to the repulsion of electrons by this group, are exerted in the degree of ionization, oxidation–reduction potential, and co-valent reactivity.

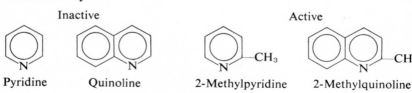

Inactive   Active

Pyridine   Quinoline   2-Methylpyridine   2-Methylquinoline

A. Homologous Series

The methyl group is a special case in the homologous series. In general they are compounds obtained through alternating the size of an alkyl group or of a polymethylene chain (5,7,10,48). They can be represented by the following formulas (48):

1. Alkane series: $C_nH_{2n+1}X$, where X is the group that defines the series.
2. Polymethylene series: $X(CH_2)_nY$, where X and Y are equal or different moieties.
3. Cyclopolymethylene series: $(CH_2)_n > X$ or $(CH_2)_n > CHX$, where the moiety X may either form part of the ring or be bound to one of the carbon atoms of the ring.

Besides these, there is the *hybrid series*, which can be represented by several formulas, such as the following:

$$\overset{\oplus}{Me_3N}C_nH_{2n+1} \qquad \overset{\oplus}{MeEt_2N}C_nH_{2n+1}$$

1. Alkane and Polymethylene Series. Although it is not possible to establish rigid rules for the pharmacological properties of homologous compounds, in the alkane and polymethylene series the following general types of change have been found:

1. Activity increases regularly until a maximum is reached, higher members being almost or entirely inactive. This can be observed particularly in structurally nonspecific drugs, such as some hypnotics, general anesthetics, volatile insecticides, and disinfectants (Table 4.22).

The same phenomenon also occurs, although seldom, in structurally specific compounds, as in the case of local anesthetics (Table 4.23) and spasmolytics (Table 4.24).

2. Activity increases irregularly, reaches a maximal value, and then decreases, again irregularly. A typical example is found among benzilic esters with atropinic properties (Table 4.25).

3. Activity increases (or decreases), reaches a relatively high (or low) value, and then remains more or less constant for a few or many higher members. One example is seen in homologous parasympathomimetics of the general formula $R\overset{\oplus}{N}Me_3$, the pharmacological properties of which are greater when the number of atoms in the chain R is five (48).

In ganglionic blocking agents of the general formula $R_3\overset{\oplus}{N}(CH_2)_n\overset{\oplus}{N}R_3$ activity is present in those in which n is 4, 5, or 6.

In the polymethylene series, corresponding to the general formula $R_3\overset{\oplus}{N}C_6H_4(CH_2)_n\overset{\oplus}{N}R_3$, activity is maximal in compounds in which n is 2.

4. Activity alternates, members with an odd number of carbon atoms being

TABLE 4.22 Phenolic Coefficients of n-Alkylphenols Tested on *Bacillus typhosus* (49)

R	p-n-Alkyl-phenols 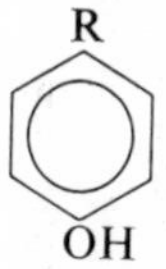	4-n-Alkyl-m-cresols 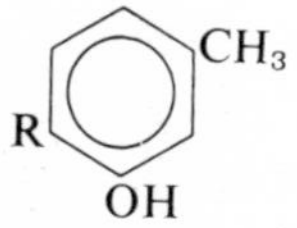	3-n-Alkyl-p-cresols 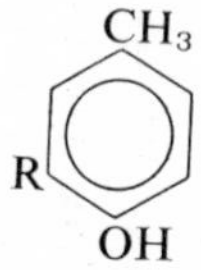	5-n-Alkyl-o-cresols 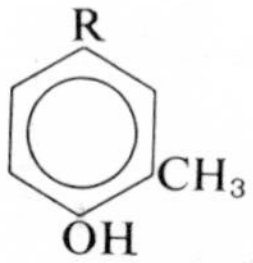	3-n-Alkyl-o-cresols 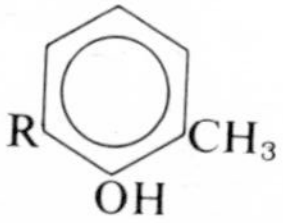	4-n-Alkyl-guaiacols 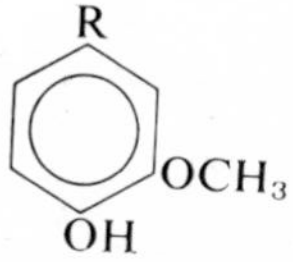
CH_3	2.5	—	—	—	—	2.7
C_2H_5	7.5	12.5[a]	12.5	15	—	2
$n\text{-}C_3H_7$	20	34	—	—	—	5
$n\text{-}C_4H_9$	70[b]	100	95	110	60	25
$n\text{-}C_5H_{11}$	104	280	250	300	250	25
$n\text{-}C_6H_{13}$	90	275	250	180	180	9
$n\text{-}C_7H_{15}$	20	30	175	100	—	—

[a] The phenol coefficient of 6-ethyl-m-cresol (Me:OH:Et = 1:3:6) was 15.
[b] The phenol coefficient of o-n-butylphenol was 75.

TABLE 4.23 Local-Anesthetic Activity in Homologous Series (*10,50*)

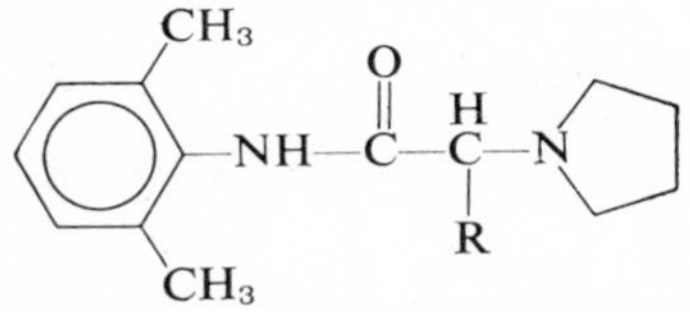

R	Duration of Anesthesia in Rabbit Cornea (min)
Hydrogen	11
Methyl	23
Ethyl	34
Propyl	49
Butyl	93

TABLE 4.24 Spasmolytic Activity in Homologous Series (*10,51*)

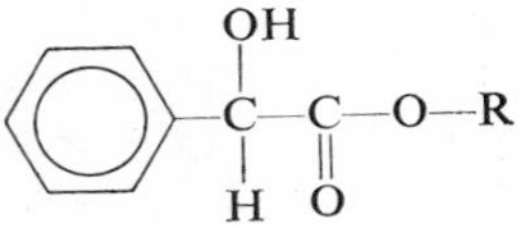

R	Spasmolytic Activity on Guinea-Pig Isolated Gut
Methyl	8
Ethyl	12
Propyl	24
Butyl	98
Pentyl	240
Hexyl	410
Heptyl	490

consistently more active than neighboring members with an even number of carbon atoms, or vice versa. This is observed with antimalarials derived from 6-methoxy-8-aminoquinoline: activity is greater in compounds in which n is an even number (range $n = 2$ to 7) (*52*).

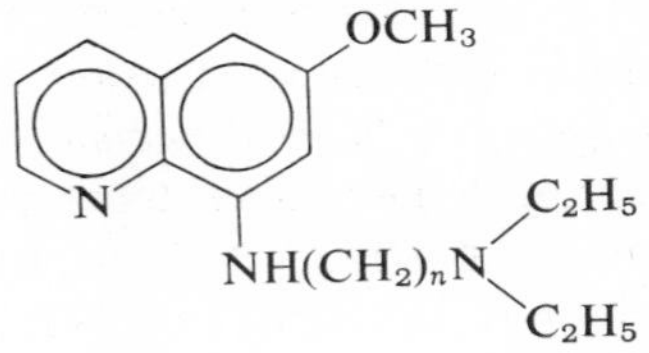

TABLE 4.25   Atropine-like Properties of Homologous Benzilic Esters (48)

$$(C_6H_5)_2C \overset{\displaystyle OH}{\underset{\displaystyle CO_2CH_2CH_2\overset{+}{N}}{\vert}} \overset{\displaystyle R}{\underset{\displaystyle R''}{\overset{\vert}{\underset{\vert}{\text{—}R'}}}}$$

Nature of the N-Alkyl Groups			Relative Molar Potencies (Atropine = 100)		
R	R′	R″	On the Salivary Gland (Cat)	On Blood Pressure (Cat)	On the Eye (Mouse)
CH_3	CH_3	H	11 ± 1.8	9.8	12.6
CH_3	CH_3	CH_3	196 ± 32	103	31
CH_3	CH_3	C_2H_5	258 ± 38	182	104
CH_3	CH_3	$n\text{-}C_3H_7$	147 ± 46	98	22
CH_3	CH_3	$n\text{-}C_4H_9$	75 ± 19	63	10.5
CH_3	CH_3	$n\text{-}C_5H_{11}$	71 ± 36	32	13
C_2H_5	C_2H_5	H	18 ± 4.6	21	6.3
C_2H_5	C_2H_5	CH_3	273 ± 49	239	64
C_2H_5	C_2H_5	C_2H_5	273 ± 44	190	83
C_2H_5	C_2H_5	$n\text{-}C_3H_7$	135 ± 30	78	22

Another example is the series of 4,4′-dimethylamino-diphenoxyalkanes tested as potential schistosomicides. Activity was found in those compounds in which $n = 2$ to 10 (53):

$$4\text{-}Me_2NC_6H_4O(CH_2)_nOC_6H_4NMe_2\text{-}4'$$

On the other hand, consideration of the classical work of Knoop and of Dakin on the metabolism of ω-phenyl fatty acids, $Ph(CH_2)_nCOOH$, shows that alternation of pharmacological properties in these series results merely from alternating rates of metabolism and excretion, and not from some peculiar properties of receptors in cells (48).

5. Activity changes, lower members possessing one type, and higher members a different type, of predominant action. Often higher members are antagonists of the pharmacological effect of lower members, and vice versa.

Such is the case in the series of N-alkyl derivatives of norepinephrine, in which alkylation reduces the hypertensive activity of the molecule in the sequence —NH_2, —NHMe, —NHEt, —NHPr-n, hypotensive effects occurring when the terminal group is —NHPr-i or —NHBu. This anomaly results from complexation of these compounds with different receptors: in the first case with α as well as with β; in the second mainly with β (Table 4.26).

TABLE 4.26 Gradual Change of Activity in a Homologous Series (*10*)

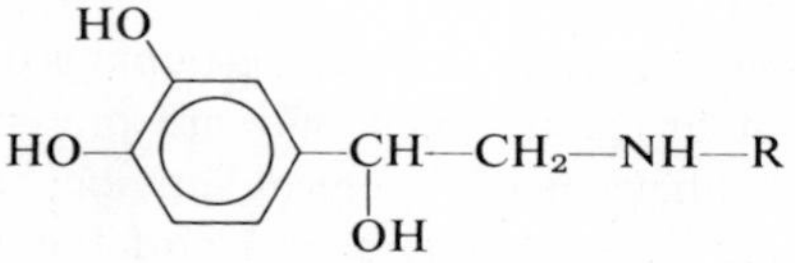

$$HO-C_6H_3(OH)-CH(OH)-CH_2-NH-R$$

	Blood Pressure of the Cat	
R	Hypertensive	Hypotensive
Hydrogen	+ +	—
Methyl	+ +	—
Ethyl	+	+
Propyl	—	+
Isopropyl	—	+ +
Butyl	—	+ +
Isobutyl	—	+ +

Analogous alternation is found in other types of compound (*10*).

2. Cyclopolymethylene Series. Few studies have been made on the cyclopolymethylene series. The best examples are antihypertensive drugs with the general formula $(CH_2)_n > NCH_2CH_2X$. In those in which X is amidoxime or guanidine greater activity is confined to compounds in which $n = 6, 7,$ or 8. In those in which X is amidine high activity is found in compounds where $n = 6$ or 7 (*48*).

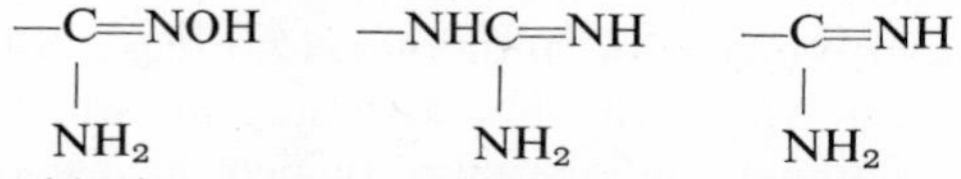

$$-C(NH_2)=NOH \qquad -NHC(NH_2)=NH \qquad -C(NH_2)=NH$$
amidoxime   guanidine   amidine

3. Hybrid Series. The classical and simplest example of hybrid series is of the blocking activity exerted at the neuromuscular junction by quaternary ammonium derivatives. It decreases when the methyl group is replaced by ethyl (*48*):

$$Me_4\overset{\oplus}{N} > Me_3\overset{\oplus}{N}Et > Me_2\overset{\oplus}{N}Et_2 \gg Me\overset{\oplus}{N}Et_3 \simeq \overset{\oplus}{N}Et_4$$

Another example is of the hybrid homologs of neostigmine: higher activity is shown by the compound in which the terminal group is $\overset{\oplus}{N}MeEt_2$ (48).

X. EFFECTS OF ACIDIC AND BASIC GROUPINGS

Because of their polarity, acidic and basic groupings determine the physico-chemical properties of drugs in which they are present, and, for this very reason, they decisively affect their biological activities. Furthermore they are often involved in drug–receptor interaction and therefore are essential to pharmacological action (5).

Acidic groups, such as —SO$_3$H and —COOH, because they are solubilizing agents, either assist in or cancel biological effect. Usually sulfonic acids, because they are strong and highly ionized and therefore cannot cross cellular membranes (which, as a rule, are permeable only to nondissociated molecules and not to ions), do not exhibit biological action; some trypanocides (trypan red, trypan blue, afridol violet, suramin) and other chemotherapeutic agents (e.g., stibophen), however, are exceptions.

Derivatives of carboxylic acids—such as esters, amides, and nitriles—can show activities that differ from those of the parent compounds. For instance, the alkyl esters of p-aminobenzoic acid, which is a vitamin for certain microorganisms, have local-anesthetic activity.

Many amides, characterized by the —CONH— group, also present in proteins and peptides, exhibit biological activity, although in general structurally nonspecific and therefore short, owing to their ability to form hydrogen bonds with organic macromolecules. This explains the narcotic action of some amides, urethanes, and cyclic substances, such as barbiturates and hydantoins (5). If, however, the drug has a great number of peptide groups, as in the polypeptides described by Law (54), the biological action may be structurally specific and therefore more prolonged, as result of the multiple interaction of such groups with similar groups that exist in proteins and nucleic acids. This happens with several polypeptide antibiotics (55) (e.g., polymyxin, colistin, tyrothricin, bacitracin, viomycin, and actinomycin, which exhibit various chemotherapeutic actions) and suramin (which has strong trypanocidal action).

Strong bases manifest reduced biological activity, as in the case of sulfonic acids—and for the same reason. However, in quaternary ammonium salts (as in cholinergic, and anticholinergic agents) protonated basic groupings play the function of attaching themselves electrostatically to groups or receptors that are negatively charged and, for this reason, are essential to pharmacological action (5).

The basic nitrogen of alkaloids is also fundamental to their affinity for enzymes on which they act. The hydrazino group not only confers basicity but also has the ability to react with carbonyl groups, and its biological action is ascribed to these two factors (5).

XI. EFFECTS OF ACYLATING GROUPS

The biological action of acyl groups—found in esters, amides, and anhydrides—can result from the acylation reaction in which they may take part. For instance, organophosphorus insecticides inhibit acetylcholinesterase through irreversible phosphorylation of serine hydroxyl, a constituent of the active site of this enzyme (56). Penicillin, owing to the steric tension of the β-lactam ring, has acylating properties, although these may be more important to its inactivation by hydrolysis catalyzed by β-lactamase than to antibacterial action (40,57–59). On the other hand, though some antibiotics and heparin, the natural anticoagulant, contain sulfamic acids formed by an acylation process, the activity of these drugs may not depend on their chemical reactivity as acylating or alkylating agents (5).

XII. EFFECTS OF HYDROXYLATION

Hydroxyl groups can affect pharmacological response in two ways: alteration of physical properties or of chemical reactivity (5). Examples of the first type of effect are those found in certain alcohols (ethanol, methylparafynol, amylene hydrate, ethchlorvynol) and simple phenols (phenol, cresol, resorcinol), which owe their narcotic and bacteriostatic activities, respectively, to physicochemical properties, since they are structurally nonspecific drugs. Examples of the second type of effect are found in hycanthone, which is 10 times as active as lucanthone (60), and certain polyhydroxylated compounds (epinephrine, norepinephrine) in which, through hydrogen bonds, hydroxy groups contribute to the binding of drug to its receptor; that is the reason why etherification and esterification decrease the activity of hydroxylated drugs (4).

Certain hydroxylated compounds owe their action to the possibility of being converted *in vivo* to a quinone form; and quinones participate in oxidative phosphorylation by acting as electron carriers (61).

XIII. EFFECTS OF THIOL AND DISULFIDE GROUPS

Several drugs and various antibiotics (bacitracin, penicillin, cephalosporin) have thiol or disulfide groups, the latter ones sometimes in cyclic form. Their biological action results partially from this peculiarity (*40,57,62,63*). Among other less important characteristics, thiol groups have the ability (*5*) to (a) interconvert to disulfides through oxidation–reduction reactions (as in the case of the antidiuretic hormone arginine vasopressin, which is attracted to the receptor site by electrostatic forces and hydrogen bonds); (b) add to double bonds, mainly to α,β-unsaturated ketonic compounds; (c) form insoluble mercaptides with heavy metals (as in cysteine, penicillin, and 2,3-dimercaptopropanol); (d) form complexes of addition with the pyridine ring of some enzymes.

XIV. EFFECTS OF ETHER AND SULFIDE GROUPS

Although the ether group has valence angles equivalent to those in C—C linkage, it manifests polar properties resulting from the unshared electronic pairs of the oxygen. For this reason ether molecules are polar: the oxygen atom is hydrophilic and hydrocarbon groups are lipophilic. This explains the orientation of ethers at the lipid–aqueous interface and, to some extent, their biological action.

Sulfides differ from ethers by being susceptible to oxidation to sulfoxides and sulfones, groups which are present in some hypnotics (sulfonmethane, sulfonethylmethane) and in several antibacterial agents (such as sulfanilamide and dapsone and their respective derivatives) (*5*).

XV. EFFECTS OF UNSATURATION

Unsaturation may cause three main effects (*5*):

1. By changing the stereochemistry of the drug, it can give rise to a compound whose activity is different from that of the saturated compound. This happens in *cis*-cinnamic acid. Unlike its dihydro derivative (β-phenylpropionic acid), it exerts a regulatory activity on plant growth. However, unsaturation does not always contribute pharmacological activity. Thus stilbestrol (unsaturated) as well as hexestrol (saturated) have approximately the same estrogenic activity.

2. By altering physicochemical properties, it can modify biological activity. This is observed in hypnotics: ethylenic hydrocarbons are slightly more active than unsaturated ones.

3. By increasing chemical reactivity, unsaturation—not only in the form of double and triple bounds but also in the form of ketone, lactone, ester, amide, nitrile, and other groups—gives rise to or intensifies biological

activity, owing to the possibility of interaction between those linkages and groups with cellular constituents. Among other examples may be cited macrolide antibiotics, such as erythromycin and oleandomycin.

XVI. EFFECTS OF METALS AND CHELATING GROUPS

Certain metals, mainly the so-called heavy metals, have the property of binding to essential groups of cellular constituents and, by this mechanism, changing their physiological function, thus producing a pharmacological response (46). For instance, mercury present in some drugs acts through binding to thiol groups of certain proteins:

$$R-Hg^{\oplus} + HS-\!\!\!\!\!\!\!\! \longrightarrow R-Hg-S-\!\!\!\!\!\!\!\! + H^{\oplus}$$

$$\!\!\!\!\!\!\!\!\!SH + HS-\!\!\!\!\!\!\!\!\quad\quad\; \longrightarrow \;\!\!\!\!\!\!\!\!-S-Hg-S-\!\!\!\!\!\!\!\! + 2\,H^{\oplus}$$
$$Hg^{2+}$$

On the other hand, some metals, being essential constituents of certain substances or enzymes, are highly important for biological activity. Such is the case with iron, copper, cobalt, molybdenum, calcium, magnesium, zinc, and other metals (46). Excess of these metals in the body can, however, be harmful. To remove undesirable or excess of necessary metals from the body, compounds are employed which have chelating groups. Among them are 8-hydroxyquinoline, ethylenediaminetetraacetic acid, trans-1,2-diamino-cyclohexanetetraacetic acid, dimercaprol, penicillamine, desferrioxamine B (26).

REFERENCES

1. B. M. Bloom and G. D. Laubach, *Ann. Rev. Pharmacol.*, **2**, 67 (1962).
2. F. N. Fastier, *Ann. Rev. Pharmacol.*, **4**, 51 (1964).
3. C. J. Cavallito, *Ann. Rev. Pharmacol.*, **8**, 39 (1968).
4. A. Burger, "Relation of Chemical Structure and Biological Activity," in A. Burger, Ed., *Medicinal Chemistry*, 3rd ed., Interscience, New York, 1970, pp. 64–80.
5. W. A. Sexton, *Chemical Constitution and Biological Activity*, 3rd ed., Spon, London, 1963.
6. N. J. Harper, *J. Med. Pharm. Chem.*, **1**, 467 (1959).
7. F. W. Schueler, *Chemobiodynamics and Drug Design*, McGraw-Hill, New York, 1960.
8. N. J. Harper, *Progr. Drug Res.*, **4**, 221 (1962).

9. F. W. Schueler, Ed., *Molecular Modification in Drug Design*, Advances in Chemistry Series, Vol. 45, American Chemical Society, Washington, D.C., 1964.

10. E. J. Ariëns, Ed., *Molecular Pharmacology*, Vol. I, Academic, New York, 1964.

11. A. Burger and A. P. Parulkar, *Ann. Rev. Pharmacol.*, **6**, 19 (1966).

12. E. J. Ariëns, *Progr. Drug Res.*, **10**, 429 (1966).

13. E. J. Ariëns, *Farmaco*, *(Pavia)*, *Ed. Sci.*, **23**, 52 (1968).

14. R. M. Levine and B. B. Clark, *J. Pharmacol. Exptl. Therap.*, **113**, 272 (1955).

15. L. Fowden, D. Lewis, and H. Tristram, *Advan. Enzymol.*, **29**, 89 (1967).

16. A. J. Glazko, W. H. Edgerton, W. A. Dill, and W. R. Lenz, *Antibiot. Chemother.*, *(Washington, D.C.)*, **2**, 234 (1952).

17. E. J. Ariëns, *Advan. Drug Res.*, **3**, 235 (1966).

18. J. Levy and B. Tchoubar, *Actualités Pharmacol.*, **5**, 143 (1952).

19. M. Martin-Smith and S. T. Reid, *J. Med. Pharm. Chem.*, **1**, 507 (1959).

20. V. B. Schatz, "Isosterism and Bio-isosterism as Guides to Structural Variations," in A. Burger, Ed., *Medicinal Chemistry*, 2nd ed., Interscience, New York, 1960, pp. 72–88.

21. I. Langmuir, *J. Am. Chem. Soc.*, **41**, 868, 1543 (1919).

22. H. G. Grimm, *Z. Elektrochem.*, **31**, 474 (1925); *ibid.*, **34**, 430 (1928).

23. H. Erlenmeyer, *Bull. Soc. Chim. Biol.*, **30**, 792 (1948).

24. T. C. Daniels and E. C. Jorgensen, "Physicochemical Properties in Relation to Biologic Action," in C. O. Wilson, O. Gisvold, and R. F. Doerge, Eds., *Textbook of Organic Medicinal and Pharmaceutical Chemistry*, 5th ed., Lippincott, Philadelphia, 1966, pp. 4–62.

25. H. L. Friedman, "Influence of Isosteric Replacements upon Biological Activity," in *First Symposium on Chemical-Biological Correlation* (May 26–27, 1950), National Academy of Sciences–National Research Council, Publication No. 206, Washington, D.C., 1951, pp. 295–358.

26. C. O. Wilson, O. Gisvold, and R. F. Doerge, Eds., *Textbook of Organic Medicinal and Pharmaceutical Chemistry*, 5th ed., Lippincott, Philadelphia, 1966.

27. R. A. Peters, *Biochemical Lesions and Lethal Synthesis*, Pergamon, Oxford, 1963.

28. E. S. Gould, *Mechanism and Structure in Organic Chemistry*, Holt, Rinehart and Winston, New York, 1959.

29. J. Hine, *Physical Organic Chemistry*, 2nd ed., McGraw-Hill, New York, 1962.

30. R. Breslow, *Organic Reaction Mechanisms*, Benjamin, New York, 1964.

31. O. Reutov, *Theoretical Principles of Organic Chemistry*, Mir Publishers, Moscow, 1967.

32. P. Sykes, *A Guidebook to Mechanism in Organic Chemistry*, 2nd ed., Longmans, London, 1967.

33. E. M. Kosower, *An Introduction to Physical Organic Chemistry*, Wiley, New York, 1968.

34. J. March, *Advanced Organic Chemistry: Reactions, Mechanisms, and Structure*, McGraw-Hill, New York, 1968.

35. C. K. Ingold, *Structure and Mechanism in Organic Chemistry*, 2nd ed., Cornell University Press, Ithaca, N.Y., 1969.

36. L. Pauling, *The Nature of the Chemical Bond*, 3rd ed., Cornell University Press, Ithaca, N.Y., 1960.

37. M. B. Chenoweth and L. P. McCarty, *Pharmacol. Rev.*, **15**, 673 (1963).

38. N. P. Buu-Hoï, *Progr. Drug Res.*, **3**, 9 (1961).

39. R. C. Fuson, *Chem. Rev.*, **16**, 1 (1935).

40. F. P. Doyle and J. H. C. Nayler, *Advan. Drug Res.*, **1**, 1 (1964).

41. F. E. Hahn, J. E. Hayes, C. L. Wisseman, Jr., H. E. Hopps, and J. E. Smadel, *Antibiot. Chemother.*, (*Washington, D.C.*), **6**, 531 (1956).

42. M. B. Chenoweth and C. L. Hake, *Ann. Rev. Pharmacol.*, **2**, 363 (1962).

43. P. Goldman, *Science*, **164**, 1123 (1969).

44. H. L. Yale, *J. Med. Pharm. Chem.*, **1**, 121 (1959).

45. J. C. Krantz, Jr., and F. G. Rudo, "The Fluorinated Anesthetics," in F. A. Smith, Sub-ed., *Pharmacology of Fluorides. Handbuch der experimentellen Pharmakologie*, Vol. XX/1, Springer, Berlin, 1966, pp. 501–564.

46. A. Albert, *Selective Toxicity*, 4th ed., Methuen, London, 1968.

47. D. R. Gilligan and N. Plummer, *Proc. Soc. Exptl. Biol. Med.*, **53**, 142 (1943).

48. H. R. Ing, *Progr. Drug Res.*, **7**, 305 (1964).

49. C. E. Coulthard, J. Marshall, and F. L. Pyman, *J. Chem. Soc.*, 280 (1930).

50. P. P. Koelzer and K. H. Wehr, *Arzneimittel-Forsch.*, **8**, 544 (1958).

51. A. B. H. Funcke, M. J. E. Ernsting, R. F. Rekker, and W. T. Nauta, *Arzneimittel-Forsch.*, **3**, 503 (1953).

52. O. J. Magidson and I. T. Strukov, *Arch. Pharm.*, **271**, 569 (1933).

53. C. G. Raison and O. D. Standen, *Brit. J. Pharmacol.*, **10**, 191 (1955).

54. H. D. Law, *Progr. Med. Chem.*, **4**, 86 (1965).

55. R. O. Studer, *Progr. Med. Chem.*, **5**, 1 (1967).

56. R. D. O'Brien, *Toxic Phosphorus Esters*, Academic, New York, 1960.

57. J. C. Sheehan, "Synthetic Penicillins," in F. W. Schueler, Ed., *Molecular Modification in Drug Design*, Advances in Chemistry Series, Vol. 45, American Chemical Society, Washington, D.C., 1964, pp. 15–24.

58. B. Lynn, *Antibiot. Chemother.*, (*Basel*), **13**, 125 (1965).

59. E. Rauenbusch, *Antibiot. Chemother.*, (*Basel*), **14**, 95 (1968).

60. D. Rosi, G. Peruzzotti, E. W. Dennis, D. A. Berberian, H. Freele, and S. Archer, *Nature*, **208**, 1005 (1965).

61. G. E. W. Wolstenholme and C. M. O'Connor, Eds., *Quinones in Electron Transport*, Churchill, London, 1961.

62. E. P. Abraham, *Quart. Rev.*, **21**, 231 (1967).

63. J. Ploquin, S. Lereste, and L. Sparfel, *Prod. Probl. Pharm.*, **23**, 258 (1968).

5

STEREOCHEMICAL
ASPECTS OF DRUGS

The receptor theory of drug action implies that the pharmacological properties of a compound are dependent not only on the nature and properties of the constituent groups within the molecule but also in the way in which these groups are distributed in space.

E. W. Gill

I. COMPLEMENTARITY BETWEEN DRUG AND RECEPTOR

The receptor is probably a limited portion of a macromolecule, usually protein in nature. For this reason it will have a specific, more or less rigid structure. In many cases it cannot undergo great conformational changes. Only by assuming this is it possible to explain the need for structurally specific drugs to possess, in many cases, a complementary conformation to that of the postulated receptor (*1–3*).

Substances with similar pharmacological activity normally contain common functional moieties—aromatic or heterocyclic (often condensed) ring; aliphatic or alicyclic chain; basic nitrogen atom; alcoholic or phenolic hydroxy group; amide, ether, or ester groups—arranged in space in an

87

analogous manner. This steric arrangement is, in the case of structurally specific drugs, of fundamental importance for the interaction of the drug with the receptor (4).

The formation of a complex between the receptor and the drug is determined by steric factors, and consequently the manifestation of medicinal action will depend on the nature of the complex. The greater the degree of complementarity, the greater the specificity, and the greater the activity of the drug. This complementarity increases with the formation of the drug–receptor complex (5). Substitution of a bulky group by a small one, spatial redisposition of groups through inversion in an asymmetric center, or change of direction of a dipole within the molecule can deeply alter the stability of the drug–receptor complex (6).

In a drug–receptor interaction and in results derived from it two values are therefore of special importance: the electronic charge distribution in the drug and in the receptor, and the conformation of drug and of receptor (5). Hence the activity of drugs depends on three structural factors: (a) stereochemistry of the molecule, (b) distance between atoms or groups, and (c) electronic distribution and configuration (7). In the case of flexible molecules the orientation of groups will change according to various factors, such as environment and pH (5). Studies in this regard have been carried out with several types of drugs (8).

II. STEREOCHEMISTRY OF DRUGS

The difference in the pharmacological activity of many stereoisomers is the best evidence for the existence of a receptor. This can be ascribed to three factors:

1. Differences in the distribution of isomers in the body.
2. Differences in the properties of drug–receptor interactions.
3. Differences in the adsorption of isomers to a complementary receptor surface (9).

In the study of the action of drugs at the molecular level it is therefore necessary to consider not only the conformation of drugs—that is, the non-superposable molecular arrangements in space—but also their configuration—that is, the arrangement of atoms that characterizes a particular stereoisomer and is determined by optical and geometric isomerism (1).

A. Conformation of Drugs

Conformers are stereoisomers that are in such a rapid state of equilibrium that they cannot be isolated under normal conditions. One conformer can be converted into another through rotation and deformation, but not through the breaking of bonds (*10–14*). For instance, cyclohexane exists in chair and boat conformations (*15*), which are not isolable, because they interconvert rapidly (10^6 times per second) and the energy barrier of conversion is small (about 10 kcal/mole). According to some authors (*13*), a boat form is not actually a conformer, since it lies at a maximum of energy, but a transition state between chair and twist conformations:

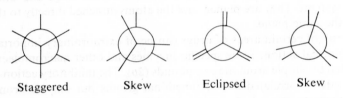

Chair	Half-chair	Twist I	Boat	Twist II
conformer		*conformer*		*conformer*

Staggered and eclipsed conformations coexist in ethane. They are transformed into one another with ease and speed, through rotation around a C—C bond:

Staggered   Skew   Eclipsed   Skew

In cyclohexane as well as in ethane, however, besides the mentioned conformations, which are extreme and well defined, there are many others, the intermediate ones. The same phenomena occur in almost all organic compounds that have single bonds: the conformations that they can assume are usually infinite in number and are called *skew* conformations. The exceptions are some cyclic compounds that have rigid structures, and compounds with bulky groups that prevent rotation around the single bond.

A very similar term to conformation, but that never should be considered as its synonym, is *configuration*. *Conformation* denotes a spatial arrangement that is in a movable equilibrium with other arrangements. *Configuration* refers to a specific, characteristic, and stable arrangement of atoms or groups; as a rule, conversion of one configuration into another is possible only through bond breakage; nevertheless, each configuration may exist in an infinite number of conformations, with the exception of compounds that have rigid structures or bulky groups. The term configuration is used to designate geometric (*cis–trans*) and optical isomers.

In the case of cyclohexane the C—H bonds of a chair conformation can occupy two different positions: (a) parallel to the axis of the general plane of the molecule (axial position); (b) radial to the same plane (equatorial position).

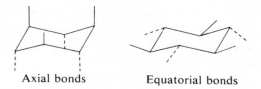

Axial bonds   Equatorial bonds

There is presently a great interest in the study of the influence of conformation on the pharmacological activity exerted by compounds that, apparently acting on the same receptors, present either rigid or flexible structures (*16–28*). This study became easier with the application of circular dichroism and optical rotatory dispersion (*29*).

Rigid molecules are the most appropriate to studies aimed at determining the drug–receptor topography. Some structures contribute heavily to the rigidity of the molecule. This happens with aromatic rings and other conjugated systems. They are planar, and the atoms attached directly to them are kept in the same plane.

Planarity of certain areas of drugs can be of extraordinary importance for their biological action. Some specific enzymes and other macromolecules can be affected by simple aromatic compounds (*26*). The inhibitory action of these compounds is correlated not to functional groups but only to aromatic or planar characteristics of the molecules (*30*). This can result, as happens in analogous cases, from π-electrons (*31*).

Often the presence of an aromatic ring enhances the pharmacodynamic action. For instance, amphetamine, which has an aromatic ring, is more active than its saturated analogs. Biological activity contributed by planar rings, such as benzene or pyridine, results from their ability to attach themselves to the receptor, if the latter has a planar surface, through van der Waals forces; 2 to 3 kcal/mole are liberated in the process of this interaction. In the case of nonplanar drugs interacting with planar receptors van der Waals forces are much weaker.

Albert (*32*) observed that the bacteriostatic activity of 9-aminoacridines is directly related to a minimal planar surface of about 38 Å². Removal of one

NH_2

9-Aminoacridine

of the external rings or substitution by a saturated (and therefore bulkier) ring results in complete loss of activity.

The adrenergic blocking action of β-haloalkylamines depends also on the coplanarity of substituents in the benzene ring. Thus such compounds as fluorene derivatives in which X is methyl or methoxy are active, but those in which X is ethyl, isopropyl, or *tert*-butyl are inactive because of the non-planarity of the substituents with the ring (33).

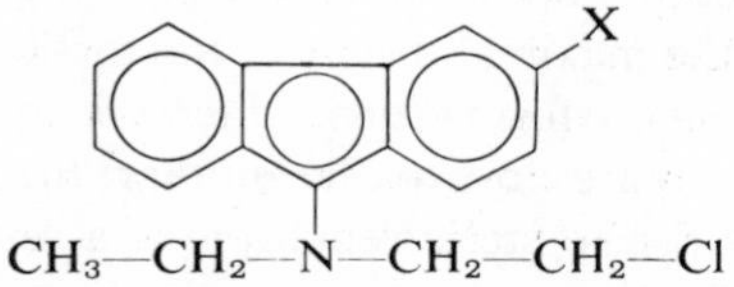

$$CH_3-CH_2-N-CH_2-CH_2-Cl$$

In nonaromatic ring systems important functional atoms or groups (e.g., phenyl) can occupy either equatorial or axial positions; other atoms or groups can occupy both positions, in proportions that are either equal or different.

In multisubstituted rings some atoms or groups will necessarily occupy an axial position: if they are bulky, this conformation can cause steric hindrance; obviously this will influence biological action. For instance, in analgetics derived from 4-phenylpiperidine the aromatic ring can take both axial and equatorial positions in relation to the piperidine ring, the equatorial one being the energetically preferred one. However, formerly it was thought that analgetics with an aromatic ring in an axial position would be more potent than those in which a phenyl group occupies an equatorial position, owing to their ability to fit better with the receptor surface, as postulated by Beckett and Casy (34, 35).

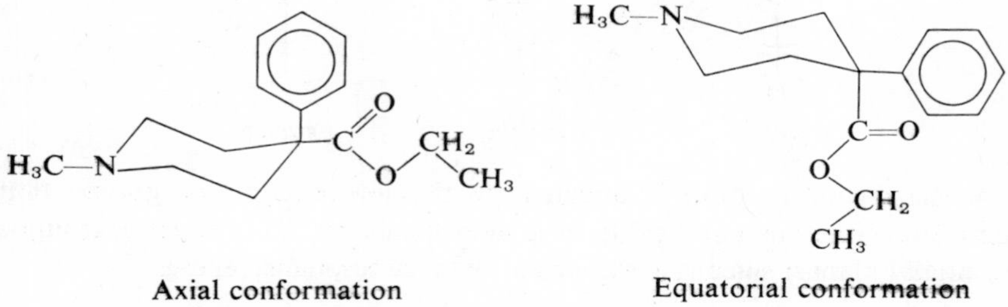

Axial conformation   Equatorial conformation

Meperidine

Later it was seen that conformational requirements in analgetics with this structure are minimal, since a preferred conformation in the ground state can be transformed during interaction with a receptor into an energetically unfavorable conformation (26,36–39).

The foregoing example indicates that, even when a bond is free so that the groups attached to it can rotate without restraint, as in a single bond, the atoms of the molecule assume various preferred positions. This is shown by infrared absorption spectra. The most common conformation is the one in which the substituents are separated by the maximal distance. This is the reason that, in solution, β-phenylethylamines, for instance, assume various conformations, three of them being extreme: one *anti* (or *trans*), and two *gauche* (or *skew*). In the *anti* conformation the phenyl group and the nitrogen atom are separated by the maximal distance; the torsion angle between them is 180°. In the two *gauche* conformations, which are equivalent, the aromatic ring and the nitrogen atom are close to one another; the torsion angle between them is 60°. This gives rise to steric repulsion as a result of van der Waals forces. A bulky group in the α-carbon compels the nitrogen atom to come closer to the ring, and this should influence the strength of bonding with the receptor (*4*).

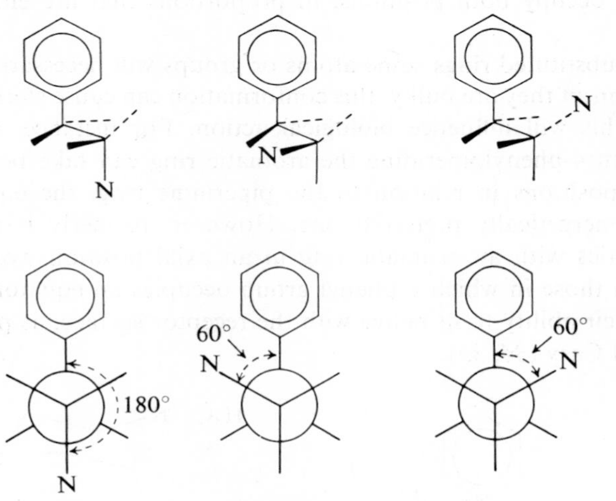

anti   gauche   gauche

A chair conformation is affected by the introduction of groups that contribute either greater rigidity or greater flexibility. Thus an ester group is essentially planar, since it is stabilized by great resonance energy:

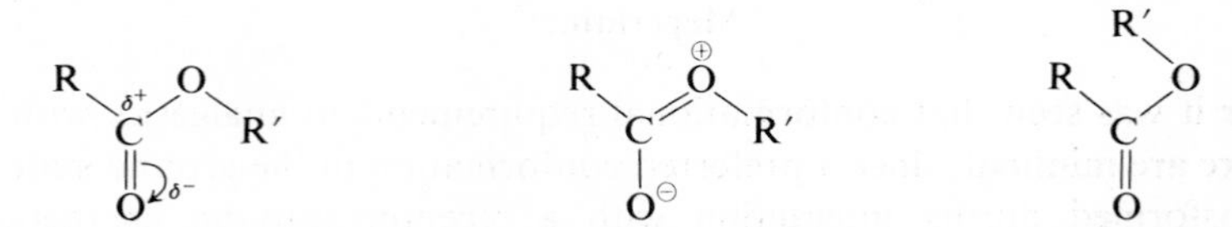

Planar form *trans*   Resonance form   Planar form *cis*

Amides are also planar, and for this very reason they are unreactive substances:

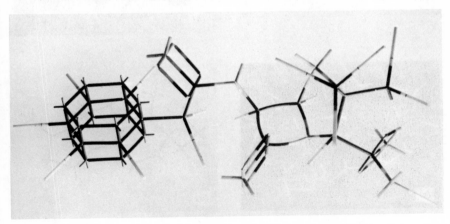

Planar form *trans*   Resonance form   Planar form *cis*

In both cases the preferred positions are *trans*. The ester and amide groups of a chain tend to maintain bulky groups in a plane and to separate them to the utmost. Hence their contribution is not only to increase the polar character of that part of the molecule to which they belong but also to compel the chains to stay completely extended (6).

Nevertheless, if a substituent is introduced into the amide group so that one of its atoms is forced out of the plane, the resonance is abolished and the resulting compound becomes reactive. For this reason four-membered β-lactams are 1000 times more readily hydrolyzed than an amide chain, such as acetamide. In penicillin a β-lactam ring is fused with the five-membered thiazolidine ring. This compels one of the carbons attached to the amide nitrogen atom to project itself even farther outside the plane of the amide group. In consequence penicillin, in regard to hydrolysis and acylating power, is about one million times more reactive than an amide of a common straight-chain acid (40).

An ether group, contrary to what happens with ester and amide groups, increases the flexibility of the hydrocarbon chain, owing to a greater freedom of rotation about the oxygen atom. For this reason the range of possible

Molecular model of penicillin G. Note the strained β-lactam ring fused with the thiazolidine ring, compelling one of the carbons attached to the amide nitrogen atom to stay away from the plane of the amide group.

conformations of ethers is far greater than that of hydrocarbons. Other groups, such as methyl, amine, and disulfide, also affect the conformation of drug molecules (6).

However, there are drugs that contain nonplanar aliphatic and alicyclic structures. These drugs are usually made up of large molecules containing bulky groups. Furthermore they can exist in several isomeric forms. Their structures at times may be totally or almost totally rigid, as in the case of amantadine, morphine, tetracyclines, and steroids. Other times, they are flexible, and the drugs can assume various spatial orientations. But, generally speaking, only one of the conformations adapts itself better to the receptor, and for this reason it causes the most intense biological effect (5), although others can also show activity.

It is difficult to ascribe a rigid conformation to compounds with flexible

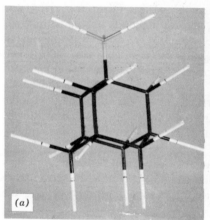
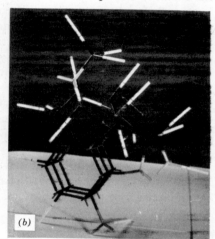
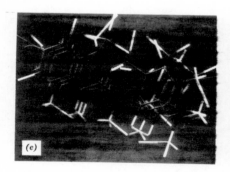
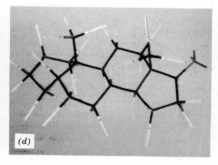

Molecular models of some drugs and chemical compounds of rigid structure: (a) amantadine, (b) morphine, (c) tetracycline, (d) androgen molecule.

structures since their functional groups can adopt different spatial orientations.

Acetylcholine can exist in many conformations, which depend on solvent effects (41). According to Smissman and co-workers (42), it can assume four main conformations:

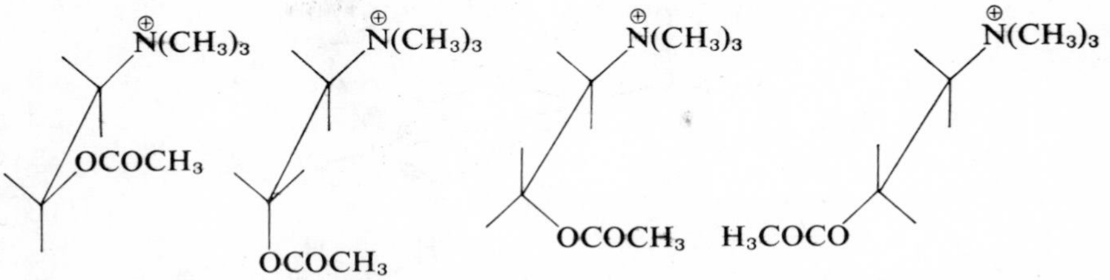

It was postulated that in solution acetylcholine exists preferentially in a cyclic form, as a result of electrostatic attraction between the polarized carbonyl group and the quaternary nitrogen (43). This, however, would lead to a very great steric compression (6), which explains the absence of this conformation in the internal medium (43):

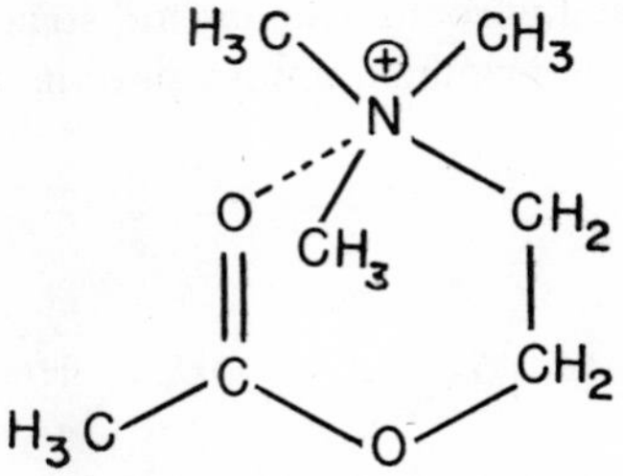

Proton-magnetic-resonance spectra showed that in aqueous solution acetylcholine is best represented as follows (44):

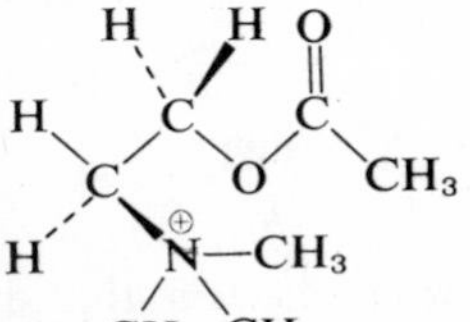

In the crystal state of acetylcholine bromide the structure of acetylcholine has the following conformation (45):

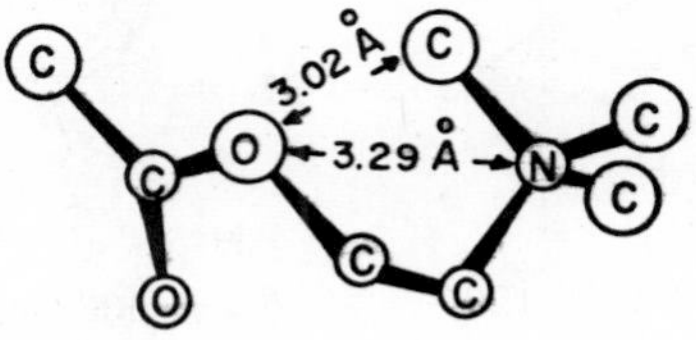

Through molecular-orbital calculations, it was shown that the preferred conformation of acetylcholine is very similar to the former one (46):

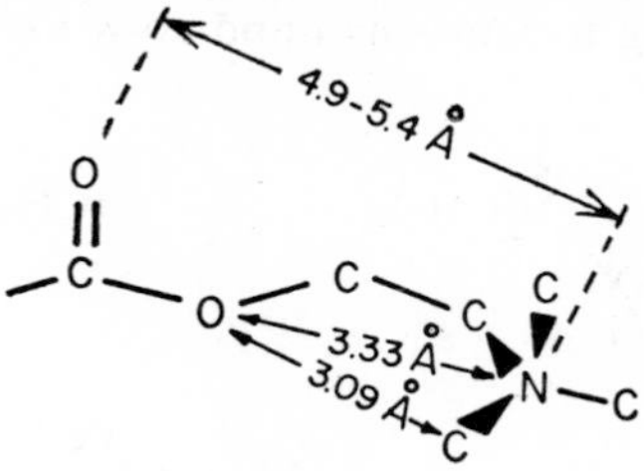

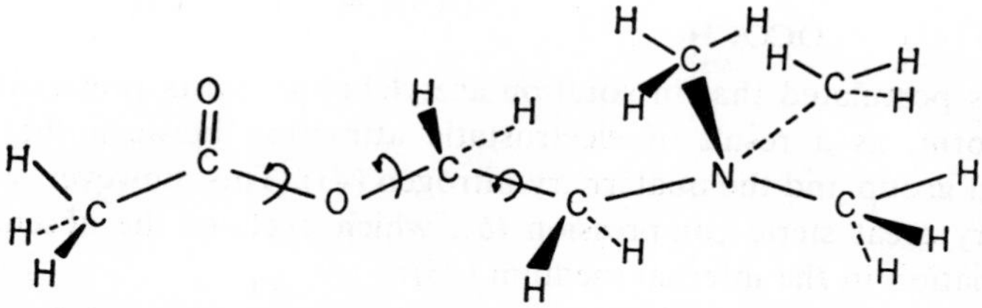

Norepinephrine, whose hydrochloride crystal structure was recently determined (47), can have three principal conformations, the preferred one being b (48):

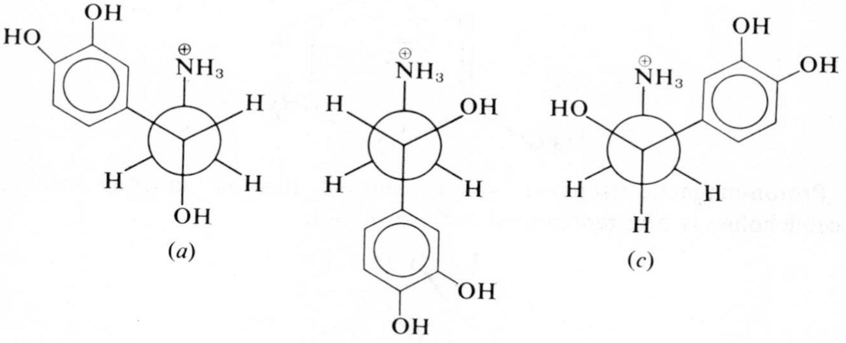

(a)

(b)

(c)

Molecular-orbital calculations showed that histamine can exist in two preferred conformations, which are in equilibrium with each other (49):

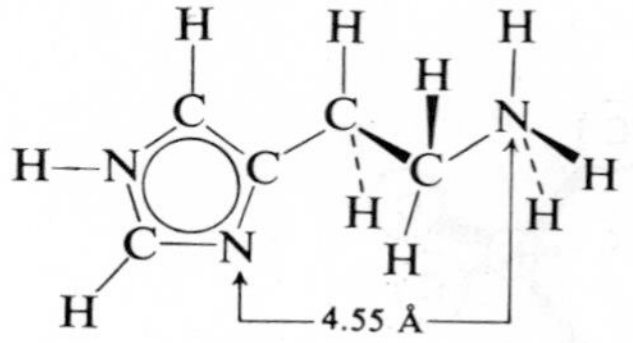

$\theta_{cc} = 180°, \theta_{ring} - C = 120°$ 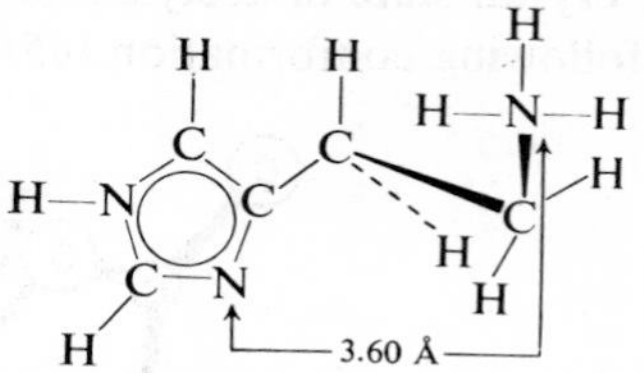 $\theta_{cc} = 300°, \theta_{ring} - C = 120°$

The preferred conformation of serotonin, according to Kier (*50*), who also proposed structural features complementary to its receptor, is the following:

$$\overset{\oplus}{N}H_3$$
$$|$$
$$CH_2$$
$$|$$
$$CH_2$$

HO. (indole ring structure with N–H)

B. Optical Isomerism in Drugs

Optical isomers, also called *optical antipodes, enantiomorphs*, and *enantiomers*, are stereoisomers in which the arrangement of atoms or groups is such that the two molecules are not superimposable (*11,13*). They are mirror images of one another and present differences similar to those that exist between a right and a left hand (*14*). Although many optical isomers have an asymmetric center, this is not an essential criterion for asymmetry.

They are called optical isomers because they rotate the plane of polarized light in opposite directions: one isomer rotates it to the right and, for this reason, is called *dextrorotatory*, or *dextrogire* (this direction is indicated by the sign +); the other one rotates it to the left and therefore is called *levorotatory*, or *levogire* (this direction is indicated by the sign −). The letters *d* and *l* are no longer employed to indicate (+) and (−) rotations. Furthermore (+) and (−) should not, for example, be mistaken for the D- and L-configurations of amino acids. Owing to the disadvantage of the DL nomenclature, the current tendency is to indicate the configuration by the RS system, which is much more precise and has wider applicability in organic chemistry (*10,11, 13,14*). A mixture of equal parts of enantiomers is called a *racemic modification*; it is optically inactive (*13*). The property of rotating the plane of polarized light per se has little bearing on the interaction of drugs with the receptor surface.

Stereoisomers that are not enantiomers—that is, do not constitute mirror images of one another—are called diastereoisomers, or diastereomers; they have two or more asymmetric centers and result from a combination of two enantiomers (*10,11*). In a pair of these isomers, as represented by projection formulas, the one that has two similar groups in the same side, as in erythrose, is called *erythro*; the name *threo* is reserved for that in which these groups are on opposite sides, as in threose. Several drugs represent such isomers, for instance, chloramphenicol (*51–53*) (Table 5.1).

By possessing the same functional groups, diastereoisomers can undergo

TABLE 5.1 Chloramphenicol and Its Stereoisomers

Formula	Isomer
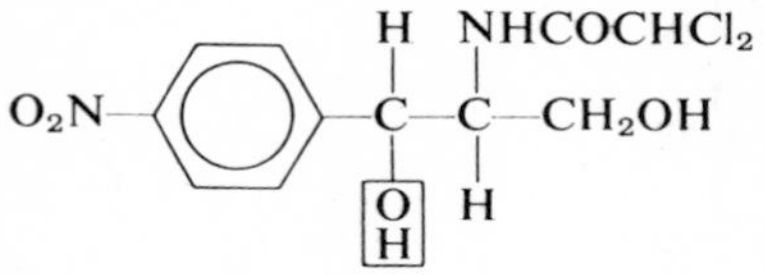	D-(−)-*threo*-Chloramphenicol (natural product)
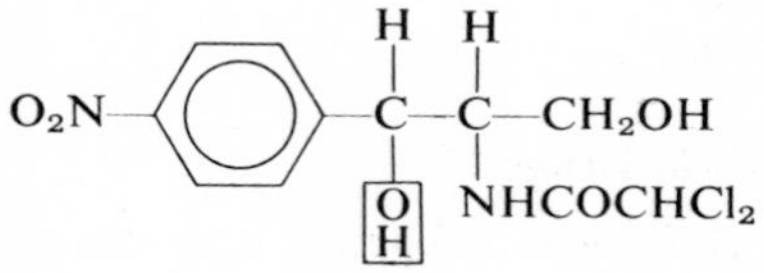	L-(+)-*erythro*-Chloramphenicol
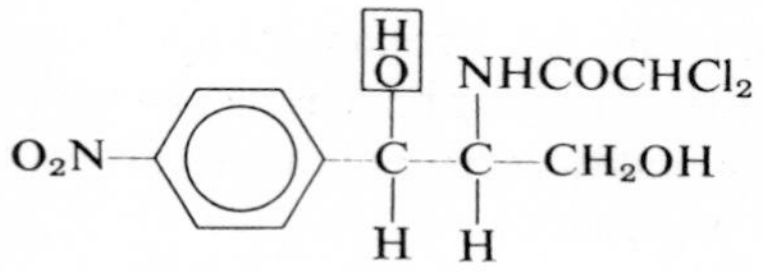	D-(−)-*erythro*-Chloramphenicol
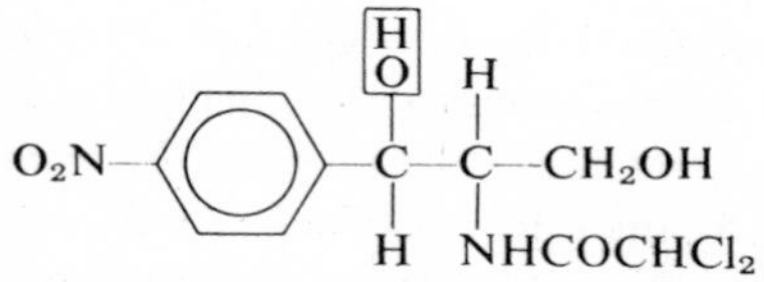	L-(+)-*threo*-Chloramphenicol

the same types of chemical reactions. However, owing to different physical properties, determined by the nonidentity of the stereochemistry of the different groups, the rates of these reactions vary. Such factors of differentiation alter the drug's distribution in the body, its metabolism, and its interaction with the receptor, affecting the biological activities of the diastereoisomers, which often vary in intensity.

The same occurs with enantiomers. With the exception that they rotate the polarization of light in opposite directions and react differently toward optically active reagents, these isomers usually possess identical physical and chemical properties (*13*). It would be expected, therefore, that the intensities of their biological action would also be identical. Such is the case in structurally nonspecific drugs (e.g., barbiturates) and also in some structurally specific ones, such as in (+)- and (−)-chloroquine, both forms having equal antimalarial activity (*54*). In the latter case it is thought that the drug–receptor interaction either does not involve an asymmetric center or, if it does involve one, it is only through two and not three points (*40*).

Nevertheless, assuming that the interaction of structurally specific drugs with biological receptors occurs at three points, it should be different for each enantiomer (Figure 5.1).

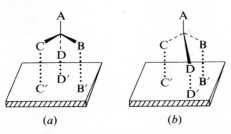

(a)   (b)

Fig. 5.1. Interaction of enantiomers (a) and (b) with a receptor surface. C, D, and B represent groups in the enantiomers and C′, D′, and B′ are three points of attachment to the receptor surface. Although both are attached to the receptor at three points, one of these (D′) in (a) does not coincide with its correspondent in (b) (9).

This explains why optical isomers exert pharmacological action with varying degrees of intensity (4,9,19,40). For instance, D-(−)-isoprenalin is 50 to 800 times more active as a bronchodilator than L-(+)-isoprenalin; (−)-norepinephrine is 70 times more active as a bronchodilator than (+)-norepinephrine; D-(−)-epinephrine is 12 to 15 times more active as a vasoconstrictor than D-(+)-epinephrine; L-(+)-acetyl-β-methylcholine is about 200 times more active in gout than D-(−)-acetyl-β-methylcholine; (−)-hyoscyamine is 15 to 20 times more active as a mydriatic than (+)-hyoscyamine; (+)-muscarine has 700 times the muscarinic activity of (−)-muscarine; L-(−)-ascorbic acid has antiscorbutic properties, whereas (+)-ascorbic acid has not; (−)-amino acids are either tasteless or bitter, but (+)-amino acids are sweet; S-(+)-isomers of indomethacin derivatives have anti-inflammatory activity, but R-(−)-isomers do not (55); natural (+)-cortisone and (+)-aldosterone are active, racemates have half this activity, and (−)-isomers are inactive (56).

Data on differences in the activity of optical isomers of cholinergic agents (57,58), adrenergic and adrenergic blocking agents (9,59), narcotic analgetics (22,35,60), and many other drugs (9,19,61,62) have been collected. Some of these data appear in Tables 5.2 and 5.3. In general the racemic compound exhibits a potency that is equivalent to the average potency of both enantiomers, and antagonism between them is infrequent.

By studying isomers of adrenergic agents, Patil and co-workers (63) have observed that molecular asymmetry exerts a deep influence on biological activity, which is related to the absolute configuration of carbons involved in the drug–receptor interaction. The D-configuration in the β-carbon of a series of adrenergic agents (isomers of epinephrine, norepinephrine, nordefrin,

TABLE 5.2 Pressor Activity of Ephedrine Isomers (*19,61*)

Isomer	Relative Pressor Activity
D-(−)-Ephedrine	36
DL-(±)-Ephedrine	26
L-(+)-Ephedrine	11
L-(+)-ψ-Ephedrine	7
DL-(±)-ψ-Ephedrine	4
D-(−)-ψ-Ephedrine	1

TABLE 5.3 Antibacterial Activity of Chloramphenicol Isomers (*51*)

Isomer	Antibacterial Activity
D-(−)-*threo*-Chloramphenicol	100
L-(+)-*erythro*-Chloramphenicol	1–2
L-(+)-*threo*-Chloramphenicol	< 0.4
D-(−)-*erythro*-Chloramphenicol	< 0.4

phenylephrine, and octopamine) favors interaction in the direct pressor receptor sites; the sole exceptions are the dextrorotatory isomers of epine-phrine and norepinephrine.

Further studies (*64*) related to the steric aspects of the same drugs seem to indicate that the β-hydroxy group of epinephrine is one of the most important groups involved in the interaction with receptors in direct sites; that is, there is a stereospecificity for the sites to which catecholamines attach. Furthermore it has been found that D-(−)-isomers are more active than L-(+)-isomers (*65*). It has also been shown that D-(−)-ephedrine blocks β-adrenergic receptors, whereas D-(−)-ψ-ephedrine does not. When one takes into account the preferred conformations of these two compounds,

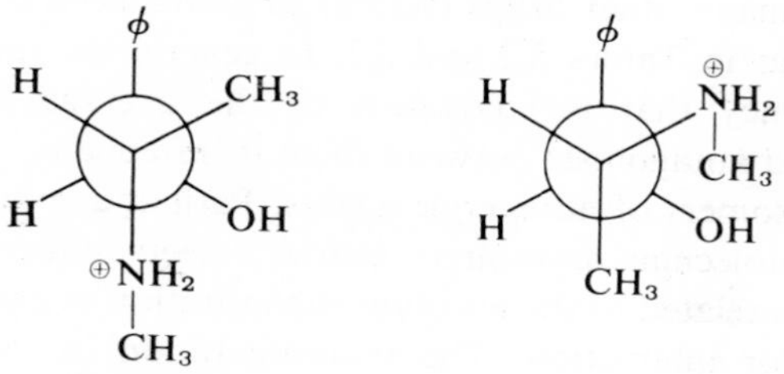

Ephedrine   ψ-Ephedrine

calculated by using the EHT (Extended Hückel Theory) (66), this difference of action can be explained by assuming that in the former case the methyl group attached to the α-carbon is projected above the plane of the phenylethylamino group, whereas in the latter case the methyl group is oriented below the plane and thus prevents efficient interaction of the drug with the receptor (67).

Because they usually display differences in biological activities, optical isomers have been much investigated in attempts to determine the nature of the drug–receptor interaction. On the basis of these studies several authors have formulated theories on this very interaction (Chapter 9) and have advanced hypotheses related to the receptor-surface topography (Chapter 8).

C. Geometrical Isomerism in Drugs

Geometric isomers (*cis–trans*), a particular kind of diastereoisomers (13), are stereoisomers of the same structures but with different spatial arrangements of atoms or groups. However, they are not mirror images of one another, as optical isomers are. Geometric isomerism is determined by a restricted rotation within a molecule, either through double bonds or through rigid or semirigid systems.

Very often geometric isomers produce differences in the intensity of biological action. This happens because, as in the case of *cis–trans* isomers, their physical and chemical properties are usually different. Contrary to the case of optical isomers, in a pair of geometric isomers the groups are separated by different distances. This makes either easier or more difficult, as the case may be, the interaction with the receptor surface and explains why the intensity of pharmacological action is not equal (Figure 5.2).

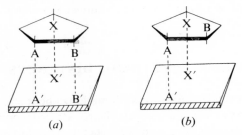

(a) (b)

Fig. 5.2. Interaction of geometric stereoisomers with a receptor surface. A, B, and X represent groups of atoms in the isomers; A′, B′, and X′ are their points of attachment to the surface. In (a) the attachment is stronger, because it is through three points; in (b), only through two, therefore it is weaker (9).

We can cite various examples of geometric isomers in which one is more potent than the other. Thus the psychotropic *trans*-chlorprothixene is 5 to 40 times as active as *cis*-chlorprothixene (68). In order to establish a connection between chemical structure and convulsive activity Jarboe and co-workers (69) have found in a series of lactones related to picrotoxinin that the four most active compounds have a lactone function binding carbons 3 and 5 of the skeleton, and the carbonyl system occupies a *cis* position in relation to the annular structure. Quantitative data regarding the *cis–trans* isomers of some cholinergic drugs are shown in Table 5.4; the formulas of these compounds are the following:

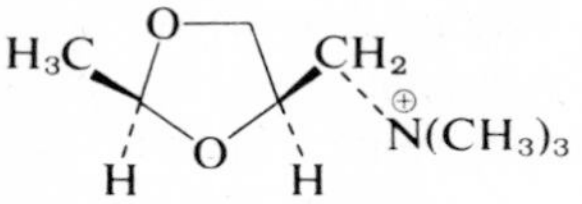

L-(+)-*cis*-2-Methyl-
4-dimethylaminomethyl-
1,3-dioxolane

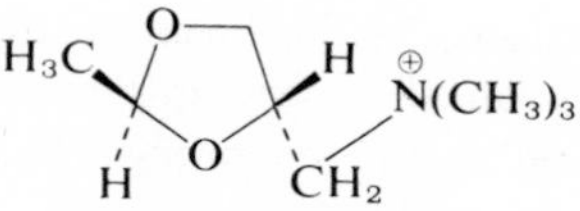

D-*trans*-2-methyl-
4-dimethylaminomethyl-
1,3-dioxolane

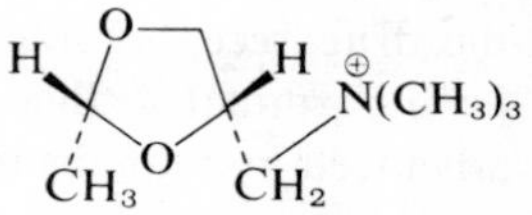

D-(−)-*cis*-2-Methyl-
4-dimethylaminomethyl-
1,3-dioxolane

TABLE 5.4   Muscarinic Activity of Isomers Derived from 4-Dimethylaminomethyl-1,3-dioxolane (70)

Compound	Relative Muscarinic Activity
DL-(±)-*cis*-2-Methyl methiodide	100
D-(−)-*cis*-2-Methyl methiodide	100
L-(+)-*cis*-2-Methyl methiodide	1
D-(+)-*trans*-2-Methyl methiodide	20

Reprinted by permission of the National Research Council of Canada.

III. INTERATOMIC DISTANCES

At this point it is convenient to say something about structure of proteins. Presently four types of structure are being studied: primary, secondary, tertiary and quaternary. The primary structure is the amino acid sequence along the backbone of the molecule. The secondary structure describes the helical coiling of polypeptide chains stabilized by hydrogen bonds. The tertiary structure means the overall conformation of the molecule as a result not only of side-chain interactions but also of interactions with the medium in which the protein may be. The quaternary structure refers to the arrangement of subunits within macromolecules.

In several proteins studied thus far, the polypeptides are coiled into a spiral.

In this spiral each amide group is linked to the third amide group beyond by an hydrogen bond, forming 13-membered rings. A complete turn of this model contains 3.6 amino acid residues. This spiral is called an α-helix.

Several examples mentioned before have pointed out the importance of the right distances between functional groups in certain drugs. In many cases these distances are critical for optimal biological activity. This substantiates the fact that such drugs are stereospecific; that is, the action produced by them results from complexation with organic receptors.

Such receptors, as described in Chapter 6, are predominantly proteins. These are made up of amino acids linked through their α-amino and α-carboxyl groups. They possess, therefore, very regular spacing between peptide bonds. Two distances are of great interest to molecular pharmacology: (a) the distance between two consecutive turns of the α-helix; (b) the distance that separates two peptide bonds when the protein is extended to the maximum. The first one was supposed to be 5.5 Å (71), but crystallographic studies have showed that it is 5.38 Å (72). The second one, usually known as the *identity distance*, is 3.61 Å.

Several drugs have, between their chemical groupings, one or another of these distances or a multiple of them. For instance, in the structure

$$R-X-C-C-NR'_2$$

where X can be nitrogen or oxygen, the distance between the X and N atoms is close to 5.5 Å (4,73). This structure is common to local anesthetics (procaine), adrenergic blocking agents (piperoxan), cholinergic agents (acetylcholine), spasmolytics (adiphenine), and antihistaminics (diphenhydramine).

The 3.61 Å distance or its multiple is found in several other drugs. Thus in some cholinergic and cholinergic blocking agents the carbonyl group of an ester is separated from a nitrogen atom by about 7.2 Å (2 × 3.61 Å) (16,74). In the curarimimetics the distance between the quaternary nitrogens is 14.5 Å (4 × 3.61 Å) (19); that is, twice the length of two molecules of acetylcholine. This seems to indicate that the receptor site of the cationic group repeats itself in a regular way. In *trans*-diethylstilbestrol the distance between

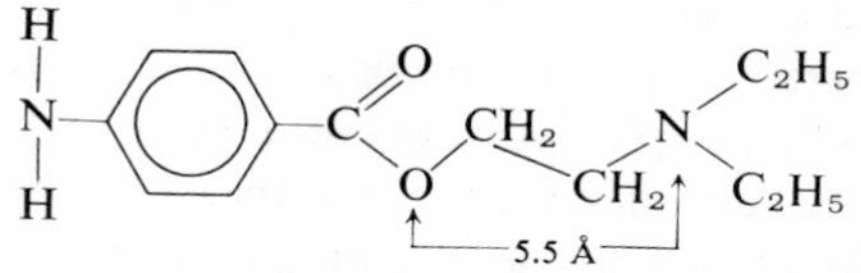

Procaine

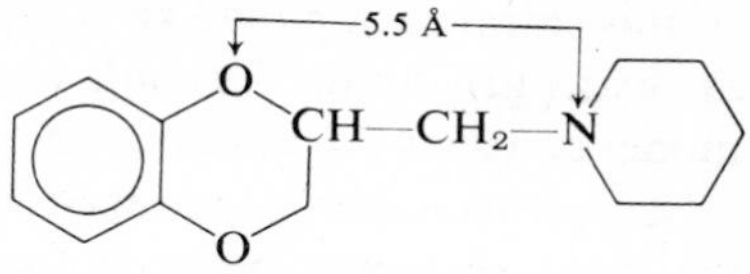

Piperoxan

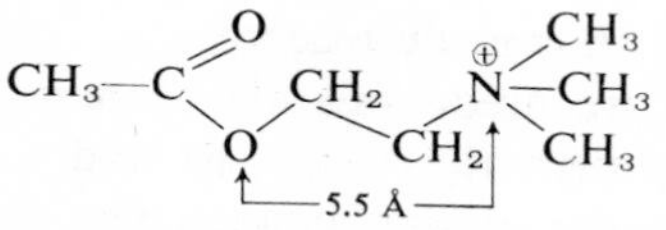

Acetylcholine

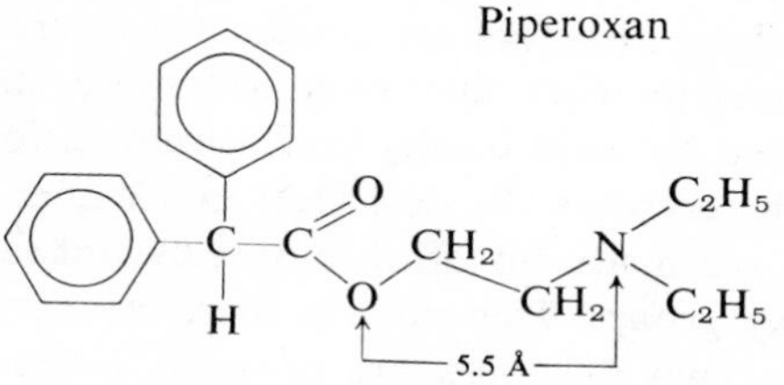

Adiphenine

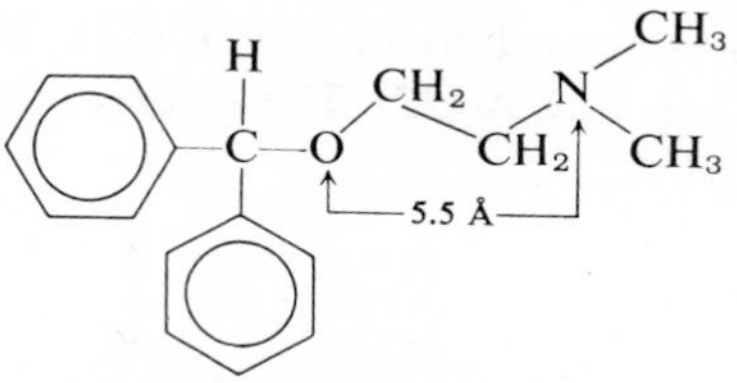

Diphenhydramine

the two hydroxy groups was believed to be 14.5 Å (4 × 3.61 Å), as in the estrogens, such as estradiol. Shortening this distance through the displacement of hydroxy groups would cause decreased estrogenic potency (16).

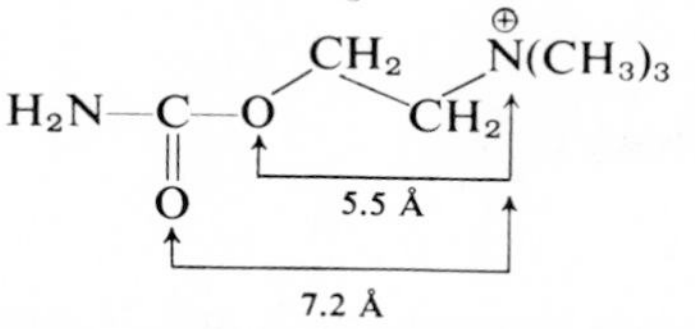

Carbachol (cholinergic)

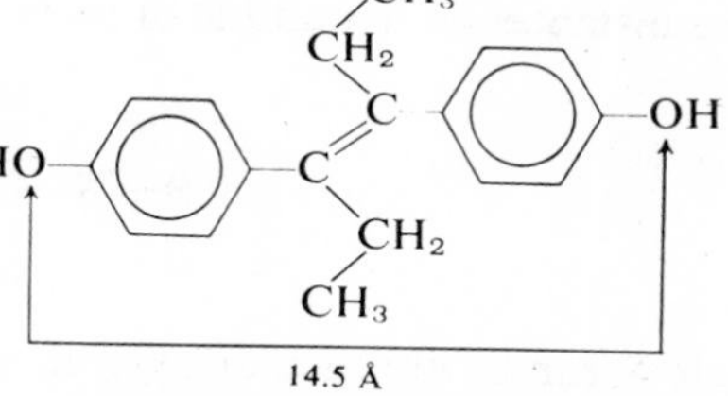

trans-Diethylstilbestrol (estrogenic)

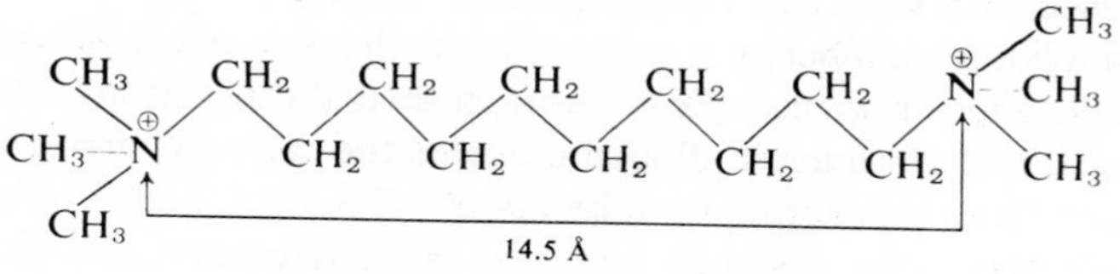

Decamethonium (curarimimetic)

Recent crystallographic measurements (72), however, showed that the average distance between the two oxygens of the phenolic hydroxy groups in estrogens is 10.98 Å, which is very close to two turns of the α-helix (2 × 5.38 Å) (Table 5.5). Since there are 3.60 amino acid residues per turn of the α-helix, it was concluded that the O—O distance in the estrogens corresponds to 7.5 residues of the α-helix.

TABLE 5.5   Intramolecular Oxygen–Oxygen Distances in the Estrogens (72)

Estrogen	O—O Distance (Å)	Distance between Hydroxyl Hydrogen Atoms (Å)
4-Bromo-17β-estradiol	10.95 ± 0.04	
4-Bromo-estrone	10.78 ± 0.04	
Estriol (3–17β), molecule 1	10.952 ± 0.007	11.66 ± 0.05
Estriol (3–17β), molecule 2	11.085 ± 0.007	11.45 ± 0.05
Estriol (3–16α), molecule 1	11.266 ± 0.007	10.92 ± 0.05
Estriol (3–16α), molecule 2	10.859 ± 0.007	11.18 ± 0.05

Although interesting, this coincidence of distances must be irrelevant, because, as Albert (40) points out, estrogens are active only on highly specific sites, whereas functional proteins of many kinds are present in all parts of the body.

When drugs act as metabolic antagonists, configuration and interatomic distances become of capital importance. The classical example is that of the sulfanilamides, which have a remarkable structural resemblance, even in interatomic distances, with p-aminobenzoic acid, of which they are antagonists (75):

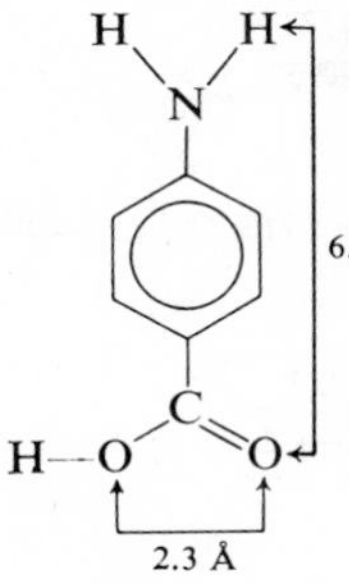

p-Aminobenzoic acid 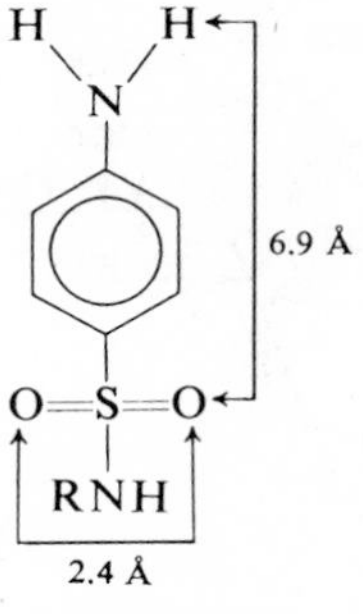   Sulfanilamides

Recent crystallographic studies of sulfanilamide (76,77) and p-aminobenzoic acid (78) prove that there are close similarities between the bond lengths and bond angles of both molecules (Figures 5.3 and 5.4).

In several types of drugs, however, the interatomic distances that are optimal for biological activity do not conform to the distances in proteins. This may be explained by the possibility that these proteins assume many different conformations (*26,79,80*), depending on (a) the medium in which they may be and (b) the ability of their normal, very coiled, structure to undergo disorganization or deep change. Consequently, alterations of their

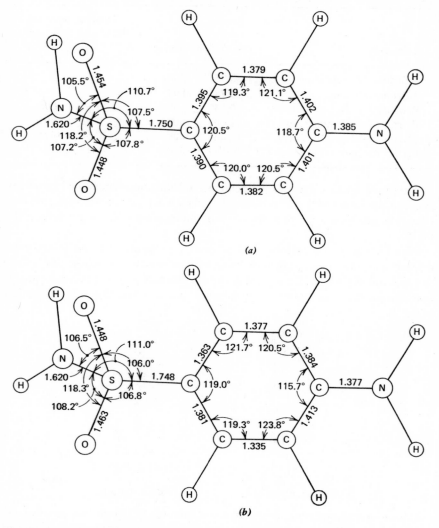

Fig. 5.3. Bond lengths and bond angles in (*a*) β-sulfanilamide; (*b*) sulfanilamide monohydrate (*77*).

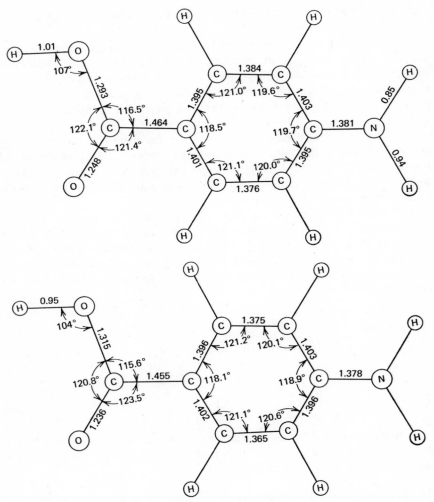

Fig. 5.4. Bond lengths and bond angles in the *p*-aminobenzoic acid dimer (*78*).

physicochemical properties as well as changes in interatomic distances may occur. Owing to this possibility interatomic distances in protein surface may become complementary to those of the drugs that interact with it.

From many studies made with the purpose of correlating the distances between functional groups with the biological activity produced by drugs it can be deduced that, though they do not usually constitute the main factor, these distances exert in many cases extraordinary influence on optimal interaction between drug and receptor.

IV. ELECTRONIC DISTRIBUTION AND CONFIGURATION

Electronic distribution in a chemical compound determines many physico-chemical properties—such as electronic charge, bond strength, interatomic distances, bond character, dissociation constants, diamagnetism, electronic absorption spectra, chemical reactivity, and ability to form complexes. It determines also to a great degree the biological action produced by the substance.

Thus, for instance, acridine compounds, in the form of cations, interact stereospecifically with a variety of cellular polyanions, binding specifically to nucleic acids (DNA and RNA), phospholipids (which are found in cellular membranes), and sulfated polysaccharides (which are found in the cell walls of certain bacteria) (81).

Polycyclic hydrocarbons, in order to produce carcinogenic activity, should contain an active K-region and an inactive L-region (82). The car-cinogenic hydrocarbon would fix itself to cellular proteins either through addition to the K-region or through Diels–Alder type of dienophilic addition to the L-region. The addition complexes thus formed would be later on eliminated from the cell.

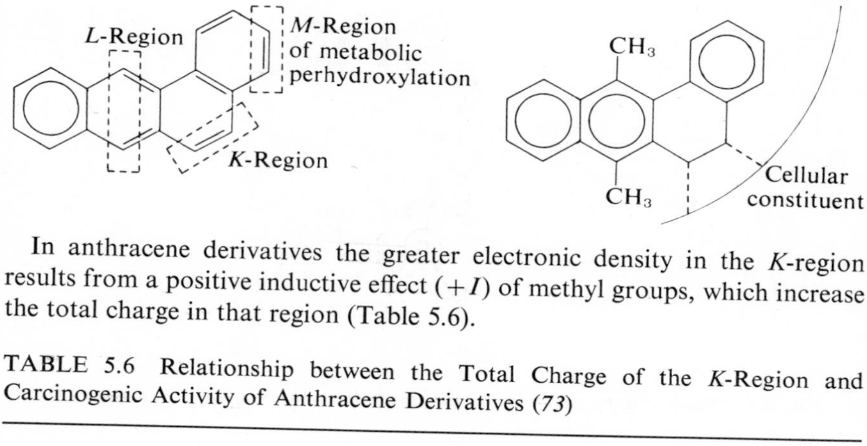

In anthracene derivatives the greater electronic density in the K-region results from a positive inductive effect ($+I$) of methyl groups, which increase the total charge in that region (Table 5.6).

TABLE 5.6   Relationship between the Total Charge of the K-Region and Carcinogenic Activity of Anthracene Derivatives (73)

Compound	Total Charge	Carcinogenic Activity
Anthracene	1.259	—
1,2-Benzanthracene	1.283	+
5-Methyl-1,2-benzanthracene	1.296	+ +
10-Methyl-1,2-benzanthracene	1.306	+ + +
5,9,10-Trimethyl-1,2-benzanthracene	1.332	+ + + +

According to Hey (*83*), the lesser the electronic density on the etheric oxygen of the esters and ethers of choline, the greater their nicotinic stimulant action. Actually, by synthesizing compounds with the following charge distribution

$$\overset{\ominus}{A}=\overset{\oplus}{O}-CH_2-CH_2-\overset{\oplus}{N}(CH_3)_3$$

he found that some of them manifested more intense action than the most potent nicotinic stimulant then known.

Sekul and Holland (*84*) discovered that a double bond introduced into the acylic side chain of choline esters enhanced the pressor effect of these drugs, probably by the formation of charges by resonance through delocalization of the π-electron cloud:

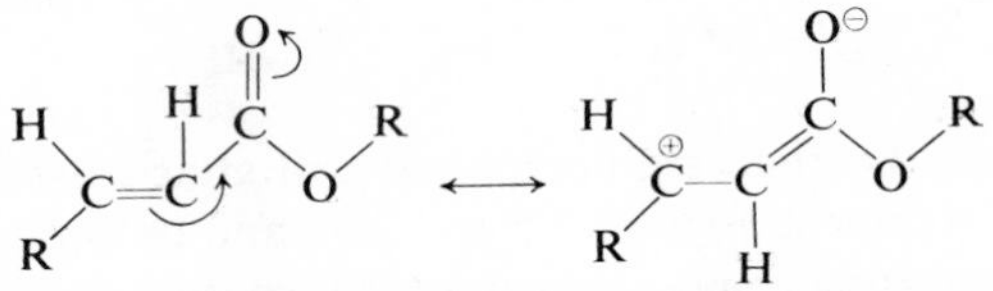

Introduction of electron-repelling groups, such as alkyl, in the α- or β-positions intensifies still more the nicotinic effects. Hence Sekul and Holland concluded that electronic density on the carbonyl oxygen was closely related to the intensity of nicotinic action. In the light of what happens with drugs at the nicotinic receptor level (Chapter 8, Section V.C) it is easy to understand the reason for this.

Local anesthetics exhibit the same phenomena. Almost all of them are related to cocaine and can be represented by the following general formula (*85*):

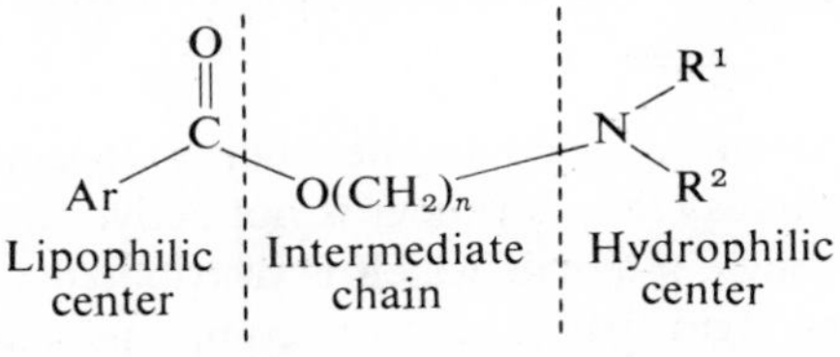

It is essential for anesthetic activity that a balance exist between the lipophilic and the hydrophilic parts of the molecule. Furthermore in all local anesthetics of the ester and amide types the carbonyl group is activated by the partially positive charge on the carbon atom. This is made possible by conjugated double bonds, which allow the π-framework over the aromatic ring to delocalize to the carbonyl oxygen:

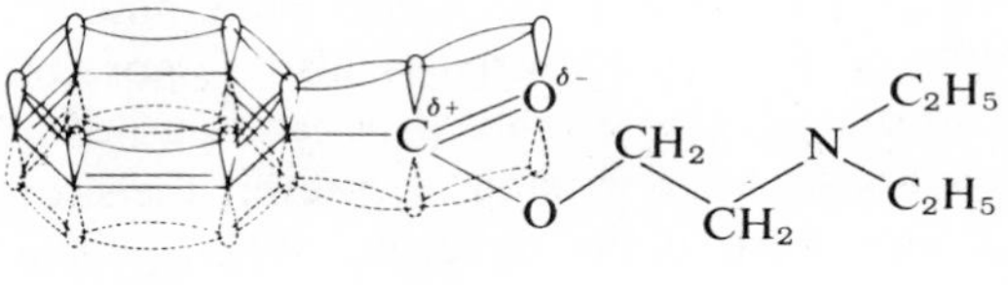

This atom, owing to its greater electronegativity, acquires a partial negative charge and gives rise to a partial positive charge on the carbonyl carbon. Introduction of a group in the *para* position of the phenyl moiety can increase this polarization if the group (as NH_2) is an electron donor, or diminish it if the group (as NO_2) is an electron acceptor (*86*):

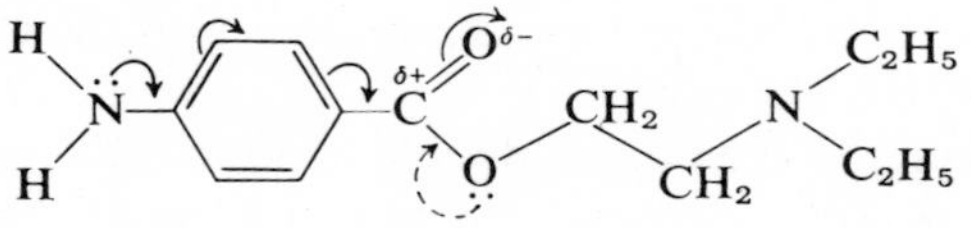

Favorable

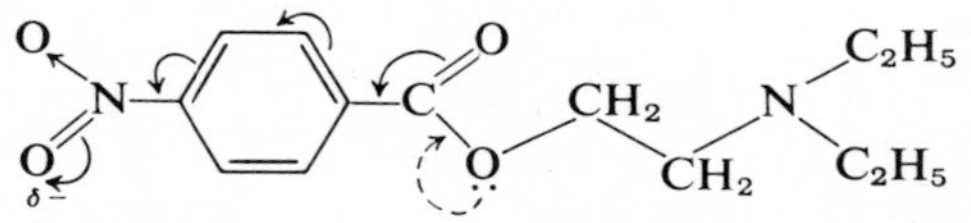

Unfavorable

In the first case the resulting compound will attach itself to the receptor more strongly (Chapter 7, Figures 7.5 and 7.6), and prolong its action. In the second case the resulting compound cannot attach itself so well to the receptor as the parent compound, and therefore its anesthetic activity will be reduced or annulled. The same result will be obtained if the conjugated system of double bonds is interrupted through introduction of a group —C— or —C—C— between the aromatic ring and the carbonyl group:

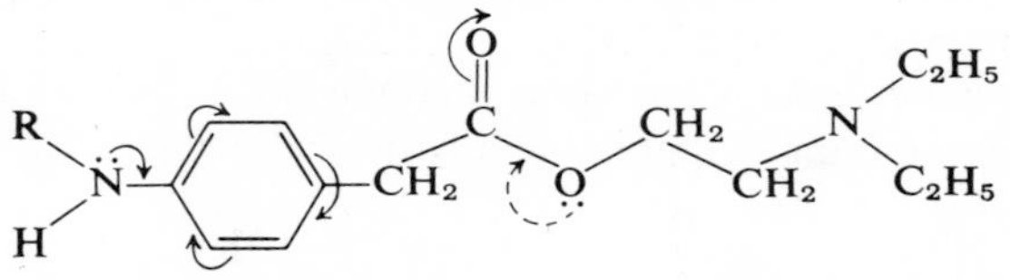

A similar explanation is given to the high estrogenic activity of *trans*-diethylstilbestrol, whereas the *cis* isomer is not active. Both have conjugated systems forming a single π-cloud, which is distributed over all atoms. This confers a planar and rigid structure to the compounds and impels the ethyl groups to adopt a definite configuration. In the *trans* isomer these groups are arranged in such a way as to form a structure very similar to that of natural estrogens. In the *cis* isomer, however, this does not happen. Hence the diversity of biological activity. Incidentally, it must be recalled that the importance of a rigid structure should not be overemphasized: hexestrol, formed by reduction of the double bond of *trans*-diethylestilbestrol, has a flexible structure, but is as active as the parent compound.

The distribution of electronic charge is also responsible for the steric arrangement of drug molecules. Should it be made up of nonpolar groups, this conformation will be quite variable. However, the situation is different when charged groups exist in the molecule. When groups have opposite charges, the electrostatic forces will attract these atoms close to one another. On the other hand, a repulsion will be observed when the groups carry the same sign, and the electrostatic forces will separate them to the maximum. Thus, in solution, the positive charges in both quaternary nitrogens of methonium compounds, of the general formula

$$\diagdown \overset{+}{\underset{\diagup}{N}}(CH_2)_n\overset{+}{\underset{\diagdown}{N}}\diagup$$

tend to separate the quaternary nitrogens and extend the alkyl chain to the maximum.

Lately the influence of π-electron charge densities on the biological activity of many substances is being extensively and deeply studied (87). Using molecular-orbital calculations (88–98), several researchers have determined in addition to π-electron charge densities other indices—such as bond order, resonance energy, and energy levels of the highest occupied molecular orbital (HOMO) and the lowest empty molecular orbital (LEMO). Significant results were obtained with fungicides (99), antibacterial agents (100,101), hallucinogens (102), cholinesterase inhibitors (103–105), and other types of drugs (105).

More recent studies have attempted to correlate the π-electron charge densities and energy levels of the HOMO and LEMO with the biological activity of antimalarials (106). Of the three quinoline antimalarials studied, it was found that chloroquine is the one with the greatest electron density on the heterocyclic nitrogen. Chloroquine base was compared with the corresponding salt, and the changes in the molecular-orbital indices that took place on protonation were examined in the light of the mechanism of action proposed for these compounds (107) in which the protonated form is thought to be the active species in forming a charge-transfer complex with DNA.

The energy level of the HOMO is taken as a measure of electron-donor ability and that of the LEMO as a measure of electron-acceptor ability (87). The smaller the HOMO, the greater are the electron-donor properties because it takes less energy to remove a π-electron from the HOMO; conversely, the closer to zero the energy level of the LEMO, the greater would be the electron affinity because the incoming electrons would be in a somewhat more stable orbital. These energy levels are very important in determining the formation of a charge-transfer complex between the drug and DNA. The base pairs in the DNA molecule, particularly the guanine–cytosine pair, are good electron donors (87). The mechanism calls for the intercalation of chloroquine salt (a good electron acceptor) between adjacent pairs of bases in the DNA molecule (Figure 5.5).

Other calculations with the omega technique have been performed on a

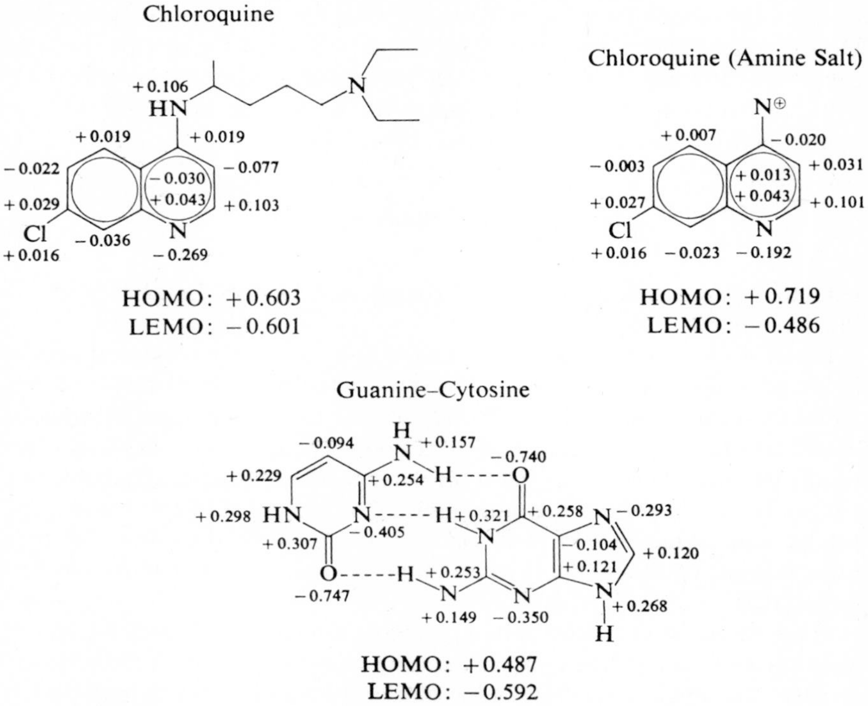

Chloroquine

Chloroquine (Amine Salt)

HOMO: +0.603
LEMO: −0.601

HOMO: +0.719
LEMO: −0.486

Guanine–Cytosine

HOMO: +0.487
LEMO: −0.592

Fig. 5.5. Electron charge densities of chloroquine base, chloroquine salt, and the guanine–cytosine pair in DNA (*106*). (Reprinted by permission of the American Chemical Society.)

different model for protonated quinoline* based on the fact that heterocyclic nitrogen compounds with an amino group attached to them add the first proton on the ring nitrogen (*108*). These results are probably more accurate, and the values of the energy levels are significantly improved.

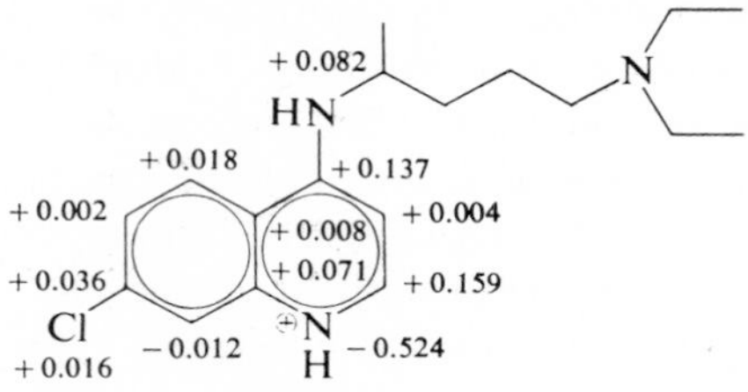

HOMO: +0.803
LEMO: −0.332

* Personal communication from V. E. Marquez-Muskus.

The surprising negative charge on the ring nitrogen in this model is a consequence of the fact that the protonated nitrogen is the most electronegative atom in the π-framework, and the calculations take into account the resonance effect:

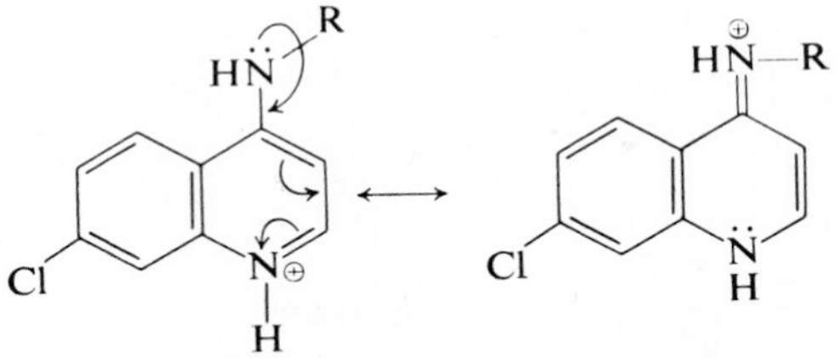

It is very likely that further studies in this field, such as those that are being performed by Kuprievich and co-workers (*109–111*), concerning the calculations of π-electron charge densities of nucleic acid bases, will lead to a deeper insight into the mechanism of action of drugs that interfere in some way with nucleic acids. These calculations are concerned not only with the ground state but mainly with the excited and ionized states, and their purpose is to relate the results obtained to particular biochemical processes.

A similar approach is being followed in attempts to explain the antibacterial action of sulfonamides at the submolecular level. For instance, in an effort to correlate the bacteriostatic activity of these drugs with the electron density of ionizing N^1, Foernzler and Martin (*112*) have recently determined the electron density of 50 sulfonamides used in 1942 by Bell and Roblin (*75*) in their studies on the influence of pK_a on chemotherapeutic action. They observed that the charge distribution of, for example, sulfanilamide is the one shown in Figure 5.6. It is enlightening to compare it with the charge distribution of *p*-aminobenzoic acid (Figure 5.7), calculated by Pullman and Pullman (*87*). On the basis of data obtained through molecular-orbital calculations, Foernzler and Martin concluded that, with few exceptions, bacteriostatic activity diminishes with decrease in the formal charge of the N^1 atom. Some of their results are shown in Table 5.7.

Improved values for electronic formal charges of sulfanilamide and *p*-aminobenzoic acid were obtained by applying the omega technique to Hückel molecular-orbital calculations (Figure 5.8).

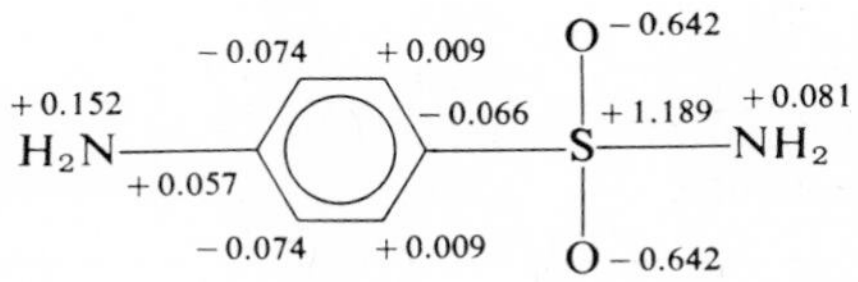

Fig. 5.6.   Electronic formal charges in sulfanilamide (*112*).

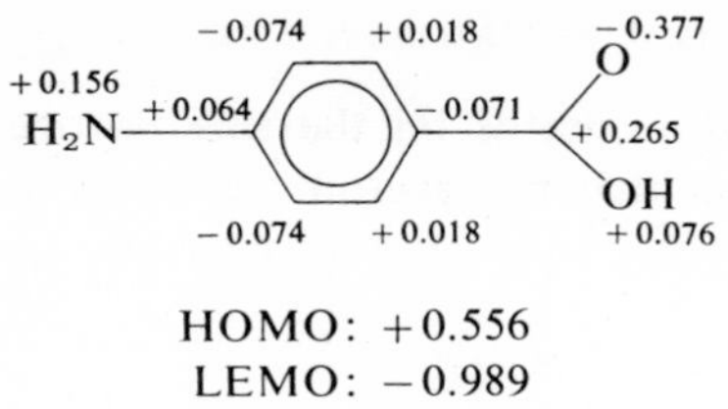

$$HOMO: +0.556$$
$$LEMO: -0.989$$

Fig. 5.7. Electronic formal charges in p-aminobenzoic acid (*87*).

TABLE 5.7 Relationship between Biological Activity and Electronic Charges in Some Sulfas (*112*)

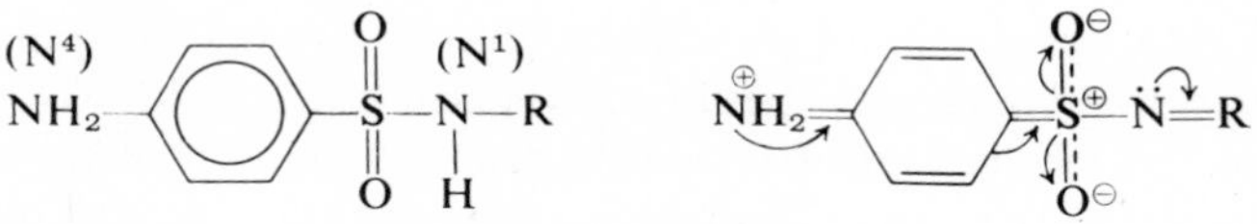

Sulfa	Activity Index $(C_R \times 10^5)^{-1}$		Formal π-Charge $f\,N^1$	
Sulfadiazine	12.5	Decreasing	(+)0.230	Decreasing
2-Sulfanilamidopyrazine	12.5	Activity	0.221	Charge
3-Sulfanilamidopyridazine	12.5		0.220	
4-S-Pyrimidine	20.0		0.232	
5-S-2-Chloropyrimidine	10.0		0.203	
3-Sulfanilamidopyridine	5.0		0.207	
5-S-Pyrimidine	5.0		0.207	
5-S-2-Bromopyridine	5.0		0.206	
2-S-5-Bromopyridine	2.0		0.219	
N⁴-Sulfanilylmetanilamide	2.0		0.210	
Sulfapyridine	1.67		0.219	
2-S-5-Aminopyridine	1.67		0.207	
N¹-Sulfanilylmetanilamide	0.50		0.208	
5-S-2-Aminopyridine	0.50		0.195	
N¹-Phenylsulfanilamide	0.33		0.206	
N¹-m-Tolylsulfanilamide	0.20		0.208	
N¹-p-Tolylsulfanilamide	0.20		0.207	
N¹-p-Aminophenylsulfanilamide	0.20		0.195	

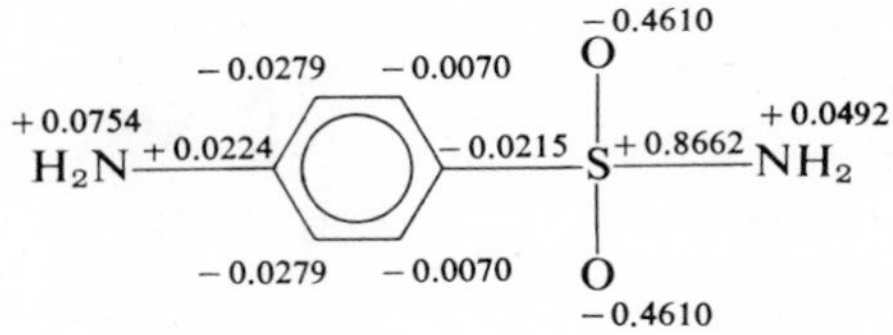

$$-0.4610$$

$$\overset{-0.0279 \quad -0.0070}{\underset{-0.0279 \quad -0.0070}{\text{[ring]}}} \quad \overset{O}{\underset{O}{\underset{-0.4610}{\overset{+0.0492}{S}}}}$$

$+0.0754$
$\text{H}_2\text{N} \overset{+0.0224}{\rule{1.2cm}{0.4pt}}$ [benzene ring] $\overset{-0.0215}{\rule{0.8cm}{0.4pt}} \underset{}{\overset{}{S}} \overset{+0.8662}{\rule{0.6cm}{0.4pt}} \text{NH}_2$

HOMO: $+0.3542$
LEMO: -1.0246

$$-0.3427$$

$+0.0845$
$\text{H}_2\text{N} \overset{+0.0460}{\rule{1.2cm}{0.4pt}}$ [benzene ring] $\overset{-0.0209}{\rule{0.8cm}{0.4pt}} \overset{O}{\underset{\underset{+0.0802}{\text{OH}}}{C}} \overset{+0.1556}{}$

$-0.0188 \quad +0.0173$

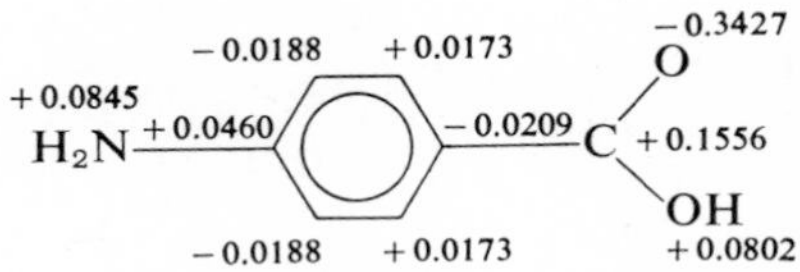

HOMO: $+0.7129$
LEMO: -0.5334

Fig. 5.8. Formal charges in sulfanilamide and *p*-aminobenzoic acid calculated by the omega technique. (Personal communication from V. E. Marquez-Muskus.)

The various features held responsible for the biological action of sulfonamides were reviewed by Seydel (*113*).

In a recent monograph, in order to establish a correlation among various types of drugs and their receptors, Perkow (*114*) pointed out that there are many drugs characterized by a lesser electronic charge on a particular atom, which he called the *biologically active center*. He postulated that the pharmacodynamic or chemotherapeutic actions that these drugs manifest result from low electron density on this center; specificity of action is conditioned by more or less secondary characteristics—such as the size of the molecule and the liposolubility—conferred by the *carrier groups*, which determine the route of transport, the distribution, and the adsorption of drugs. A similar study was also carried out by Ariëns (*115*).

Among various other drugs, whose action he ascribed to the presence of the *biologically active center*, Perkow (*114*) mentioned derivatives of diphenylmethane, a group that includes spasmolytics, antihistaminics, psychotonics, analgetics, antitussives, insecticides, and bactericides:

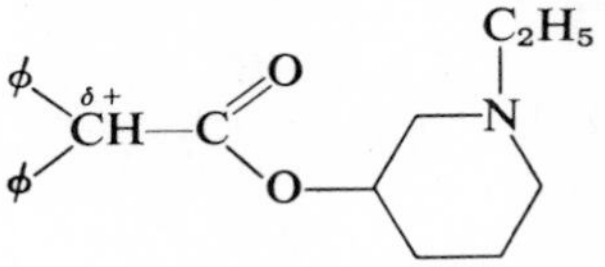

Piperidolate
(spasmolytic)

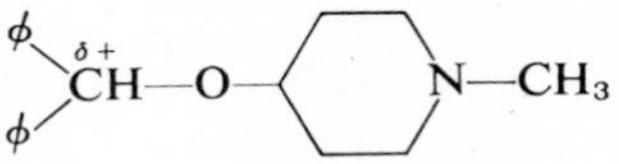

Diphenylpyraline
(antihistaminic)

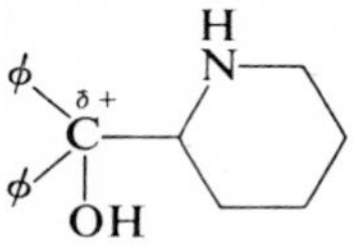

Pipradrol
(psychotonic)

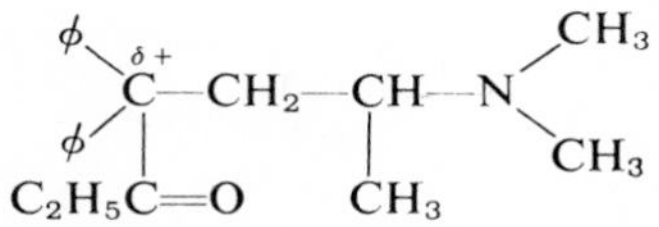

Methadone
(analgetic)

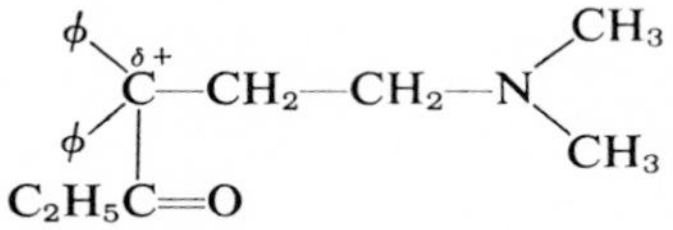

Normethadone
(antitussive)

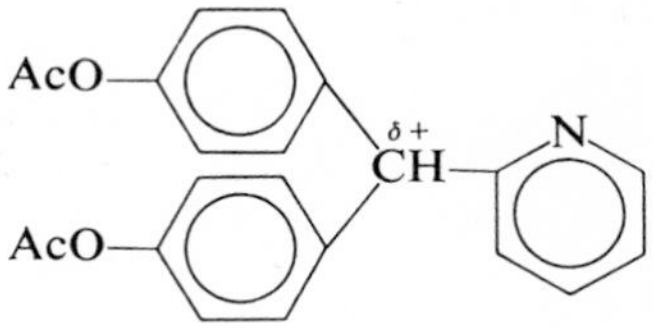

Bisacodyl
(cathartic)

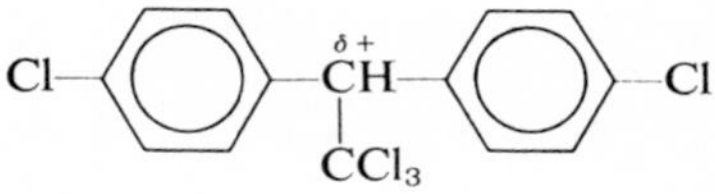

DDT
(insecticide)

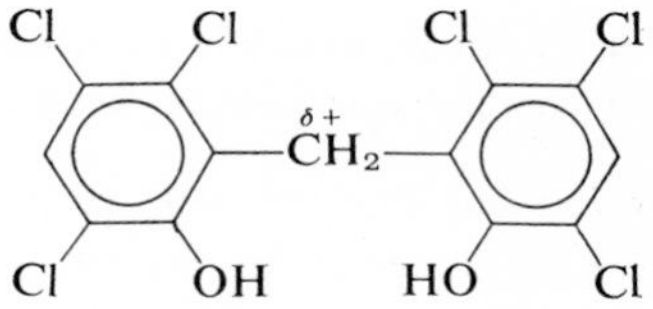

Hexachlorophene
(bactericide)

In another interesting series (namely, the hypnotics) Perkow stressed the presence of a quaternary carbon that is attached to electronegative groups and thus has low electron density:

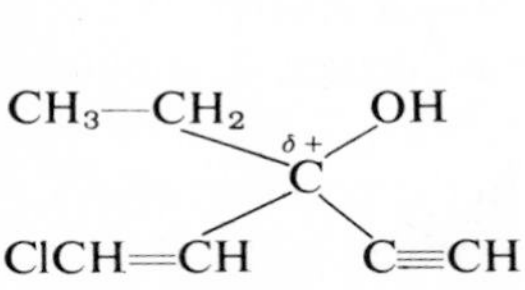

Ethchlorvynol

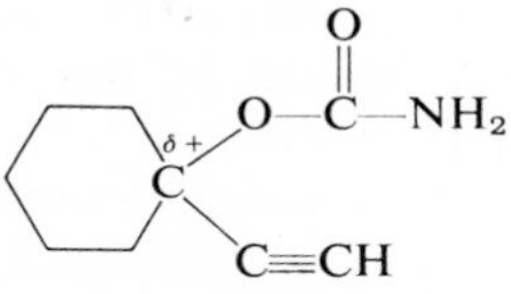

Ethinamate

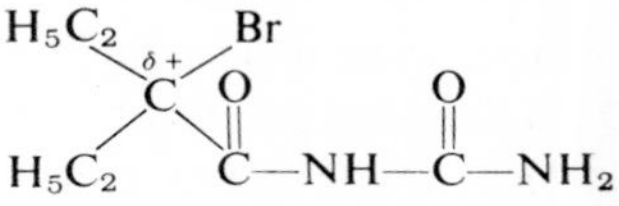

Carbromal

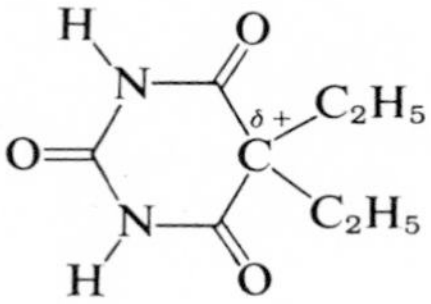

Barbital

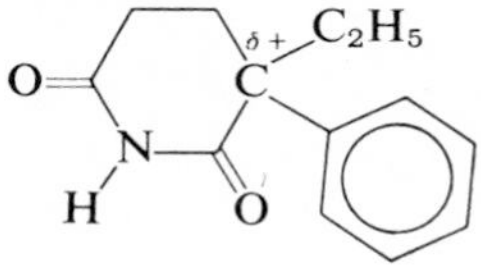

Glutethimide

Still according to Perkow, the activity of sulfonamides is explained in a similar manner: they owe their pharmacodynamic or chemotherapeutic action to their having a lower electron density on the sulfur atom:

Cl—⟨benzene⟩—$\overset{\delta+}{\underset{O_2}{S}}$—NH—$\overset{O}{\overset{\|}{C}}$—NH—$C_3H_7$ Chlorpropamide (antidiabetic)

H_2N—⟨benzene⟩—$\overset{\delta+}{\underset{O_2}{S}}$—NH—⟨thiazole⟩   Sulfathiazole (bacteriostatic)

Cl—⟨benzene⟩—$\overset{\delta+}{\underset{O_2}{S}}$—⟨benzene⟩—Cl   Di-(p-chlorophenyl)-sulfone **(acaricide)**

In order to compare the charges at Perkow's biologically active center with anticonvulsant activity, Andrews (*116*) calculated the atomic charges on a number of anticonvulsant drugs and related compounds by using EHT and CNDO (Complete Neglect of Differential Overlap) methods. His research showed that there is no direct correlation between the two. He concluded, therefore, that the net charge at that center does not determine the type or degree of the central nervous system activity exhibited by the drugs studied.

Very recently, in research aimed at determining the preferred conformation of histamine, Kier (*49*) observed through molecular-orbital calculations that, although the C—NH_3 group has a net charge of $+0.811$, the quaternary nitrogen atom, contrary to the usual representation, bears a *negative*, and not a positive, charge (Figure 5.9).

To test the validity of his apparently unexpected result, Kier further examined the charge on the nitrogen of the simplest quaternary amine, the ammonium ion NH_4^+. He showed that in this symmetrical ion also the

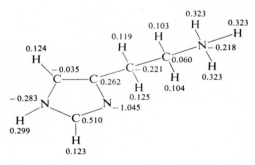

Fig. 5.9. Histamine monocation total ($\sigma + \pi$) net charges (*49*). (Reprinted by permission of the American Chemical Society.)

nitrogen atom bears a negative charge (-0.36, on the average) and the hydrogen atoms, a positive charge ($+0.34$, on the average). This leaves the ammonium ion with the positive charge $+1$. Hence he concluded that the nitrogen atom of a quaternary alkyl salt would also be negatively charged. The discrepancy between the usual representation (positive nitrogen) and Kier's finding (negative nitrogen) can be reconciled if we consider that a positively charged atom has a tendency to attract electrons and thus can become negative; and a negatively charged atom, due to its tendency to repel electrons, can become positive.

The interesting results obtained through molecular-orbital calculations, nuclear magnetic resonance, optical rotatory dispersion, circular dichroism, and other techniques in attempts to elucidate the structure and function of drug–receptor complexes have encouraged researchers to proceed on this course of investigation.

REFERENCES

1. R. Croxatto and F. Huidobro, *Arch. Intern. Pharmacodyn.*, **106**, 207 (1956).
2. N. Robinson, *J. Pharm. Pharmacol.*, **12**, 129, 193 (1960).
3. D. R. H. Gourley, *Progr. Drug Res.*, **7**, 11 (1964).
4. T. C. Daniels and E. C. Jorgensen, "Physicochemical Properties in Relation to Biologic Action," in C. O. Wilson, O. Gisvold, and R. F. Doerge, Eds., *Textbook of Organic Medicinal and Pharmaceutical Chemistry*, 5th ed., Lippincott, Philadelphia, 1966, pp. 4–62.
5. E. J. Ariëns, Ed., *Molecular Pharmacology*, Vol. I, Academic, New York, 1964.
6. E. W. Gill, *Progr. Med. Chem.*, **4**, 39 (1965).
7. J. Levy and B. Tchoubar, *Actualités Pharmacol.*, **5**, 143 (1952).
8. K. J. Brunings, Ed., *Modern Concepts in the Relationship Betweeen Structure and Pharmacological Activity*, Pergamon, Oxford, 1963.
9. A. H. Beckett, *Progr. Drug Res.*, **1**, 455 (1959).
10. E. L. Eliel, *Stereochemistry of Carbon Compounds*, McGraw-Hill, New York, 1962.
11. E. L. Eliel, N. L. Allinger, S. J. Angyal, and G. A. Morrison, *Conformational Analysis*, Interscience, New York, 1965.
12. K. Mislow, *Introduction to Stereochemistry*, Benjamin, New York, 1966.
13. R. T. Morrison and R. N. Boyd, *Organic Chemistry*, 2nd ed., Allyn and Bacon, Boston, 1966.
14. J. D. Roberts and M. C. Caserio, *Modern Organic Chemistry*, Benjamin, New York, 1967.
15. D. L. Robinson and D. W. Theobald, *Quart. Rev.*, **21**, 314 (1967).
16. F. W. Schueler, *Chemobiodynamics and Drug Design*, McGraw-Hill, New York, 1960.
17. J. Büchi, *Grundlagen der Arzneimittelforschung und der synthetischen Arzneimittel*, Birkhauser, Basel, 1963.

18. J. B. Stenlake, *Progr. Med. Chem.*, **3**, 1 (1963).
19. R. B. Barlow, *Introduction to Chemical Pharmacology*, 2nd ed., Methuen, London, 1964.
20. J. C. Kellett and C. W. Hite, *J. Pharm. Sci.*, **54**, 883 (1965).
21. J. M. van Rossum, *J. Pharm. Pharmacol.*, **17**, 202 (1965).
22. P. S. Portoghese, *J. Pharm. Sci.*, **55**, 865 (1966).
23. G. L. Szendey, *Arzneimittel-Forsch.*, **16**, 77 (1966).
24. K. W. Bentley, D. G. Hardy, B. Meek, et al., *J. Am. Chem. Soc.*, **89**, 3267, 3273, 3281, 3293, 3303, 3312 (1967).
25. P. D. Armstrong, J. G. Cannon, and J. P. Long, *Nature*, **220**, 65 (1968).
26. P. S. Portoghese et al., *J. Med. Chem.*, **11**, 12, 219 (1968).
27. P. S. Portoghese and D. L. Larson, *J. Pharm. Sci.*, **57**, 711 (1968).
28. A. F. Casy and A. P. Parulkar, *J. Med. Chem.*, **12**, 178 (1969).
29. G. Snatzke, *Angewandte Chemie, Intern. Ed.*, **7**, 14 (1968).
30. W. H. Vogel, R. Snyder, and M. P. Schulman, *J. Pharmacol. Exptl. Therap.*, **146**, 66 (1964).
31. R. S. Schnaare and A. N. Martin, *J. Pharm. Sci.*, **54**, 1707 (1965).
32. A. Albert, *The Acridines*, 2nd ed., Arnold, London, 1966.
33. J. D. P. Graham, *Progr. Med. Chem.*, **2**, 132 (1962).
34. A. H. Beckett and A. F. Casy, *J. Pharm. Pharmacol.*, **6**, 986 (1954).
35. A. H. Beckett and A. F. Casy, *Progr. Med. Chem.*, **4**, 171 (1965).
36. I. N. Nazarov, N. S. Prostakov, et al., *J. Gen. Chem. USSR* (Eng. Transl.), **26**, 3117, 3131, 3139, 3153 (1956).
37. O. I. Sorokin, *Izv. Akad. Nauk SSSR, Otd. Khim. Nauk*, 460 (1961); through *Chem. Abstr.*, **55**, 22310c (1961).
38. N. J. Harper, C. F. Chignell, and G. Kirk, *J. Med. Chem.*, **7**, 726 (1964).
39. E. E. Smissman and M. Steinman, *J. Med. Chem.*, **9**, 455 (1966).
40. A. Albert, *Selective Toxicity*, 4th ed., Methuen, London, 1968.
41. J. H. Fellman and T. S. Fujita, *Nature*, **211**, 848 (1966).
42. E. E. Smissman, W. L. Nelson, J. B. LaPidus, and J. L. Day, *J. Med. Chem.*, **9**, 458 (1966).
43. A. W. Solter, *J. Pharm. Sci.*, **54**, 1755 (1965).
44. C. C. J. Culvenor and N. S. Ham, *Chem. Commun.*, 537 (1966).
45. F. G. Canepa, P. Pauling, and H. Sörum, *Nature*, **210**, 907 (1966).
46. L. B. Kier, *Mol. Pharmacol.*, **3**, 487 (1967).
47. D. Carlström and R. Bergin, *Acta Cryst.*, **23**, 313 (1967).
48. L. B. Kier, *J. Pharm. Pharmacol.*, **21**, 93 (1968).
49. L. B. Kier, *J. Med. Chem.*, **11**, 441 (1968).
50. L. B. Kier, *J. Pharm. Sci.*, **57**, 1188 (1968).
51. R. E. Maxwell and V. S. Nickel, *Antibiot. Chemother.*, (*Washington, D.C.*), **4**, 289 (1954).
52. M. M. Shemyakin and M. N. Kolosov, *Pure Appl. Chem.*, **6**, 305 (1963).
53. F. E. Hahn, "Chloramphenicol," in D. Gottlieb and P. D. Shaw, Eds., *Antibiotics*, Vol. I, Springer, New York, 1967, pp. 308–330.
54. B. Riegel and L. T. Sherwood, Jr., *J. Am. Chem. Soc.*, **71**, 1129 (1949).
55. T. Y. Shen, *Topics Med. Chem.*, **1**, 29 (1967).

56. I. E. Bush, *Pharmacol. Rev.*, **14**, 317 (1962).

57. E. J. Ariëns, *Advan. Drug Res.*, **3**, 235 (1966).

58. E. J. Ariëns and A. M. Simonis, *Ann. N.Y. Acad. Sci.*, **144**, 842 (1967).

59. E. J. Ariëns, *Ann. N.Y. Acad. Sci.*, **139**, 606 (1967).

60. P. S. Portoghese, *J. Med. Chem.*, **8**, 609 (1965).

61. C. O. Wilson, O. Gisvold, and R. F. Doerge, Eds., *Textbook of Organic Medicinal and Pharmaceutical Chemistry*, 5th ed., Lippincott, Philadelphia, 1966.

62. A. Burger, Ed., *Medicinal Chemistry*, 3rd ed., Interscience, New York, 1970.

63. P. N. Patil, A. Tye, and J. B. LaPidus, *J. Pharmacol. Exptl. Therap.*, **149**, 199 (1965).

64. P. N. Patil, J. B. LaPidus, A. Tye, and D. Campbell, *J. Pharmacol. Exptl. Therap.*, **155**, 1, 13, 24 (1967).

65. P. N. Patil, *J. Pharmacol. Exptl. Therap.*, **160**, 308 (1968).

66. L. B. Kier, *J. Pharmacol. Exptl. Therap.*, **164**, 75 (1968).

67. P. S. Portoghese, *J. Med. Chem.*, **10**, 1057 (1967).

68. P. V. Petersen and I. Møller-Nielsen, "Thiaxanthene Derivatives," in M. Gordon, Ed., *Psychopharmacological Agents*, Vol. I, Academic, New York, 1964, pp. 301–324.

69. C. H. Jarboe, L. A. Porter, and R. T. Buckler, *J. Med. Chem.*, **11**, 729 (1968).

70. D. J. Triggle and B. Belleau, *Can. J. Chem.*, **40**, 1201 (1962).

71. A. Gero and V. J. Reese, *Science*, **123**, 100 (1956).

72. A. Cooper, D. A. Norton, and H. Hauptman, *Acta Cryst.*, **B25**, 814 (1969).

73. N. J. Doorenbos, "Physical Properties and Biological Activity," in A. Burger, Ed., *Medicinal Chemistry*, 2nd ed., Interscience, New York, 1960, pp. 46–71.

74. C. C. Pfeiffer, *Science*, **107**, 94 (1948).

75. P. H. Bell and R. O. Roblin, Jr., *J. Am. Chem. Soc.*, **64**, 2905 (1942).

76. A. M. O'Connell and E. N. Maslen, *Acta Cryst.*, **22**, 134 (1967).

77. M. Alléaume and J. Decap, *Acta Cryst.*, **B24**, 214 (1968).

78. T. F. Lai and R. E. Marsh, *Acta Cryst.*, **22**, 885 (1967).

79. S. N. Timasheff and M. J. Gorbunoff, *Ann. Rev. Biochem.*, **36**, 13 (1967).

80. M. F. Perutz, *European J. Biochem.*, **8**, 455 (1969).

81. S. D. Silver, "Acridine Dye Action at Cellular and Molecular Levels," in R. J. Schnitzer and F. Hawking, Eds., *Experimental Chemotherapy*, Vol. IV, Academic, New York, 1966, pp. 505–511.

82. J. C. Arcos and M. Arcos, *Progr. Drug Res.*, **4**, 407 (1962).

83. P. Hey, *Brit. J. Pharmacol.*, **7**, 117 (1952).

84. A. A. Sekul and W. C. Holland, *J. Pharmacol. Exptl. Therap.*, **133**, 313 (1961).

85. S. Wiedling and C. Tegnér, *Progr. Med. Chem.*, **3**, 332 (1963).

86. A. M. Galinsky, J. E. Gearien, A. J. Perkins, and S. V. Susina, *J. Med. Chem.*, **6**, 320 (1963).

87. B. Pullman and A. Pullman, *Quantum Biochemistry*, Interscience, New York, 1963.

88. R. Daudel, R. Lefebvre, and C. Moser, *Quantum Chemistry*, Interscience, New York, 1959.

89. A. Streitwieser, *Molecular Orbital Theory for Organic Chemists*, Wiley, New York, 1961.

90. J. D. Roberts, *Notes on Molecular Orbital Calculations*, Benjamin, New York, 1962.

91. C. A. Coulson, *Valence*, 2nd ed., Oxford University Press, London, 1961.

92. K. B. Wiberg, *Physical Organic Chemistry*, Wiley, New York, 1964.

93. K. Higasi, H. Baba, and A. Rembaum, *Quantum Organic Chemistry*, Interscience, New York, 1965.

94. J. N. Murrell, S. F. A. Kettle, and J. M. Tedder, *Valence Theory*, Wiley, London, 1965.

95. L. Salem, *The Molecular Orbital Theory of Conjugated Systems*, Benjamin, New York, 1966.

96. C. W. N. Cumper, *Wave Mechanics for Chemists*, Academic, New York, 1966.

97. R. Daudel, *The Fundamentals of Theoretical Chemistry*, Pergamon, Oxford, 1968.

98. R. L. Flurry, *Molecular Orbital Theories of Bonding in Organic Molecules*, Dekker, New York, 1968.

99. K. Fukui, A. Imamura, and C. Nagata, *Bull. Chem. Soc. Japan*, **33**, 122 (1960).

100. F. Yoneda and Y. Nitta, *Chem. Pharm. Bull.*, **12**, 1264 (1964).

101. K. Hirano, S. Yoshina, K. Okamura, and I. Suzuka, *Bull. Chem. Soc. Japan*, **40**, 2229 (1967).

102. S. H. Snyder and C. R. Merril, *Proc. Natl. Acad. Sci. U.S.*, **54**, 258 (1965).

103. K. Fukui, K. Morokuma, C. Nagata, and A. Imamura, *Bull. Chem. Soc. Japan*, **34**, 1224 (1961).

104. W. B. Neely, *Mol. Pharmacol.*, **1**, 137 (1965).

105. A. Cammarata and R. L. Stein, *J. Med. Chem.*, **11**, 829 (1968).

106. J. A. Singer and W. P. Purcell, *J. Med. Chem.*, **10**, 754 (1967).

107. F. E. Hahn, R. L. O'Brien, J. Ciak, J. L. Allison, and J. G. Olenick, *Mil. Med.*, Suppl. 9, **131**, 1071 (1966).

108. H. C. Longuet-Higgins, *J. Chem. Phys.*, **18**, 275 (1950).

109. V. A. Kuprievich, V. I. Danilov, and O. V. Shramko, *Theoret. Exptl. Chem.* (Eng. Transl.), **2**, 535 (1966).

110. V. A. Kuprievich, *Int. J. Quantum Chemistry*, **1**, 561 (1967).

111. V. A. Kuprievich, V. I. Danilov, and O. V. Shramko, *Mol. Biol.*, **1**, 343 (1967).

112. E. C. Foernzler and A. N. Martin, *J. Pharm. Sci.*, **56**, 608 (1967).

113. J. K. Seydel, *J. Pharm. Sci.* **57**, 1455 (1968).

114. W. Perkow, *Arzneimittel-Forsch.*, **16**, 1287 (1966).

115. E. J. Ariëns, *Progr. Drug Res.*, **10**, 429 (1966).

116. P. R. Andrews, *J. Med. Chem.*, **12**, 761 (1969).

6

DRUG RECEPTORS

Contemporary ideas of drug action and drug specificity are all based
on the assumption that the initial process in drug action is the formation of a reversible complex between the drug and a cell component
generally known as the drug receptor.

A. S. V. Burgen

I. NATURE OF RECEPTORS

Some drugs, as discussed in Chapter 2, exhibit biological activity in minute
concentrations. For this reason they are described as *structurally specific.*
The effect produced by them is attributed to interaction with a specific
receptor substance (*1,2*). As a result of this interaction the drug forms a
complex with a cellular component (*3,4*), which is named *receptor* (*5,6*). A
chemist refers to the receptor in terms of chemical structural components,
but the biologist prefers to treat it in microanatomic terms (*7*).

It is assumed that structurally specific drugs present a high degree of
molecular complementarity toward the site at which they act (*8,9*). The interaction of a drug of this type with its receptor would therefore be similar to the
interaction of a substrate with the active site of an enzyme (*10*), as shown in
Figure 6.1, or of a haptene with an antibody (*11*), as represented in Figure
6.2.

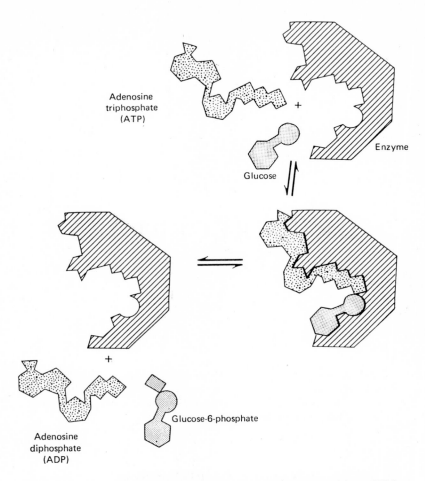

Fig. 6.1. Formation of enzyme–substrate complex. [Adapted from (*12*).]

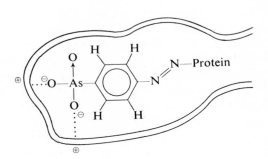

Fig. 6.2. Interaction of haptene with antibody (*13*).

Experimental evidence seems to indicate that receptors are localized in macromolecules most of which have proteinlike properties and exhibit the specific ability to interact at least with natural substrates at their active sites (*14,15*). Their nature is probably similar to that of the active site or allosteric site of enzymes, and they approximate in size the drug molecule that is able to form a complex with them (*16*).

Complexation of a drug with special chemical groups on the receptor results in a sequence of chemical or conformational changes that either cause or inhibit biological reactions. Nowadays it is acknowledged that such changes in biopolymers actually occur as an effect of the action of small molecules (*17–27*). A drug's ability to adapt itself to a receptor depends on the structural, configurational, and conformational characteristics of both drug and receptor (*28*).

A theoretical basis of drug–receptor complex formation was expounded recently by Burgen (*29*), who calculated that the association rate of drug with receptor, when limited only by diffusion, is equal to 2.5×10^9 l/mole-sec, with a net activation energy of 3 to 4 kcal/mole. Complex formation results from drug stabilization in the force field generated by electrostatic interactions, both dispersive and hydrophobic.

According to Smith and Williams (*30*), some drugs, rather than interacting directly with receptors, are able to alter biochemical processes in the proximity of these receptors and, as a consequence, promote modifications in physiological function, particularly in those cases in which, owing to their ionic nature, the drugs can act as catalysts.

Mackay (*31,32*) has proposed a new method for analyzing drug–receptor interactions; it consists in comparing dose–response curves. In the study of adrenergic receptors Bloom and Goldman (*33*) have suggested the hypothesis of a *dynamic receptor*. They regard such receptors not as simple enzymes but as *enzyme–substrate complexes*. Interaction of these with a catecholamine results in destruction of the substrate and, by extension, of the receptor. However, owing to the very nature of the destructive process, regeneration of the receptor is fast, while in the biophase there is unbound nucleotide substrate—hence the qualifying *dynamic* receptor. To their hypothesis they have given mathematical expressions and proposed planar and spatial representations both of α- and β-agonism (Chapter 8, Section VI).

Another conception of drug–receptor interaction has been suggested by Watkins (*34*). It is related to membrane permeability. Resembling closely the dynamic-receptor hypothesis, it is based on similarities between several pharmacodynamic agents and the polar chains of certain phospholipids. Association of an appropriate drug with the protein of a phospholipid–protein complex in the cell membrane causes dissociation of the original complex, as Figure 6.3 illustrates. Then protein, which in this process undergoes

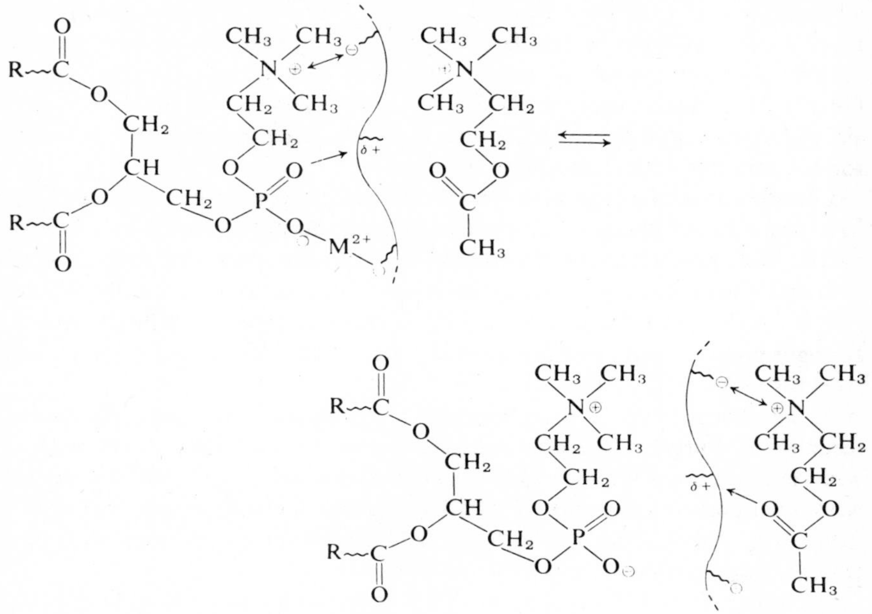

Fig. 6.3. Interaction between a phospholipid complex and an appropriate drug (*34*).

conformational change, combines with the drug and transports it into the cell, where it dissociates from the drug. Afterward, the protein is able to associate again with the phospholipid and form with it a complex, which is ready to function once more as an active receptor (*35*).

Presently it is assumed that certain proteins—apparently only those called allosteric (*36–39*), which usually are oligomers built up by subunits or protomers (*40*)—contain at least two noninterpenetrating and stereospecifically different receptor sites: the active site and the allosteric site. The first one binds to the substrate, triggering the biological activity. The second one is complementary to the structure of the protein–substrate complex, and it binds to this complex specifically and reversibly (*36*). This causes a slight reversible change—called *allosteric transition*—in the protein's structure, which modifies the properties of its active site and alters its function. It is likely that structural change is actually caused by a distortion in association of the protein's component subunits, as shown in Figure 6.4. Details on conformational changes are given in Chapter 9.

Therefore, when the action of a certain drug results from its association with an enzyme, the receptor to which it binds needs not necessarily be its active site; it may be the allosteric site (*16,21,36*), as represented in Figure 6.5.

With the assumption that a macromolecule that interacts with the drug

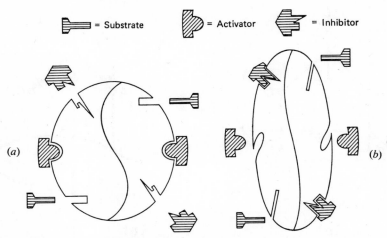

Fig. 6.4. Schematic representation of regulatory changes in an allosteric molecule. As shown at the left (*a*), when the polymeric protein binds to an activator, its conformation is such that its active site, which binds to the substrate, is able to be attached to it. In the picture to the right (*b*) it is seen that, when the same protein binds to an inhibitor, its conformation undergoes change so that the site that attaches to the substrate is sterically hindered. [Adapted from (*41*).]

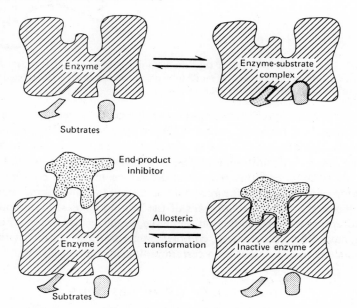

Fig. 6.5. Inhibition of enzyme through binding of a drug to its allosteric site. [Adapted from (*12*).]

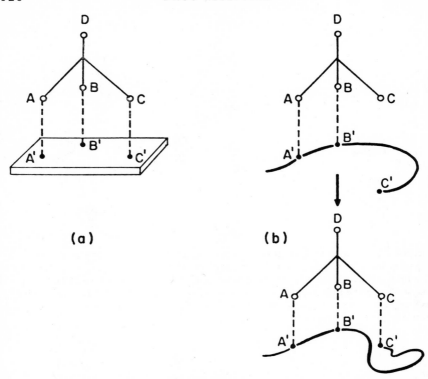

Fig. 6.6. Schematic illustration of (*a*) "three-point attachment" of a drug to a rigid receptor and (*b*) "two-point attachment" to a plastic receptor (*21*). (Reprinted by permission of the Williams and Wilkins Company.)

may undergo stereospecific conformational change, drug–receptor association may be through three points, or two (*42*), or even only one (Figure 6.6).

Actually, it was shown (*21*) that some drugs are as active as their prototypes, although their configuration is different or even inverse from that of the prototype (*43,44*). For this reason medicinal chemists are considering introduction of the concept of *isoreceptors*, in keeping with the term *isoenzymes* of the biochemists and *isoantibodies* of the immunologists. Isoreceptors are those receptors that, depending on the tissue, organ, or species to which they belong, have different structures, complementary to those of drugs with which they associate in order to cause a certain biological action (*36*).

II. CONCEPT OF RECEPTORS

First introduced by Langley (*45*), the concept of the receptor was developed by Ehrlich, who created the term *toxophoric* (carrier of toxic substance) and uttered the famous phrase: "Corpora non agunt nisi fixata" (Drugs do not act unless they bind) (46).

Clark (47) and Gaddum (48) gave a quantitative basis to the receptor concept. Clark claimed that intensity of drug action is proportional to the number of occupied receptors. In attempts to explain the mode of action of drugs, lately other theories have been proposed by Ariëns, Stephenson, Paton, Croxatto and Huidobro, Koshland, and Belleau. Their theories, which are modifications of Clark's to a greater or lesser degree, are discussed in Chapter 9.

III. STRUCTURE OF RECEPTORS

Until recently little was known about three-dimensional structures of macromolecules to which drugs would attach. From 1960 on, however, this

TABLE 6.1   Proteins Solved to Nearly Atomic Resolution (49)

Hydrolases	Number of Residues
Ribonuclease A and S (bovine pancreatic)	124
Lysozyme (hen's egg white)	129
Papain (SH-protease from papaya latex)	212
α-Chymotrypsin (bovine; serine protease)	241
Carboxypeptidase A (bovine; metal protease)	307
Elastase (porcine)	230[a]
Subtilisin BPN'	275
Rubredoxin (*Clostridium pasteurianum*)	

Oxygen Carriers	
Myoglobin (sperm whale)	153
Oxyhemoglobin (horse)	2 × 287

Other proteins	
Glucagon	
Cytochrome C (horse heart)	
Erythrocruorin (larva of *Chironomus thummi*)	
Carbonic anhydrase (human erythrocyte)	

[a] Approximate.

subject has been widely studied (*8*). Modern techniques have made possible the determination of three-dimensional structures of some proteins and a few very complex enzymes, such as ribonuclease, carboxypeptidase, carbonic anhydrase, α-chymotrypsin, egg white lysozyme, and papain (Table 6.1). The basic feature of these proteins is the exclusion of polar residues from the interior, except for special purposes connected with function (*49*). According to Bernhard (*50*), these enzymes present certain common characteristics:

1. A single, highly folded polypeptide chain of nearly spherical shape.

2. A cavity that is at least partially bounded by regions of polypeptide involved in substrate binding and catalysis.

3. Only a small fraction of the folded polypeptide chain has the α-helical configuration, which is unlike the case in myoglobin and hemoglobin.

Studies of certain enzymes have afforded evidence that polar groups of amino acids—such as lysine, arginine, histidine, serine, threonine, tyrosine, tryptophan, glutamic acid, aspartic acid—are almost all situated in the external part of the protein molecules (*12,21,23,49–51*). Some of these amino acids, represented in Figure 6.7 as ions, are able to form complexes with drugs by attaching to them through electrostatic forces and establishing

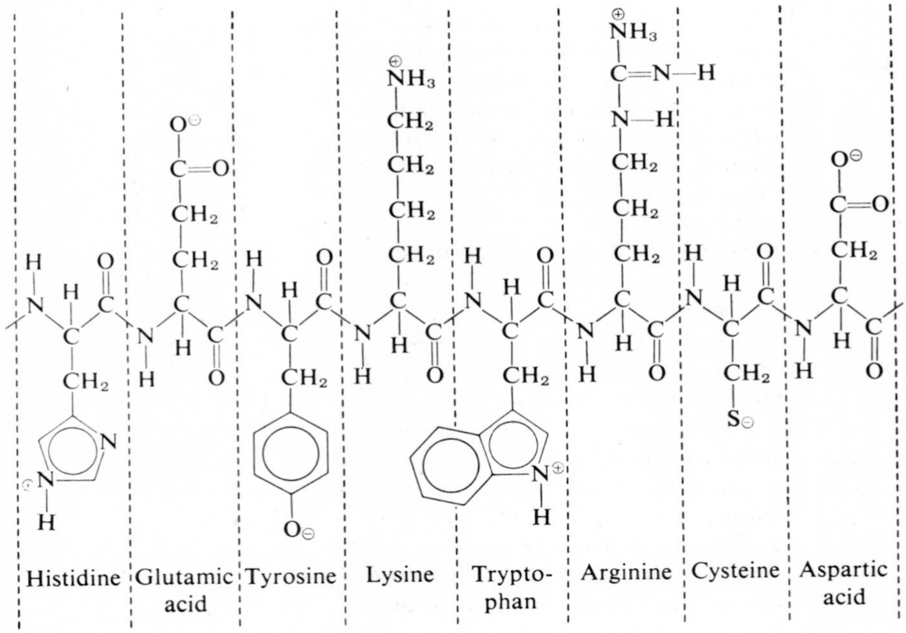

Fig. 6.7. Protein amino acids that have ionic charges.

covalent and hydrogen bonds, in addition to hydrophobic and van der Waals interactions.

Through the use of labeling substances that are stereospecific for the active sites of the enzymes and containing a chemically reactive group able to form a covalently stable derivative with one or more amino acid residues, the catalytic sites of several enzymes were determined (Table 6.2). Many other examples are listed elsewhere (50–53). Drugs that act on enzymic systems attach themselves to active sites equal or analogous to these and produce their specific effects.

In 1967, by X-ray diffraction methods, Fridborg and co-workers (54) determined the three-dimensional structure of the complex formed between human carbonic anhydrase C (Figure 6.8) and acetoxymercurisulfonamide, which is a modified inhibitor of this enzyme (Figure 6.9). They observed that the inhibitor inserts itself into a narrow slit in the enzyme's cavity and,

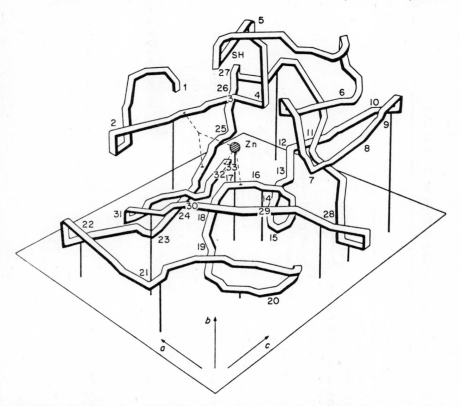

Fig. 6.8. Drawing of a model of human carbonic anhydrase C showing the proposed tertiary structure (54).

TABLE 6.2 Specific Chemical Labeling of Catalytic Residues (50)

Enzyme	Labeling Agent	Chemical Reaction Involved	Amino Acid Residue Labeled
Mammalian pancreatic proteases (chymotrypsin, trypsin, thrombin, elastase) Esterases (cholinesterase, liver esterases) Bacterial proteases (subtilisin)	$[(CH_3)_2CHO]_2{-}\overset{O}{\overset{\|}{P}}{-}F$ (bracket = R)	$R_2{-}\overset{O}{\overset{\|}{P}}{-}F + EOH \longrightarrow R_2{-}\overset{O}{\overset{\|}{P}}{-}OE + HF$	Serine ($-CH_2OH$)
Chymotrypsin, subtilisin	p-NO_2 phenyl acetate Acetyl imidazole 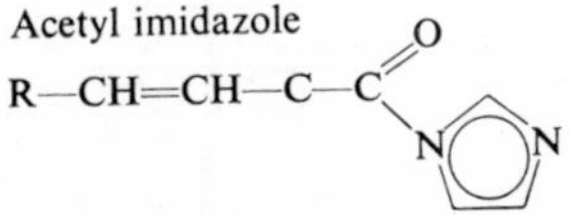 $R{-}CH{=}CH{-}\overset{O}{\overset{\|}{C}}{-}N\langle\text{imidazole}\rangle$	$R{-}\overset{O}{\overset{\|}{C}}{-}X + EOH \xrightarrow{\text{denature}} R{-}\overset{O}{\overset{\|}{C}}{-}OE + HX$	Serine
Phosphoglucomutase	Glucose-6-PO_4	$ROPOH + EOH \xrightarrow{\text{denature}} EOPOH + ROH$	Serine
Alkaline phosphatase	$H_2PO_4^{\ominus}$	$HOPOH + EOH \xrightarrow{\text{denature}} EOPOH + H_2O$	Serine
Phosphorylase, glutamate-aspartate transaminase	Pyridoxal phosphate	$E{-}NH_2 + RCHO \rightleftharpoons E{-}\overset{H}{\underset{\|}{N}}{=}CR \xrightarrow{NaBH_4} E{-}\overset{H}{\underset{\|}{\overset{\|}{N}}}{}^{\oplus}{-}CH_2R$	Lysine ($-(CH_2)_4{-}NH_2$)

Enzyme	Reaction	Residue
Acetoacetate decarboxylase	$$CH_3\overset{O}{\overset{\|}{C}}CH_2CO_2^{\ominus} + ENH_3^{\oplus} \rightleftharpoons$$ $$\underset{HNE^{\oplus}}{CH_3CH_2\!-\!CO_2^{\ominus}} \longrightarrow \underset{HNE^{\oplus}}{CH_3CCH_3} + CO_2$$ $$\Big\downarrow \text{NaBH}_4$$ $$\underset{H_2NE^{\oplus}}{CH_3CHCH_3}$$	Lysine
Aldolase	$$CH_3\overset{H}{\overset{\|}{C}}{=}O + ENH_3^{\oplus} \rightleftharpoons CH_3\overset{H}{\underset{\oplus}{C}}{=}\overset{H}{NE}$$ $$\Big\downarrow \text{NaBH}_4$$ $$CH_3CH_2NH_2E$$	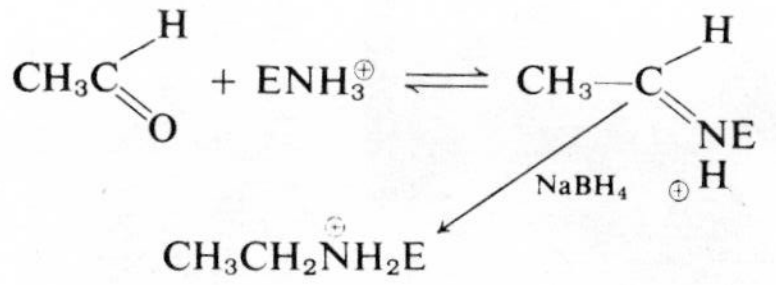 Lysine
Glyceraldehyde-3-phosphate dehydrogenase, lactic dehydrogenase, alcohol dehydrogenase	$$ICH_2CO_2^{\ominus} + ESH \longrightarrow ES\!-\!CH_2CO_2^{\ominus}$$ $$ICH_2CO_2^{\ominus}$$	Cysteine (—CH$_2$SH)
Glyceraldehyde-3-phosphate dehydrogenase, papain	$$ESH + CH_3\overset{O}{\overset{\|}{C}}\!-\!O\!-\!\underset{}{\text{NO}_2} \longrightarrow$$ $$ES\overset{O}{\overset{\|}{C}}\!-\!CH_3 + \text{nitrophenol} \xrightarrow{\text{denature}}$$	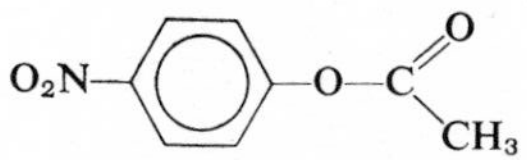 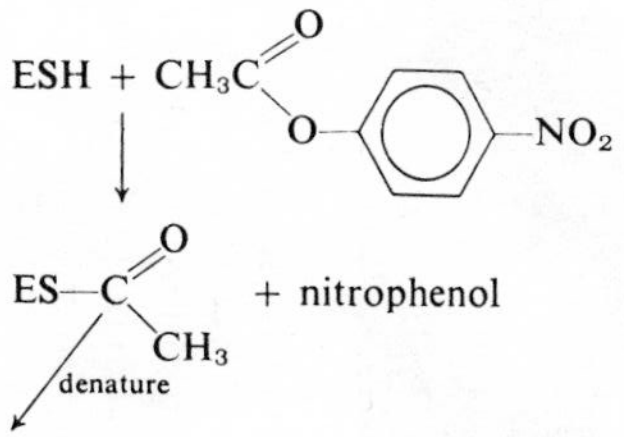 Cysteine
Chymotrypsin, trypsin	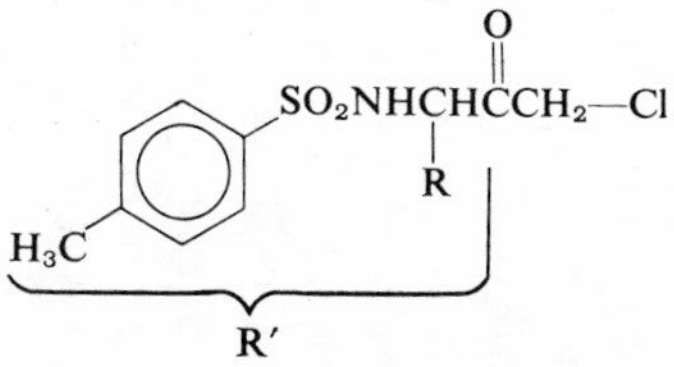 $$R'\overset{O}{\overset{\|}{C}}\!-\!CH_2\!-\!Cl + \underset{E}{\overset{H}{\underset{\|}{N}}}\overset{N}{\diagdown} \longrightarrow$$ $$\overset{O}{\overset{\|}{C}}\!-\!CH_2CR' + HCl$$	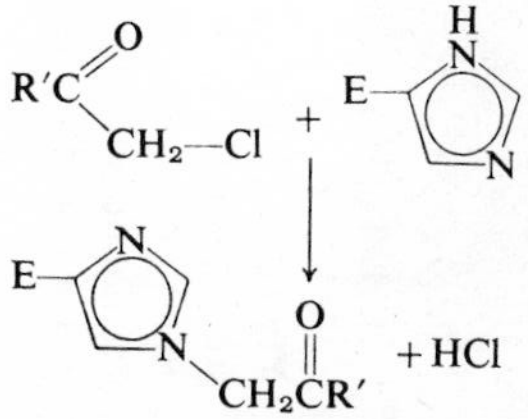 Histidine

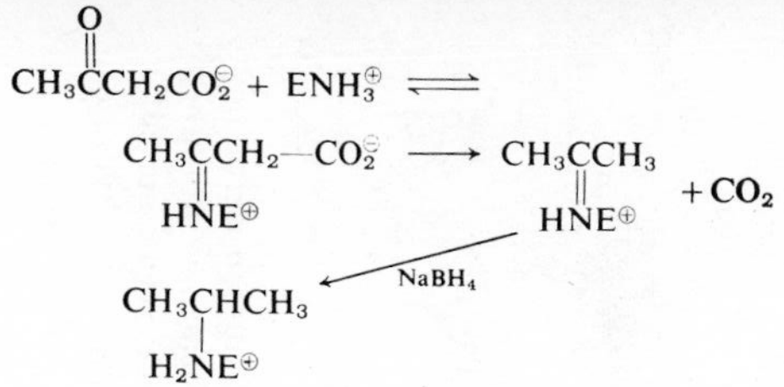

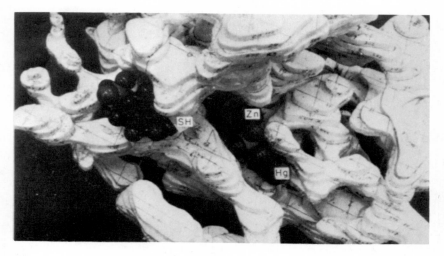

Fig. 6.9. Acetoxymercurisulfanilamide bound to the active site of human carbonic anhydrase C (*54*). The benzene ring is with great probability almost vertical. The inhibitor is bound to the zinc atom through the sulfonamide group. Another acetoxymercurisulfanilamide molecule is bound to the only sulfhydryl group of human carbonic anhydrase C through the mercury atom.

through the sulfonamide group, is bound to the zinc present in carbonic anhydrase. Another molecule of the same inhibitor binds to the only sulfhydryl group of the enzyme through the mercury atom. This work gives factual evidence of drug–receptor complexation. On the other hand, on the basis of chemical and crystallographic data, Chipman and Sharon (*55*) presented recently a picture of the mechanism of lysozyme action, making clear, for the first time, the relation between an enzyme structure and its function.

Several direct and indirect attempts to isolate receptors, in order to study their interactions with drugs *in vitro*, have been made in recent times (*6*). Unfortunately these attempts have not succeeded. The difficulties in separating the receptor from tissue proteins are great, because during the process of extraction the forces that unite both entities—drug and receptor—are broken. Concomitantly, owing to changes in the structural shape of the macromolecule of which the receptor is an integral part, the functionality of this macromolecule can be destroyed (*6,56*). Furthermore in the isolation process the receptor undergoes changes in its natural spatial arrangement and charge distribution, and both of these factors are essential to its interaction with the drug (*35*).

In short, in spite of the little that is known about the subject, it is generally accepted that a receptor is an elastic three-dimensional entity, consisting perhaps in most cases of protein-constituent amino acids, whose stereo-chemical structure is often complementary to that of the drug and which, sometimes after undergoing conformational change, is able to interact with it, usually in its preferred conformation, in order to form a complex held together by various binding forces. As result of this drug–receptor complexation a stimulus is generated and, in turn, causes a biological action or effect.

REFERENCES

1. C. Heymans, *Actualités Pharmacol.*, **5**, 111 (1952).
2. R. F. Furchgott, *Ann. Rev. Pharmacol.*, **4**, 21 (1964).
3. J. M. van Rossum, "Drug–Receptor Theories," in J. M. Robson and R. S. Stacey, Eds., *Recent Advances in Pharmacology*, 4th ed., Little, Brown, Boston, 1968, pp. 99–133.
4. H. O. Schild, "A Pharmacological Approach to Drug Receptors," in D. H. Tedeschi and R. E. Tedeschi, Eds., *Importance of Fundamental Principles in Drug Evaluation*, Raven, New York, 1968, pp. 257–276.
5. P. N. Campbell, Ed., *The Interaction of Drugs and Subcellular Components in Animal Cells*, Little, Brown, Boston, 1968.
6. S. Ehrenpreis, J. H. Fleisch, and T. W. Mittag, *Pharmacol. Rev.*, **21**, 131 (1969).
7. C. J. Cavallito, *Ann. Rev. Pharmacol.*, **8**, 39 (1968).
8. C. C. Porter and C. A. Stone, *Ann. Rev. Pharmacol.*, **7**, 15 (1967).
9. G. Kuschinsky and H. Lüllmann, *Kurzes Lehrbuch der Pharmakologie*, Thieme, Stuttgart, 1967.
10. R. E. Dickerson and I. Geis, *The Structure and Action of Proteins*, Harper and Row, New York, 1969.
11. B. M. Bloom and G. D.Laubach, *Ann. Rev. Pharmacol.*, **2**, 67 (1962).
12. J. D. Watson, *Molecular Biology of the Gene*, Benjamin, New York, 1965.
13. D. Pressman and A. L. Grossberg, *The Structural Basis of Antibody Specificity*, Benjamin, New York, 1968.
14. A. Burger and A. P. Parulkar, *Ann. Rev. Pharmacol.*, **6**, 19 (1966).
15. P. G. Waser, *Arzneimittel-Forsch.*, **19**, 260 (1969).
16. J. M. van Rossum, *Advan. Drug Res.*, **3**, 189 (1966).
17. D. Nachmansohn, "Chemical control of the permeability cycle in excitable membranes during activity", in B. Shapiro and M. Prywes, Eds., *Impact of Basic Sciences on Medicine*, Academic, New York, 1966, pp. 123–141.
18. T. M. Birshtein and O. B. Ptitsyn, *Conformations of Macromolecules*, Interscience, New York, 1966.
19. J.-P. Changeux, *Mol. Pharmacol.*, **2**, 369 (1966).
20. W. J. O'Sullivan and M. Cohn, *J. Biol. Chem.*, **241**, 3116 (1966).
21. H. G. Mautner, *Pharmacol. Rev.*, **19**, 107 (1967).
22. G. N. Ramachandran, Ed., *Conformation of Biopolymers*, Vols. I and II, Academic, London, 1967.
23. G. N. Ramachandran and V. Sasisekharan, *Advan. Protein Chem.*, **23**, 283 (1968).

24. C. Tanford, *Accounts Chem. Res.*, **1**, 161 (1968).
25. W. B. Gratzer and D. A. Cowburn, *Nature*, **222**, 426 (1969).
26. F. W. Studier, *J. Mol. Biol.*, **41**, 189, 199 (1969).
27. O. B. Ptitsyn and T. M. Birshtein, *Biopolymers*, **7**, 435 (1969).
28. D. R. Waud, *Pharmacol. Rev.*, **20**, 49 (1968).
29. A. S. V. Burgen, *J. Pharm. Pharmacol.*, **18**, 137 (1966).
30. H. J. Smith and H. Williams, *J. Pharm. Pharmacol.*, **17**, 529, 601 (1965).
31. D. Mackay, *Advan. Drug Res.*, **3**, 1 (1966).
32. D. Mackay, *J. Pharm. Pharmacol.*, **18**, 201 (1966).
33. B. M. Bloom and I. M. Goldman, *Advan. Drug Res.*, **3**, 121 (1966).
34. J. C. Watkins, *J. Theoret. Biol.*, **9**, 37 (1965).
35. R. E. Rice, *J. Chem. Educ.*, **44**, 565 (1967).
36. J. Monod, J.-P. Changeux, and F. Jacob, *J. Mol. Biol.*, **6**, 306 (1963).
37. J. Monod, J. Wyman, and J.-P. Changeux, *J. Mol. Biol.*, **12**, 88 (1965).
38. J. Wyman, *J. Am. Chem. Soc.*, **89**, 2202 (1967).
39. Federation of European Biochemical Societies, *Regulation of Enzyme Activity and Allosteric Interactions*, edited by E. Kvamme and A. Pihl, Universitetsforlaget, Oslo, and Academic, London, 1968.
40. D. E. Green and R. F. Goldberger, *Molecular Insights into the Living Process*, Academic, New York, 1967.
41. J.-P. Changeux, *Scientific American*, **212** (4), 36 (1965).
42. A. Gero, "Mathematical Treatment of Two-Point Attachment Between Drug and Receptor," in E. J. Ariëns, Ed., *Physico-Chemical Aspects of Drug Action*, Pergamon, Oxford, 1968, pp. 261–269.
43. P. G. Waser, *Experientia*, **17**, 300 (1961).
44. P. S. Portoghese, *J. Med. Chem.*, **8**, 147, 609 (1965).
45. J. N. Langley, *J. Physiol.*, **33**, 374 (1905).
46. P. Ehrlich, *Ber.*, **42**, 17 (1909).
47. A. J. Clark, *The Mode of Action of Drugs on Cells*, Williams and Wilkins, Baltimore, 1933.
48. J. H. Gaddum, *J. Physiol.*, **89**, 7P (1937).
49. M. F. Perutz, *European J. Biochem.*, **8**, 455 (1969).
50. S. A. Bernhard, *The Structure and Function of Enzymes*, Benjamin, New York, 1968.
51. B. R. Baker, *Design of Active-Site-Directed Irreversible Enzyme Inhibitors*, Wiley, New York, 1967.
52. S. J. Singer, *Advan. Protein Chem.*, **22**, 1 (1967).
53. J. F. Moran, M. May, H. Kimelberg, and D. J. Triggle, *Mol. Pharmacol.*, **3**, 15 (1967).
54. K. Fridborg, K. K. Kannan, A. Liljas, J. Lundin, B. Strandberg, R. Strandberg, B. Tilander, and G. Wirén, *J. Mol. Biol.*, **25**, 505 (1967).
55. D. M. Chipman and N. Sharon, *Science*, **165**, 454 (1969).
56. E. J. Ariëns, *Advan. Drug Res.*, **3**, 235 (1966).

DRUG–RECEPTOR
INTERACTIONS

Ionic forces, hydrogen bonding and van der Waals' forces are probably involved in the "combination" of drugs and receptor. It is not implied that combination alone produces the response, but that a suitable combination may initiate, modify or block a series of interdependent chemical processes.

Arnold H. Beckett

I. TYPES OF BONDING

In order to understand the mode and mechanism of drug action, it is of the utmost importance to know the forces of interaction that bind drugs to their receptors (*1–4*). However, the determination of these forces by experimental methods is very difficult. Nonetheless, on the basis of facts already known on this subject, it is assumed that structurally specific drugs attach themselves to their receptors through the same forces that are involved in interactions between simple molecules (*5–8*). The majority of these forces are identical to the ones that stabilize the structure of a protein (*9–11*), as shown in Figure 7.1.

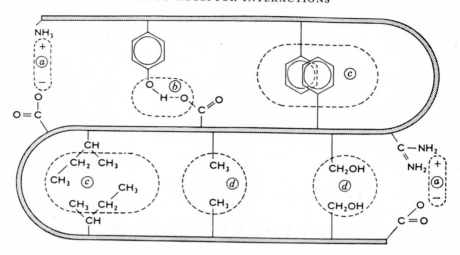

Fig. 7.1. Some types of noncovalent bonds that stabilize protein structure: (a) electrostatic interaction; (b) hydrogen bonding between tyrosine residues and carboxylate groups on side chains; (c) hydrophobic interactions; (d) van der Waals interactions (9).

Table 7.1 not only lists the forces responsible for the formation of the drug–receptor complex but also presents some typical examples of their effects. Weak interactions between the drug and the receptor are usually possible only when the molecular surfaces have complementary structures, in such a way that the salient group (or positive charge) on one surface corresponds to a cavity (or negative charge) on the other surface. In other words, between molecules that interact there must be, in many cases, a relationship analogous to the one that exists between a key and a lock (12), although the phenomenon is much more complex.

Bond strength depends on the distance that separates two particular atoms; at the optimal distance the strongest bond is formed. The spontaneous formation of a bond between atoms occurs with a decrease of free energy; that is, ΔG shows a negative value. The quantity of free energy thus released, which is converted into another form of energy, will increase with increasing bond strength. During the formation of covalent bonds there is a decrease in free energy of 40 to 110 kcal/mole, whereas in van der Waals interactions the release of free energy is only on the order of 0.5 to 1 kcal/mole. The higher the variation of free energy, the higher the proportion of atoms in bonded form. This can be deduced from the following equation:

$$\Delta G^{\circ} = -RT \ln K_{eq} \quad \text{or} \quad K_{eq} = e^{-\Delta G^{\circ}/RT} \tag{I}$$

where ΔG° represents the standard free energy; K_{eq}, an equilibrium constant; R, the universal gas constant; T, the absolute temperature; and $\ln K$, the

TABLE 7.1 Some Types of Drug–Receptor Interactions (*13*)

Bond Type	Interaction Energy (kcal/mole)	Examples
Covalent bond	$-(40-110)$	CH_3—OH
Reinforced ionic bond	-10	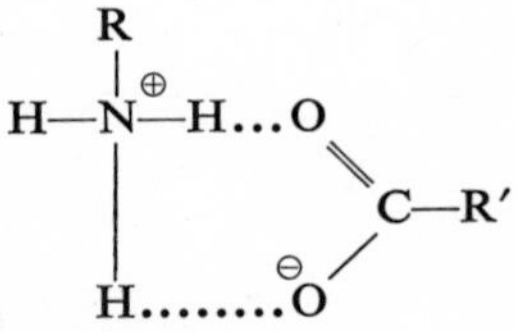 (see structure)
Ionic bond	-5	$R_4N^{\oplus}...^{\ominus}I$
Ion–dipole bond	$-(1-7)$	$R_4N^{\oplus}...:NR_3$
Dipole–dipole bond	$-(1-7)$	$O{=}C^{\delta+}...:NR_3$
Hydrogen bond	$-(1-7)$	—OH...O=
Charge transfer	$-(1-7)$	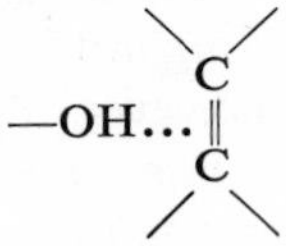 (see structure)
Hydrophobic interaction	-1	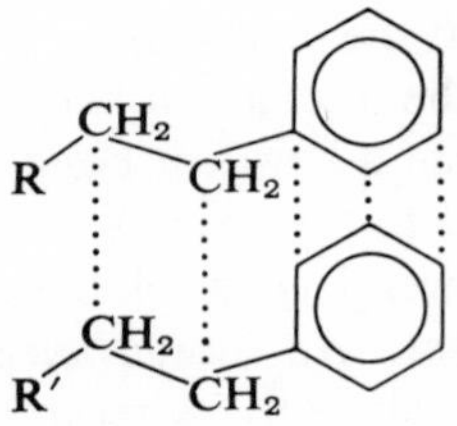 (see structure)
Van der Waals interaction	$-(0.5-1)$	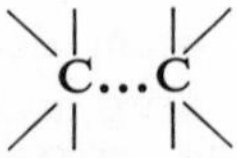 $C...C$

natural logarithm of K to the base e (equal to 2.718). This equation permits us to calculate that, at physiological temperatures, energies on the order of 2 to 3 kcal/mole are sufficient to force the majority of molecules to establish the maximum number of good secondary bonds (*12*). Table 7.2 shows some values for the equilibrium constant K_{eq} and the corresponding change in free energy.

In general bonds formed between a drug and a receptor are relatively weak: ionic, polar, hydrogen, hydrophobic, van der Waals. Consequently the effects produced are reversible; that is, the drug–receptor bond is cleaved,

TABLE 7.2 Numerical Relationship between the Equilibrium Constant and Change in Standard Free Energy at 25°C (*14*)

K_{eq}	$\Delta G°$ (kcal/mole)
0.001	4.089
0.01	2.726
0.1	1.363
1.0	0
10.0	−1.363
100.0	−2.726
1000.0	−4.089

and the drug ceases to act as soon as its concentration in the extracellular fluids decreases. In most cases, especially when pharmacodynamic agents are involved, this is exactly what is looked for: it is desired that the effect caused by the drug last for only a limited time.

Sometimes, however, the effect produced by a drug should persist and even be irreversible. For instance, it is absolutely desirable that a chemotherapeutic agent form an irreversible complex with the receptor sites in a parasite, so that the drug can exert its toxic action for a prolonged period (*13*). In this case the interaction between the drug and the receptor should be established through a covalent bond, which is the strongest.

Due to the reasons given above it is appropriate to consider in more detail the several types of bonds that can be established between a drug and its receptor. We should keep in mind that in the internal medium, as a drug comes close to its receptor, until complexation occurs, the amount of free energy of the system decreases, because the water molecules that were surrounding the drug and the receptor take a less ordered orientation, as discussed in Section VIII of this chapter. This disordering means an increase in entropy and results in a force that helps the drug–receptor complex to stay together. A similar phenomenon occurs also in the antigen–antibody complex (*15*).

II. COVALENT BOND

The strongest bond that can be established between a drug and its receptor, the covalent bond, is seldom formed and is not easily cleaved. Its energy is on the order of 40 to 110 kcal/mole (*16*). From this it can be derived, based on

Equation I, that the equilibrium constant of the binding reaction will also be high.

The covalent bond is formed by the sharing of electrons between the atoms involved, such as carbon, hydrogen, nitrogen, and oxygen. Although in an external medium most of the covalent bonds can be cleaved only by the use of heat and strong chemical agents, some of them cleave through the action of milder reagents at the temperature of living tissue (*13*). In the internal medium, however, many of them are formed and cleaved through enzymic processes.

In the case of insecticides, chemotherapeutic agents, and some other types of drugs it is desirable that the combination between the receptor and the drug, in the parasite or human being, be formed through a covalent bond, so that the toxic or healing action will be prolonged. This is what occurs in a reaction between organophosphorus insecticides and the esteratic site of cholinesterase (*17*). This site involves in part serine, and not the imidazole ring of histidine, as was thought earlier. The function of the imidazole ring, located in another fold of the enzyme protein, perhaps consists in contributing to the hydrolysis of the acetylated serine moiety. Accordingly this interaction was often represented as shown in Figure 7.2, where G stands for glyoxaline, a synonym of imidazole. The evidence that organophosphorus compounds combine with serine was brought about through the use of labeled phosphorus. After the reaction of ribonuclease with an organophosphorus ester of the following type,

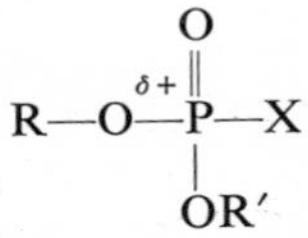

$$R-O-\overset{\overset{\displaystyle O}{\|}}{\underset{\underset{\displaystyle OR'}{|}}{P}}-X$$

an equivalent of radioactive phosphorus was found firmly bound to it.

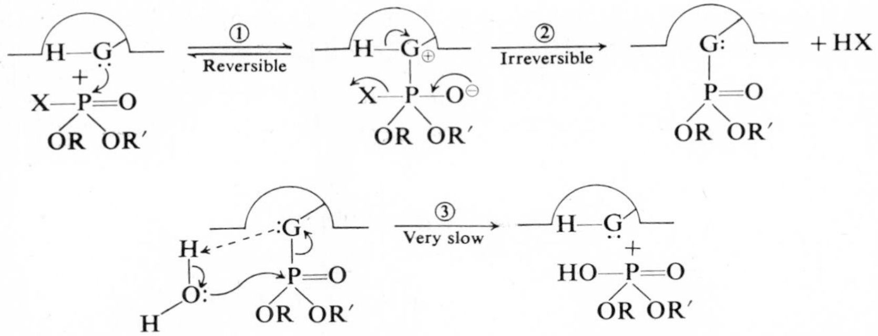

Fig. 7.2. Reaction of an organophosphorus compound with the esteratic site of cholinesterase (*18*).

Denaturation and dissociation of this complex produced a stable peptide including ^{32}P-phosphoserine:

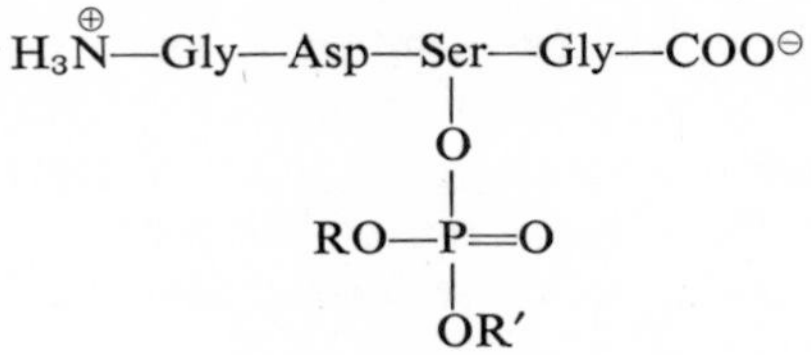

$$H_3\overset{\oplus}{N}\text{—Gly—Asp—Ser—Gly—COO}^{\ominus}$$

$$\begin{array}{c} | \\ O \\ | \\ RO\text{—}P\text{=}O \\ | \\ OR' \end{array}$$

This is the first example in which it was possible to identify chemically the participation of an amino acid side chain in a covalent interaction (*19,20*). It is assumed that the same occurs in chymotrypsin and acetylcholinesterase (*13,21*).

An analogous mechanism explains the cholinergic activity of carbamic esters, such as neostigmine, pyridostigmine, and physostigmine. Their action is due to the irreversible inhibition of acetylcholinesterase, through a covalent bond with this enzyme, by forming the corresponding carbamyl acetylcholinesterase (*22*). The complexation of pyridostigmine with acetylcholinesterase may be represented as shown in Figure 7.3.

The chemotherapeutic and toxic action of the arsenicals, mercurials, and antimonials results from the combination of these compounds, also by covalent bonds, with the sulfhydryl groups of the essential enzymes:

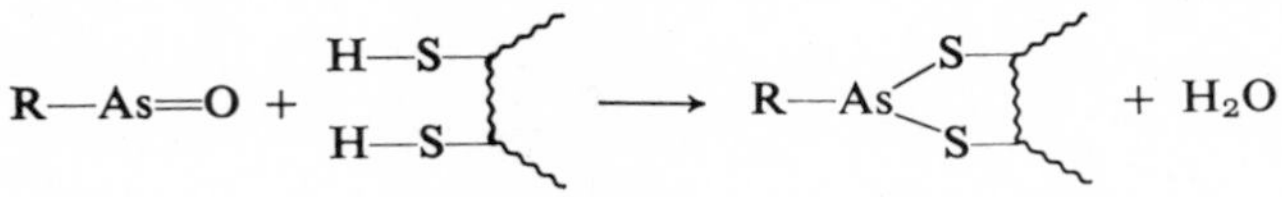

An identical mechanism is postulated to explain the action of an organomercurial diuretic. It is assumed that the active species is the mercuric ion, which is combined with two receptor sites, one being a sulfhydryl and the other another sulfhydryl or a phenolic hydroxy group, amino group, carboxy group, or imidazole ring (*23*).

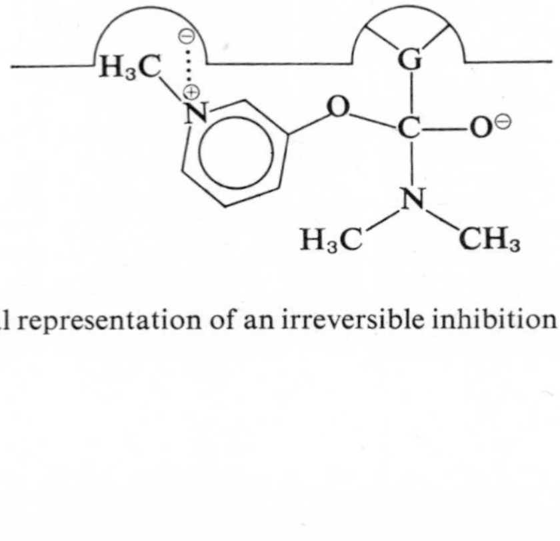

Fig. 7.3. Hypothetical representation of an irreversible inhibition of acetylcholinesterase by pyridostigmine.

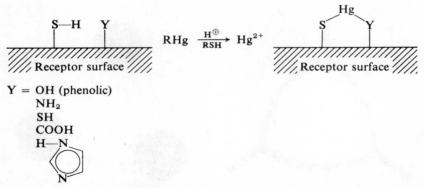

Y = OH (phenolic)
   NH₂
   SH
   COOH
   H—N

The antiseptic action of chlorine compounds is ascribed to covalent-bond formation. By reacting with water, they are converted into hypochlorous acid. Once formed, this acid reacts with the amino group of the bacterial protein and attaches itself by a covalent bond:

$$Cl_2 + H_2O$$

$$OCl^\ominus + H_2O \longrightarrow HOCl \xrightarrow{\substack{O\ H\\\|\ |\\R-C-N-R''}} R-C-N-R'' + H_2O$$

$$R-N-Cl + H_2O$$
$$\quad\ |$$
$$\quad R'$$

Many fungicides owe their action to covalent-bond formation (24); this is true specially of compounds that contain highly strained rings, such as epoxides. Examples are ethylene oxide, which is used as a fumigant, and butadiene epoxide, which has been employed as an antitumor agent:

$$A{:}^\ominus + H_2C\text{---}CHR \longrightarrow A{:}CH_2\text{---}CH\text{---}O^\ominus$$
$$\qquad\qquad \diagdown O \diagup \qquad\qquad\qquad |$$
$$\qquad\qquad\qquad\qquad\qquad\qquad\qquad R$$

The specific acylation or alkylation of the receptor groups by covalence might be generalized to explain the biological action of drugs that have either a three- or four-membered highly strained ring, which is therefore easily cleaved (three- and four-membered rings are strained, as can be seen in molecular models in the next page).

This is true of certain lactones (depsidones) and lactams (penicillins). The chemotherapeutic action of penicillin is ascribed to its ability to form a covalent bond with transpeptidase, one of the enzymes involved in the bacterial cell wall biosynthesis (25,26). Once the drug is fixed to the substrate binding site of the transpeptidase, the enzyme can open the highly reactive amide bond in penicillin's β-lactam ring to form a penicilloyl-enzyme, thus inactivating

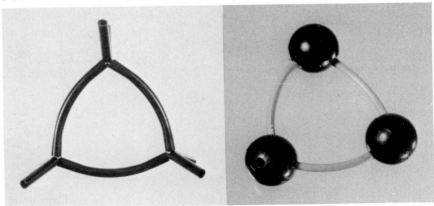

the transpeptidase (25). A similar reaction of penicillin can also take place with small molecules:

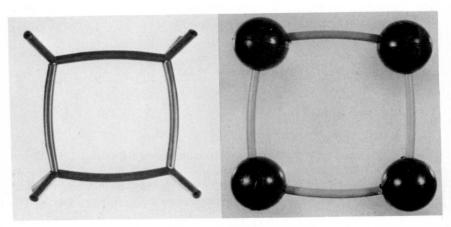

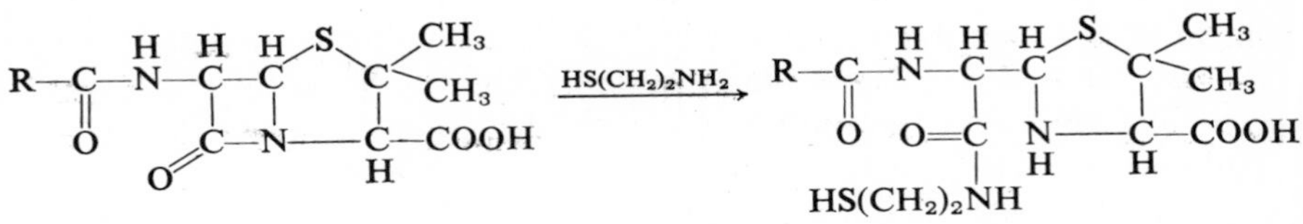

The anticancerous alkylating agents constitute another example of drugs that, it is thought, owe their biological activity to the establishment of covalent bonds with some proteins or certain nucleic acids and consequently obstructing their normal participation in cellular division (27). This covalent bond establishes itself as shown in the following diagram:

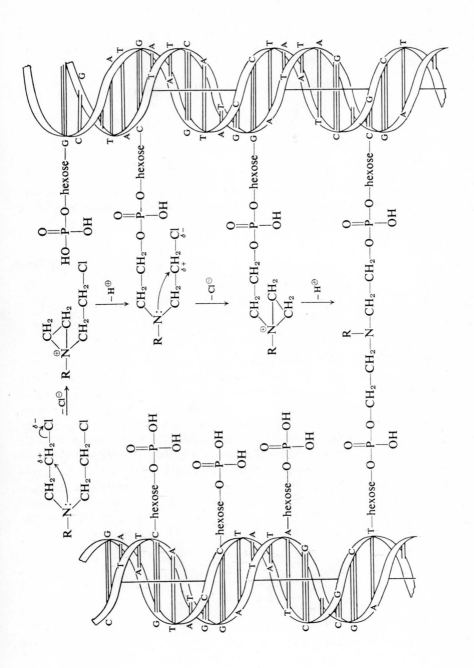

A covalent bond can also be formed between alkylating agents and nucleic acid bases. For instance, mechlorethamine binds covalently to one or two molecules of guanine (27):

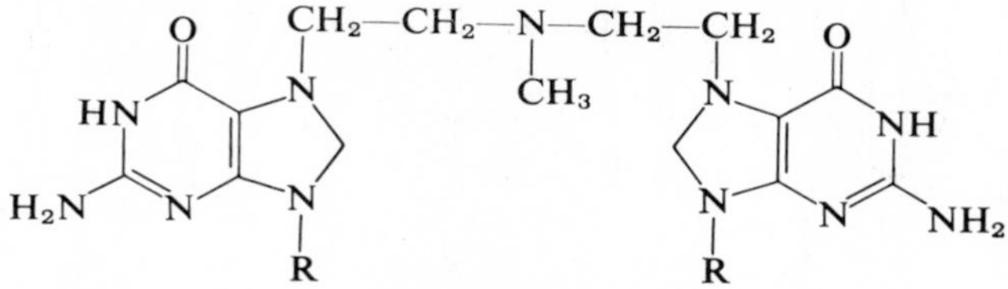

The chemotherapeutic action of mitomycin is ascribed to a similar mechanism: it prevents replication of the DNA duplex by alkylating and cross-linking its complementary strands (28):

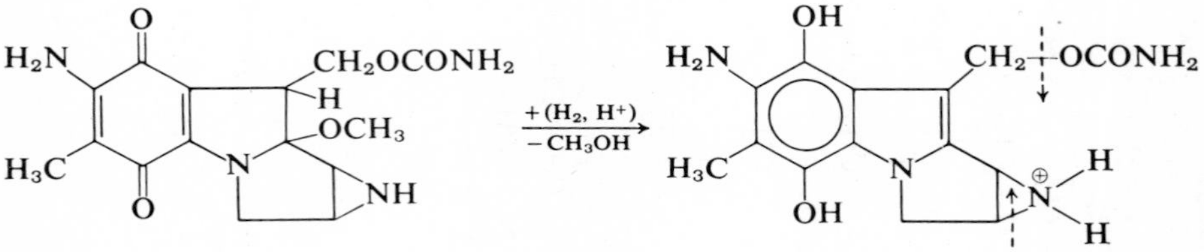

An analogous case occurs by an identical mechanism with some β-halo-alkylamines. Through an intramolecular cyclization, these can form, with extreme rapidity (29), an immonium ion that will act as an alkylating agent (30). A three-membered ring, due to its strain, cleaves easily and combines covalently with the receptors of the receptor substance; however, in the presence of water this ion undergoes solvolysis; likewise it can react with many other nucleophiles that are present in the blood or the tissues instead of reacting with only one receptor (30). According to Belleau (31), the pharmacodynamic action of ethylenimmonium ions derives from the fact that they alkylate phosphate anions (encountered in nucleotides) or carboxylate anions that exist in proteins by forming labile esters. These, depending on the adjacent basic groups, would be hydrolyzed, either rapidly or slowly.

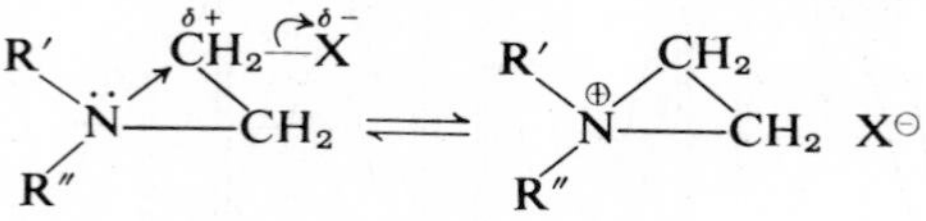

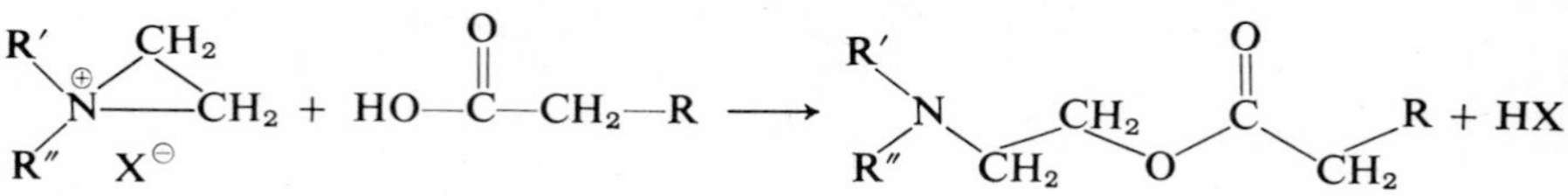

The formation of covalent bonds between the drug and the receptor constitutes the basis of Baker's work on the active-site-directed irreversible enzyme inhibitors. His first results in this field were compiled into a book (*32*), and the subsequent results are being published regularly, especially in the *Journal of Medicinal Chemistry* and the *Journal of Pharmaceutical Sciences*. The following facts served as the basis:

1. Enzymes are polypeptide macromolecules that can form complexes with substrates and inhibitors.

2. These enzymes have functional groups on their surfaces—such as the sulfide of methionine, the hydroxyl of tyrosine—besides some rings, as the imidazole of histidine, that can be attacked by chemical reagents, with the formation of a covalent bond.

3. Reactions in which neighboring groups participate can be accelerated as much as 10,000 times over the same chemical reaction proceeding by a bimolecular process (*32*).

From this Baker derived the following concept: "The macromolecular enzyme has functional groups on its surface which logically could be attacked selectively in the tremendously accelerated neighboring group reactions capable of taking place within the reversible complex formed between the enzyme and an inhibitor substituted with a properly placed neighboring group" (*33*).

According to Baker (*32*), an irreversible inhibition of enzymes can occur by two mechanisms: endomechanism and exomechanism. The first one has little specificity. The second one, however, is quite specific and is represented in Figure 7.4.

By using compounds that contain especially alkylating and acylating groups capable of forming a covalent linkage with appropriate groups—not

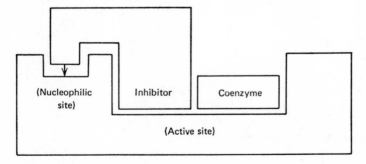

Fig. 7.4. A schematic diagram of an active-site-directed irreversible inhibitor operating by formation of a covalent linkage with an enzymic nucleophilic group situated outside the "active site"; the arrow represents the covalent-bond-forming group on the inhibitor (*34*).

necessarily at the active site—of certain enzymes, Baker and co-workers demonstrated that his concept was valid. Baker and other authors have succeeded in preparing irreversible inhibitors of several enzymes, although these experiments have not yet resulted in the introduction of new drugs for therapeutic use (32). Recently Baker and co-workers became interested in the synthesis of active-site-directed irreversible inhibitors of dihydrofolic reductase (35), α-chymotrypsin (36), and xanthine oxidase (37). Compounds synthesized with this goal in mind form covalent bonds with the above-mentioned enzymes through chloro acetyl and sulfonyl fluoride groups, which are set free after the reaction of the compounds with the active site of the enzymes. In the case of α-chymotrypsin sulfonyl fluoride attacks rapidly the hydroxy group of the serine or threonine within the inhibitor–enzyme complex. Among the innumerable compounds prepared by Baker and collaborators, the following showed interesting activities:

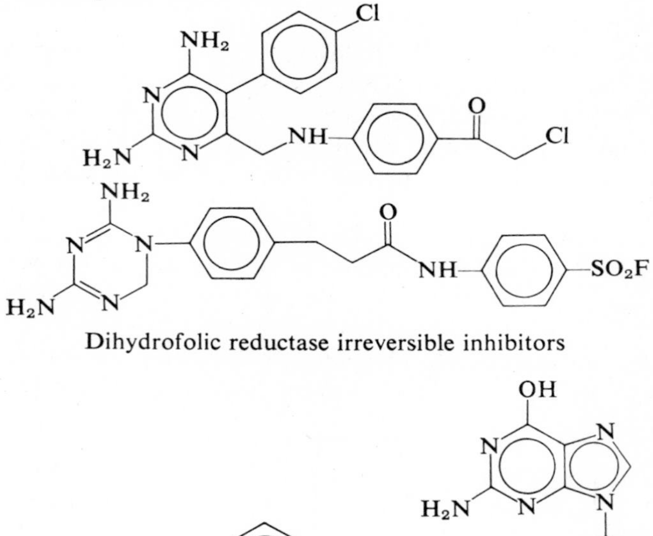

Dihydrofolic reductase irreversible inhibitors

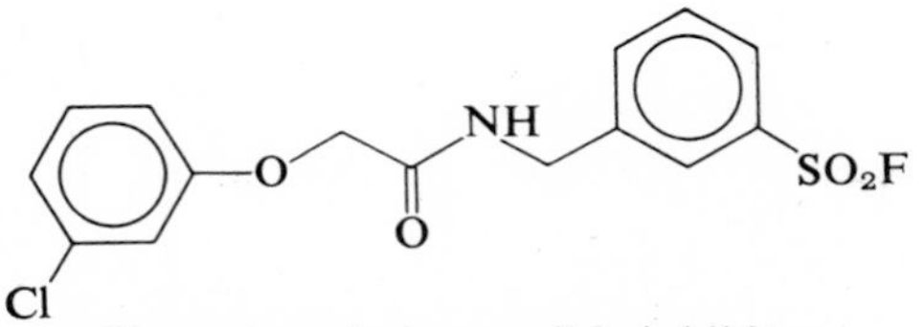

α-Chymotrypsin irreversible inhibitor

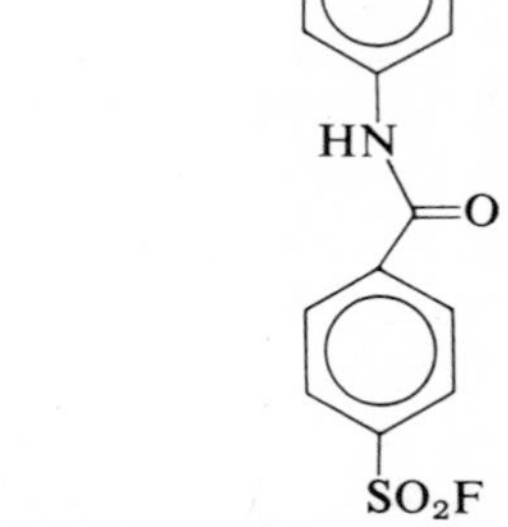

Xanthine oxidase irreversible inhibitor

Trypsin irreversible inhibitor

III. IONIC ATTRACTION

It was seen that chemotherapeutic agents (and some other compounds) form covalent linkages with the receptor that are strong and quite often irreversible. Because of this property they have a prolonged action: a toxic effect on parasites, but a healing effect on man. However, in the case of pharmacodynamic agents, such as central nervous system stimulants and depressors, a prolonged action is highly harmful. Therefore the medicinal action of pharmacodynamic agents is sought to be exercised during a relatively short period. And this really occurs, since the combination between them and their respective receptors is established through ionic or even weaker forces, which, however, are strong and stable enough for the drugs to be not too easily removed from their site of action.

At physiological pH several groups that are present in the drug—such as carboxyl, sulfonamide, and aliphatic amino—become ionized. An analogous phenomenon can be observed, at any pH, with a quaternary ammonium group. Almost all drugs capable of carrying charges are cations; only a very few are anions (*38*). On the other hand, the receptors, being constituted mainly of proteins, which in turn are made up of amino acids, also have groups that can be ionized. Thus the basic groups of arginine and lysine become completely protonated at the physiological pH, giving cationic groups. The same phenomenon, but to a lesser degree, depending on the environment, occurs in the imidazole ring of histidine. Aspartic and glutamic acids, at physiological pH, usually ionize completely, forming anionic groups, although environmental conditions may weaken them. Figure 6.7 represents amino acids that can undergo ionization, forming cations or anions.

Drug and receptor ions may be mutually attracted, provided they have opposite charges, thus forming a kind of linkage known as ionic bond. This bond is relatively strong. From the viewpoint of electrostatic interactions, it is the most important one. In the case of two charges, q' and q'', separated by a distance r in a medium with a dielectric constant D, the energy of the ionic bond is given by the following equation:

$$E = \frac{q'q''}{Dr} \tag{II}$$

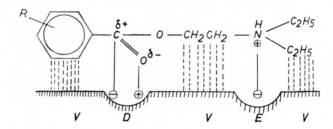

Fig. 7.5. Model of binding of local-anesthetic molecule to the receptor by E, electrostatic forces; D, dipole–dipole interaction; V, van der Waals forces (39, 40).

When q', q'', and r remain constant, the magnitude of interaction will depend on the dielectric constant. The value of the dielectric constant for water is 80 (20), but at physiological conditions it is 28, as found experimentally (38).

In the internal medium the cationic–anionic interaction lasts only a fraction of a second (10^{-5} sec) because of the quantity of ionic salts present and of the possibility this offers for ion exchange (13). However, if this bond is reinforced, as it is assumed, through the simultaneous presence of other interactions (hydrophobic, hydrogen bonding, charge transfer, dipole, van der Waals), it becomes stronger and is able to last much longer (13).

An example of the drug–receptor complexation through ionic and secondary bonds is found in local anesthetics and their respective receptor sites. Anesthetics are linked to the receptor site by weak bonds (39–41), as can be seen in Figure 7.5, and this explains why the effect they produce is reversible and of only short duration.

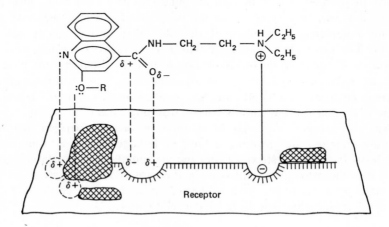

Fig. 7.6. Interaction of dibucaine ($R = C_4H_9$) with receptor (42).

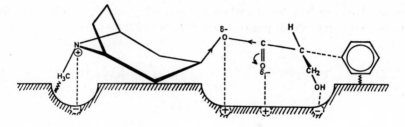

Fig. 7.7. Attachment of (−)-S-hyoscyamine to the muscarinic receptor (43).

In the case of local anesthetics derived from cinchoninic acid the interaction between them and the receptor will be stronger, since bonding will be possible at more sites (Figure 7.6).

The combination of (−)-S-hyoscyamine with a muscarinic receptor may be represented as in Figure 7.7.

Figure 7.8 indicates the manner in which acetylcholine is attached to two active sites of acetylcholinesterase.

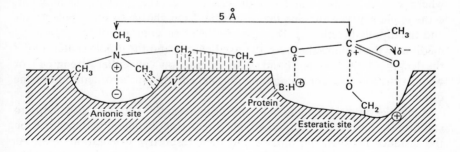

Fig. 7.8. Attachment of anionic and esteratic sites of acetylcholinesterase to complementary parts of acetylcholine. In the esteratic site two nucleophilic species play a role: the oxygen atom of a serine, and the imidazole ring (B) of a histidine, which will accept a proton released in the reaction (43).

IV. ION–DIPOLE AND DIPOLE–DIPOLE INTERACTIONS

Differences in the electronegativity between carbon and other atoms— such as nitrogen and oxygen—found in drugs and also in receptors result in an asymmetric distribution of electrons, with the formation of electronic dipoles. This can be seen in carbonyl, ester, ether, amide, nitrile, and other groups that carry partial positive and negative charges (*16*):

$$R \underset{R'}{\overset{R}{>}}\overset{\delta+}{C}\overset{\delta-}{=}O \qquad R\overset{\delta+}{-}\overset{\delta-}{C}\overset{O}{<}_{OR'} \qquad R\overset{\delta+}{-}CH_2\overset{\delta-}{-}O\overset{\delta+}{-}CH_2\overset{}{-}R'$$

$$R\overset{\delta+}{-}C\overset{\overset{\delta-}{O}}{<}_{NHR'} \qquad R\overset{\delta+}{-}C\overset{\delta-}{\equiv}N$$

As long as the charges are of opposite signs and properly aligned, the dipoles thus formed can be attracted by ions or other dipoles present in the receptor. The same phenomenon occurs in an aqueous solution, and hydrated ions are formed (*13*).

The energy of interaction (E_i) between one fixed charge and a dipole is given by the following equation (*38*):

$$E_i = \frac{Ne\mu \cos \phi}{D(r^2 - d^2)} \tag{III}$$

where N is Avogadro's number, e the electrical charge, μ the dipole moment, ϕ the angle between the line that binds the fixed charge to the dipole center and the dipole direction, D the effective dielectric constant of the separating medium, r the distance between the fixed charge and the dipole center, and d the length of the dipolar bond. This interaction can either strengthen or weaken the drug–receptor combination, depending on the orientation of the dipole.

A dipole–dipole interaction in the drug–receptor complex also helps to stabilize it, but less than an ion–dipole interaction, being quite dependent on the distance between the dipoles and their respective orientations (*38*). As far as magnitude is concerned, the dipole–dipole interaction lies between the ion–dipole interaction and the induced ion–dipole interaction, which is stronger than van der Waals bonds.

The ion–dipole and dipole–dipole interactions appear frequently in drug–receptor complexes.

V. HYDROGEN BONDING

A hydrogen bond or hydrogen bridge is formed when a hydrogen atom is linked to two or more other atoms (*44–46*). In most cases one of the two or more bonds formed by hydrogen is stronger than the others. To the weaker of the two bonds is given the name of hydrogen bond, in order to distinguish it from the stronger bond, which is assumed to be covalent. This situation is represented as X—H···Y. However, sometimes both of the hydrogen bonds have the same strength and length; in such a case the bonds are represented in the following way: X—H—Y. This is what occurs in the difluoride ion (F—H—F) and also in acid salts of various monobasic acids (O—H—O).

A hydrogen bond is formed every time there is a simultaneous presence of an acidic hydrogen and a basic acceptor, with the following distribution of charges: $A^{\ominus}$—$H^{\oplus}$···$B^{\ominus}$. For instance, the hydrogen atom of the imino group (N—H) is attracted by the ketonic oxygen atom, which is negatively charged (C=$\overset{\frown}{O}^{\ominus}$).

Therefore hydrogen bonding consists of an attraction between two nearby electronegative atoms with a proton between them. If the partial positive charge of the hydrogen is not well shielded, it can be attracted by a pair of unshared electrons that belongs to another neighboring electronegative atom, as shown in Figure 7.9.

In the formation of hydrogen bonds the molecules or molecular segments that most commonly are involved in donation of protons are F—H, O—H, and N—H; Cl—H, S—H, and P—H groups come next, but the bonds formed in this case are much weaker (47); there is evidence that the C—H group can be a donor (48), and this occurs when the whole C—H group has a net positive charge (46). The capacity of the C—H group to donate protons decreases with the change of the carbon hybridization [$C_{(sp)}$—H > $C_{(sp^2)}$—H > $C_{(sp^3)}$—H] and increases with the number of adjacent groups that withdraw electrons (48).

Atoms in a molecule able to be proton acceptors must have at least one lone electron pair in a complete octet. They are fluorine, oxygen, nitrogen, and, to a lesser degree, chlorine, sulfur, and phosphorus. Other halogen atoms can also function as acceptors; however, F^-, Cl^-, Br^-, and I^- ions are better acceptors.

Being weaker than a covalent bond, but stronger than van der Waals

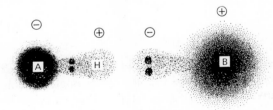

Fig. 7.9. Hydrogen bonding results from the attraction between two dipoles: one formed by the A—H bond and the other produced by atom B and an unshared pair of its valence electrons. [Adapted from (19).]

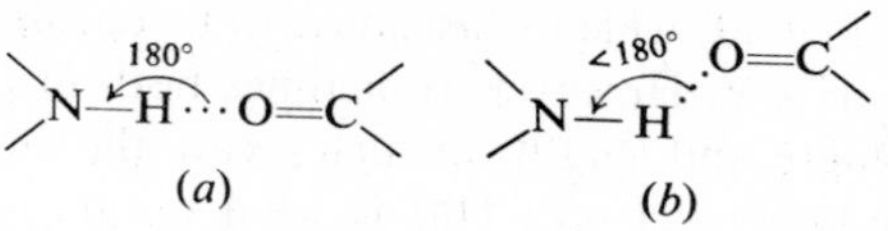

Fig. 7.10. Directional properties of hydrogen bonds. In (*a*) the vector along the covalent O—H bond points directly at the acceptor oxygen, thereby forming a strong bond. In (*b*) the vector points away from the oxygen atom, resulting in a much weaker bond. [Adapted from (*12*).]

forces, a hydrogen bond links two atoms closer together than the sum of their van der Waals radii, but not as close as a covalent bond. The strength of hydrogen bonding is inversely proportional to the distances between the atoms (*12*), as in common chemical bonding. As distinct from what occurs with van der Waals forces, hydrogen bonding is highly directional; that is, the more it points toward the acceptor, the stronger it is (Figure 7.10).

Although from an energetic viewpoint linear hydrogen bonding is preferred, linearity does not constitute the rule but rather the exception (*46,49*). There is not much correlation between the length of the hydrogen bond and its deviation from strict linearity (*50*). In fact, hydrogen bonding has great flexibility (*48*). For instance, there are many bifurcated hydrogen bonds, where the covalently bound hydrogen participates in two weaker hydrogen bonds (*49,51,52*):

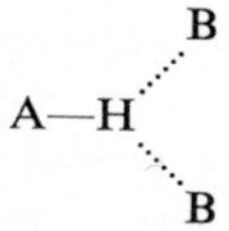

The flexibility of the hydrogen bond can also be shown by comparing H—O—H angles of the water molecule with O···O···O angles in systems that can be represented as follows:

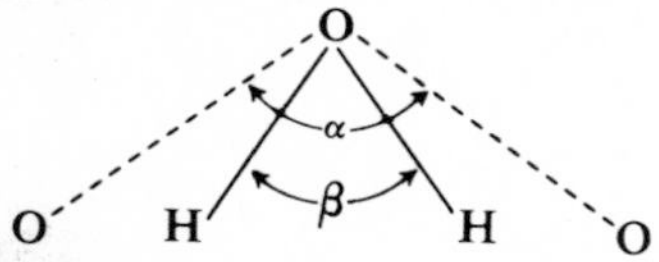

It was found that the variations of the O···O···O angles (from 81 to 147°) are much larger than variations of the H—O—H angles (from 106 to 114°), which are relatively constant (about 110°). This variation in the so-called acceptor angle indicates that the A—H···B bond does not have to be linear (*49*).

More evidence in favor of the flexibility of hydrogen bonding is the deviation from linearity of the O—H···O bond in all compounds studied by the neutron-diffraction method: instead of the O—H···O angle systematically being 180°, great deviations have been observed, and an average value of 165° has been found (*49*). Deviations from 10 to 20° are common (*50*).

The most common hydrogen bonds and their respective distances are listed in Table 7.3, where A···B (calc) and H···B (calc) refer to the calculated

TABLE 7.3 Van der Waals Contact Distances and Hydrogen-Bond Distances Observed (Given in Angstroms) in Some Common Hydrogen Bondings (*46*)

Bond Type	A···B (calc)	A···B (obs)	H···B (calc)	H···B (obs)
F—H—F	2.7	2.4	2.6	1.2
O—H···O	2.8	2.7	2.6	1.7
O—H···F	2.8	2.7	2.6	1.7
O—H···N	2.9	2.8	2.7	1.9
O—H···Cl	3.2	3.1	3.0	2.2
N—H···O	2.9	2.9	2.6	2.0
N—H···F	2.9	2.8	2.6	1.9
N—H···Cl	3.3	3.3	3.0	2.4
N—H···N	3.0	3.1	2.7	2.2
N—H···S	3.4	3.4	3.1	2.4
C—H···O	3.0	3.2	2.6	2.3

sum of van der Waals radii (*5*), whereas A···B (obs) and H···B (obs) are values determined by diffraction methods. It is accepted that a hydrogen bond is formed when the distance between two heavy atoms and a hydrogen atom is less than the sum of the van der Waals radii (*46*).

In biological systems the most important hydrogen bonds are those formed between hydrogen atoms covalently bound to oxygen (O—H) or nitrogen (N—H) and nitrogen or oxygen atoms. Hydrogen bonding stabilizes a protein in its helical arrangement and assists in stabilizing the double helical structure of deoxyribonucleic acid (Figure 7.11).

The geometry of hydrogen bonds between peptide units can be represented as shown in Figure 7.12.

Some examples of hydrogen bonds encountered in biological systems and in drug–receptor interactions are shown in Figure 7.13.

Many drugs contain groups—such as hydroxyl, carbonyl, amino, and imino—that can form hydrogen bonds either as donors or as acceptors of protons. On the other hand, biological macromolecules where drug receptors are situated also contain such groups. Among others the following amino

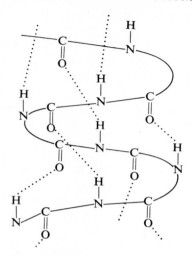

Fig. 7.11. Schematic representation of a protein in a right α-helical conformation of L-amino acids.

acids can act as proton donors: arginine, lysine, and cysteine; as proton acceptors, the following: aspartic acid, glutamic acid, methionine, and cystine. Other amino acids can act at one time as donors and at another time as acceptors or as donors and acceptors simultaneously; to the first group belongs histidine, which, when protonated, is a donor and, when non-protonated, is an acceptor. Asparagine, glutamine, serine, threonine, hydroxy-proline, tyrosine, and others belong to the second group (32). From this it can be deduced that hydrogen bonds intervene in the formation of drug–receptor linkages, contributing to the stability of the drug–receptor complex, which increases with the number of bonds formed.

By considering that in the internal medium the drug as well as the receptor are already linked to water by hydrogen bonds, these should be broken before new bonds can be formed, this time between drug and receptor. Designating as D the electron-donor group of the receptor (R) and as A the acceptor group of the drug (F), the interactions that take place in the internal medium—that

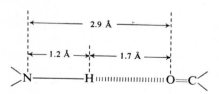

Fig. 7.12. Geometry of hydrogen bonds between peptide units. [Adapted from (20).]

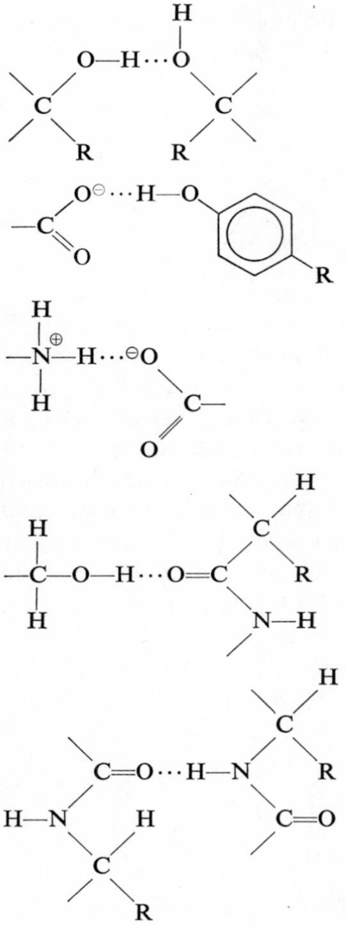

$$\begin{array}{c} \text{H} \\ | \\ \text{O—H}\cdots\text{O} \end{array}$$

Hydrogen bond between two hydroxy groups

$$-\text{C} \overset{\text{O}^{\ominus}\cdots\text{H—O}}{\underset{\text{O}}{}}$$

Hydrogen bond between a charged carboxy group and the hydroxy group of tyrosine

$$\begin{array}{c} \text{H} \\ | \\ -\overset{\oplus}{\text{N}}\text{—H}\cdots\overset{\ominus}{}\text{O} \\ | \\ \text{H} \end{array}$$

Hydrogen bond between a charged amino group and a charged carboxy group

Hydrogen bond between a hydroxy group of serine and a peptide group

Hydrogen bond between two peptide groups

Fig. 7.13. Examples of hydrogen bonds established in biological systems. [Adapted from (12).]

is, in an aqueous phase—can be represented by the following equations (32):

$$\text{R—D:} \longrightarrow \text{H—O} \quad + \text{F—A} \longleftarrow \text{:O—H} \rightleftharpoons$$

$$\text{R—D:} \longrightarrow \text{A—F} + \quad \text{O—H} \longleftarrow \text{O—H}$$

However, this exchange is favorable (20) and occurs with very little change in free energy.

Hydrogen bonds can be intramolecular or intermolecular. The former are stronger than the latter. Some molecules, such as salicylic acid, can have both types of hydrogen bonds (5):

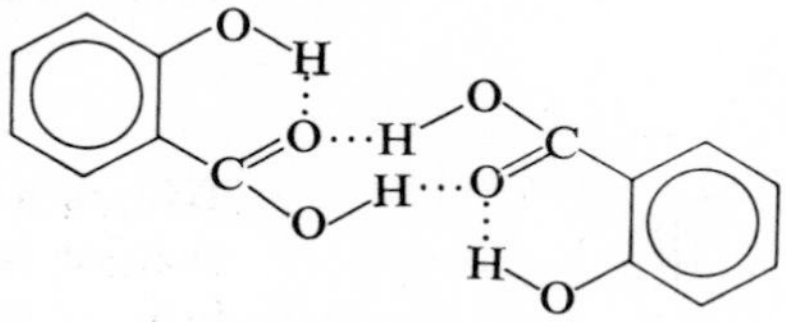

Salicylic acid

The presence or absence of biological action in some compounds is ascribed, in some cases, to their capacity for forming or not forming hydrogen bonds. This fact has substantial influence on their physicochemical properties and therefore on their pharmacodynamic activity. Thus, whereas 1-phenyl-2,3-dimethyl-5-pyrazolone (antipyrine), which is soluble in water and moderately soluble in ether, has analgetic properties, its demethylated analog, the 1-phenyl-3-methyl-5-pyrazolone, being insoluble in water and only slightly soluble in ether, has no analgetic activity. This discrepancy seems to derive from the fact that the former compound does not form intermolecular hydrogen bonds, whereas the latter compound does (53).

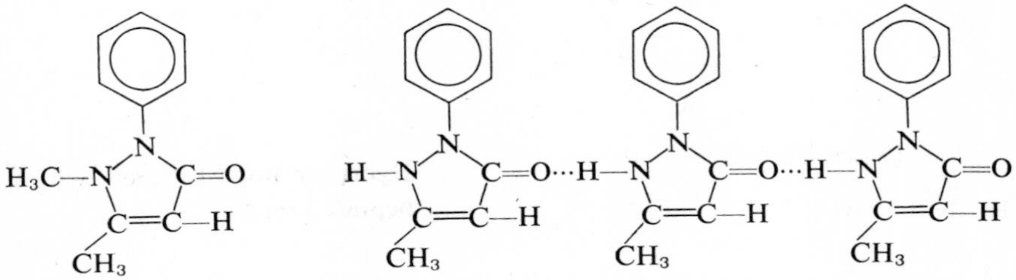

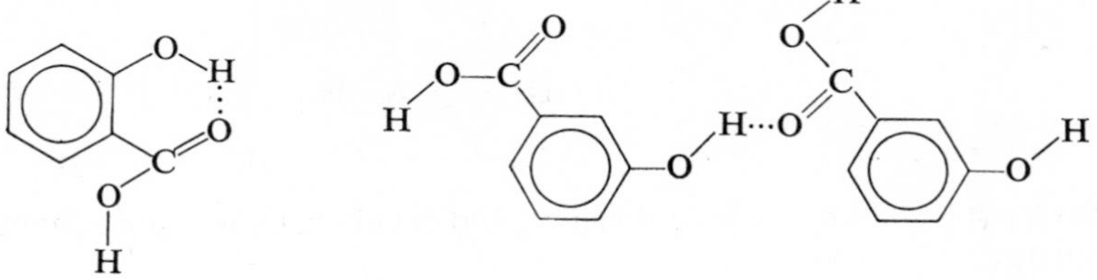

Another example is salicylic acid (o-hydroxybenzoic acid), which has antibacterial activity, whereas its isomers p-hydroxybenzoic acid and m-hydroxybenzoic acid have none. This difference in biological action is ascribed to the fact that only the salicylic acid is capable of establishing intramolecular hydrogen bonds, which, although masking the phenolic hydroxy group, leave the carboxy group free; as a result of this phenomenon, salicylic acid can function as an antibacterial agent. The two other isomers cannot form intramolecular but only intermolecular hydrogen bonds. These result in a high degree of association of the compounds and could account for the pronounced reduction of their biological activity (53).

The opposite occurs with the respective esters: methyl salicylate possesses an extremely weak antibacterial action, whereas methyl-*p*-hydroxybenzoate (Nipagin) manifests this activity to an appreciable degree. This fact is due to the possibility of the latter compound's functioning as a phenol: when the dimers are formed, through *intermolecular* hydrogen bonds, the phenolic hydroxy group is set free. Methyl salicylate is unable to function as a phenol because in the establishment of *intramolecular* hydrogen bonds the phenolic hydroxy group is masked.

Derivatives of isatin-β-thiosemicarbazone and of benzimidazole with a high antiviral activity have, as a common characteristic, an intramolecular hydrogen bond (54).

Likewise, it is postulated that sulfamido as well as benzothiadiazino diuretics, which function as carbonic anhydrase inhibitors by a competitive mechanism with carbonic acid, attach themselves to the active site of the enzyme through hydrogen bonding, as shown in Figure 7.14. If this bond is

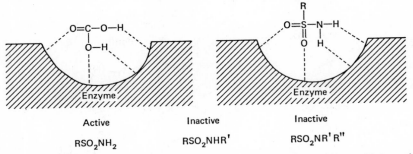

Fig. 7.14. Combination of activator and inhibitors of carbonic anhydrase with its active site through hydrogen bonding.

weakened through the substitution of hydrogens of the amino group, the compounds lose their activity.

Tetracyclines establish intramolecular hydrogen bonds and can chelate with metallic ions. However, their antibiotic action does not result solely from such properties.

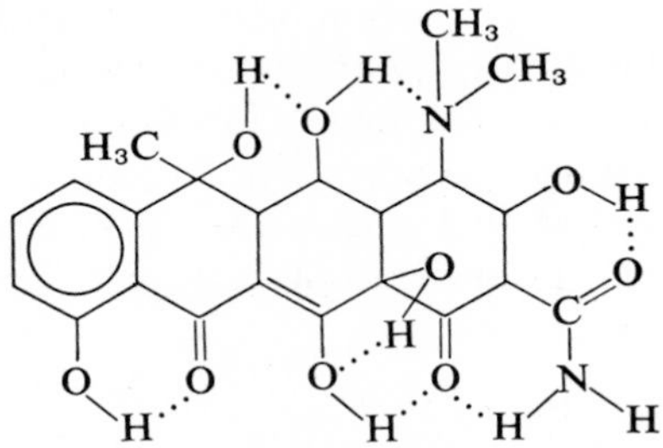

As has been shown above, there are many molecules in biological systems that are linked among themselves by hydrogen bonds. Examples are the four nitrogen bases—cytosine (C), thymine (T), adenine (A), and guanine (G)— constituents of DNA. In RNA uracil takes the place of thymine.

The interaction energies of these bases are shown in Table 7.4.

Hydrogen bonds play an important role in the process of replication. They maintain the structural integrity of the constituent pairs of DNA bases and are responsible for the interactions between amino acids, messenger RNA, and transfer RNA that finally result in the synthesis of specific polypeptide chains. This throws light on the mechanism of action of mutagenic and chelating agents, as well as of some antimetabolites. Through hydrogen

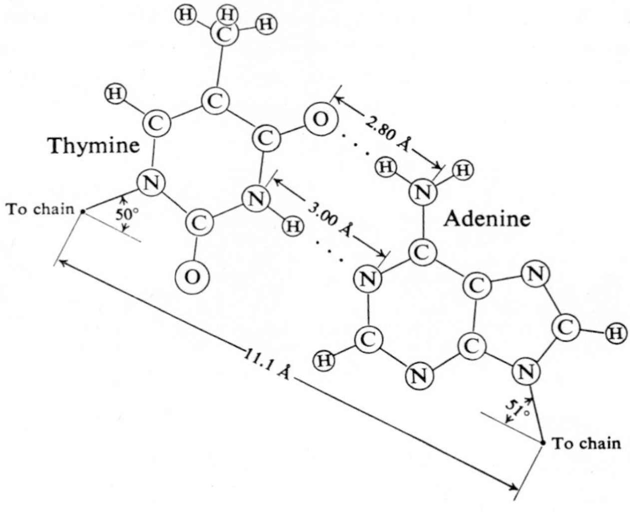

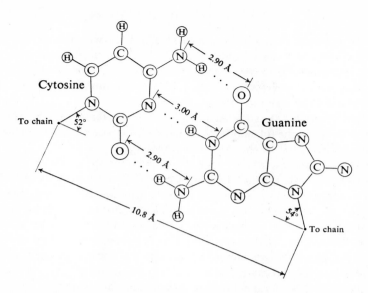

TABLE 7.4 Interaction Energies in Pairs of Bases Linked by Hydrogen Bonding in DNA (8)

Pair of Bases	Interaction Energy (kcal/mole)	Pair of Bases	Interaction Energy (kcal/mole)
A—A T—T	−5.8 −5.2	A—T	−7.0
G—G C—C	−14.5 −13	G—C	−19.2
A—A C—C	−5.8 −13	A—C	−7.8
G—G T—T	−14.5 −5.2	G—T	−7.4
C—C T—T	−13 −5.2	C—T	−6.5
A—A G—G	−5.8 −14.5	A—G	−7.5

$$A—T > \frac{A—A}{T—T} \qquad \begin{array}{l} A—C < C—C \\ G—T < G—G \end{array}$$

$$G—C > \frac{G—G}{C—C} \qquad \begin{array}{l} C—T < C—C \\ A—G < G—G \end{array}$$

A = Adenine, C = cytosine, G = guanine, T = thymine.

161

bonds these compounds initially establish a linkage with the site of action. Then they take the place of the constituent bases of nucleic acids, by interrupting, unleashing, or altering some vital process. In the case of chelating agents this action is irreversible, due to their ability to establish strong covalent bonds with the receptor.

Sax and Pletcher (55) suggested that a common feature in the action of local anesthetics is the formation of a hydrogen-bonded complex between the drug and an acceptor on the neural membrane.

Cammarata and Stein (56) indicate a method for investigating drug–receptor interactions through hydrogen bonds. It consists in the determination of σ- and π-charges of certain atoms in a drug through simple molecular-orbital calculations and of the influence of these charges on interaction with receptors. By using this method to study the interaction of 3-hydroxyphenyl-trimethylammonium derivatives with acetylcholinesterase, they concluded that it is through hydrogen bonds formed with the hydroxy group attached to the carbon 3 of the aromatic rings that this interaction occurs.

On the basis of experimental data Jarboe and co-workers (57) postulated that in the interaction of compounds analogous to picrotoxinin with its receptor hydrogen bonding is involved between the hydroxy group in the bridgehead and the π-electrons of the isopropenyl group.

VI. CHARGE TRANSFER

The complex formed between two molecules through hydrogen bonding is a special case of the general phenomenon of donor-acceptor complexes (32), which are established through an electrostatic attraction between an electron-donating molecule (D) and an electron-accepting molecule (A). Although resonance form $D^{\oplus}A^{\ominus}$ contributes only slightly to the formal resonance hybrid of these complexes, such a form increases the stability of the complex. Details on charge transfer can be found elsewhere (58–60).

An example of a charge-transfer complex is the one derived from N-methylpyridinium iodide; another example is the benzene–iodine complex (32,61,62).

These complexes can be regarded as ionic pairs, with the property of undergoing an observable transition of charge transfer.

According to Baker (*32*), for a particular charge-transfer complex there are two classes of donors and two classes of acceptors. The donors are the following:

1. Those that are rich in π-electrons, such as alkenes, alkynes, and aromatic compounds with electron-donating substituents.

2. Those that have an unshared electron pair, such as

$$
\begin{array}{cccccc}
\text{R—O:,} & \text{R—S:,} & \text{R—I:,} & \text{R}_3\text{N:,} & \text{R—O:,} & \text{R—S:} \\
| & | & & & | & | \\
\text{H} & \text{R} & & & \text{R} & \text{R—S}
\end{array}
$$

that is, the same groups that act as proton acceptors in hydrogen bonds.

The acceptors are the following:

1. Those that, being deficient in π-electrons—such as *sym*-trinitrobenzene, tetracyanoethylene, and chloranil (tetrachlorobenzoquinone)—have groups that withdraw electrons very strongly and can be regarded as π-acids.

2. Weakly acidic hydrogens of molecules, such as Br_3C—H, alkyl—O—H, Ar—O—H, R—S—H, imidazole—H; that is, the same groups that in hydrogen bonding act as proton donors.

The ability of a given compound to be a donor of electrons can be experimentally calculated from the wavelength of maximal absorption of the charge-transfer complexes. Electron-donating ability will increase with increase in the wavelength of the charge-transfer band. Although it is difficult to measure the electrostatic-bond energy in the ground state, there is evidence that charge-transfer complexes are formed in water, which gives a hint of the degree of electron-donating ability. For certain acceptors wavelengths are inversely proportional to the ionization potential of the donors (*63*). The ionization potential is related to the energy of the highest occupied molecular orbital (HOMO). This energy can be calculated by using the simple Hückel molecular-orbital theory.

Cilento and Zinner observed that three classes of donors act as catalysts in auto-oxidation reactions: the monoanion of catechol and catecholamines (*64*), the protonated form of *p*-phenylenediamines (*65*), and the iodide ion (*66*). Cilento and Sanioto showed that polycyclic hydrocarbons, including the carcinogenic ones, form charge-transfer complexes with the pyridinium ring (*67*) and some quinones (*68*), although apparently there is no correlation between carcinogenic activity and complexation.

Macromolecules of biological systems that act as receptor components have various protein groups that in complex formation by charge transfer can function as (a) electron donors, (b) electron acceptors, and (c) electron donors and acceptors. Among the first group are aspartate, glutamate, cystine, methionine, and tyrosine (aromatic ring only). Among the second group are cysteine, and probably arginine and lysine. In the third group are histidine, asparagine, glutamine, polyamide backbone, serine, threonine, hydroxyproline, tyrosine (OH only), phenylalanine (aromatic ring only), and tryptophan (32).

Drugs also have the same abilities. Among those that act as electron donors are the following:

1. Those that have anionic groups [$RCOO^-$, $RCOS^-$, RSO_3^-, RSO_2^-, $RCSS^-$, $RPO(O^-)_2$, $RAsO(O^-)_2$].

2. Certain weak bases (R_3N, $R_3N \rightarrow O$).

3. Some neutral sulfur compounds (R_2S, $RSSR$, $ROSO_2R$).

4. Several neutral nitrogen compounds ($RONO$, $RONO_2$, R_3CNO_2, R_3CNO, $R—N{=}N—R$).

5. Certain neutral phosphorus compounds [R_3P, $(RO)_3P$, $RP(OR)_2$].

6. Various neutral oxygen compounds [R_2O, $R_2C(OR)_2$].

7. Halogen compounds ($R—Hal$).

Among the electron acceptors, the following may be indicated:

1. Weak acids (RSH, $RNHCSNR_2$, $RCSNHR'$, $R_2C{=}NOH$, $RNHC{\equiv}N$).

2. Some neutral phosphorus compounds

$$\left(\begin{array}{c} R_3P \rightarrow O,\ R_2P—NH_2 \\ \downarrow \\ O \end{array} \right).$$

3. Perhaps those compounds that present cationic groups

$$\left(R_3NH^+,\ R_4N^+,\ RNHNH_3^+,\ \overset{\overset{\displaystyle NH_2}{|}}{RC}{=}NH_2^+,\ RNH\overset{\overset{\displaystyle NH_2}{|}}{C}{=}NH_2^+,\ \overset{\overset{\displaystyle OR'}{|}}{RC}{=}NH_2^+, \right.$$

$$\left. Ar\overset{+}{N}{\equiv}N,\ \overset{\overset{\displaystyle SR'}{|}}{RC}{=}NH_2^+,\ R_3S^+ \right).$$

Among those that simultaneously function as donors and acceptors are the following:

1. Some that contain anionic groups [$ROPO(O^-)_2$].

2. Certain weak bases (RNH_2, $RCONHNH_2$).

3. Several weak acids ($ArOH$, $RCONHOH$, R_2CHNO_2, $RNHNO_2$).

4. Various neutral nitrogen compounds

$$(RCONHR,\ RCONR_2,\ ROCONH_2,\ RCON_3).$$

5. Many neutral phosphorus compounds

$$\left[(RO)_3P \rightarrow O,\ \underset{\downarrow O}{RP(OH)_2},\ \underset{\downarrow O}{(RO)_2PNH_2},\ \underset{\downarrow O}{(RO)_2PNR_2} \right].$$

6. Various neutral oxygen compounds

[ROH, RCOOR, (RO)$_2$CO, RCH=O, R$_2$C=O].

7. A number of miscellaneous compounds (R$_2$C=CR$_2$, aromatic) (32).

The following monocyclic heterocycles can act concomitantly as electron donors and acceptors: imidazole, thiophene, triazole, pyridine, pyrimidine, and *sym*-triazine. On the other hand, furan, pyrrole, and pyrazol function solely as donors.

Certain antimalarial drugs such as acridine and aminoquinoline derivatives appear to act through intercalation between adjacent base pairs of DNA, thus inhibiting DNA-primed synthesis of DNA and RNA (69). The complexation

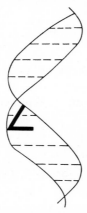

of aminoquinolines with DNA is thought to occur through both ionic attraction between the side chain of these drugs and the phosphate groups of the companion strands of DNA across the minor groove and a more specific interaction involving the aromatic ring portions of aminoquinolines and DNA bases (Figure 7.15).

Fig. 7.15. Hypothetical complexation between antimalarial aminoquinolines and DNA. The figure shows superimposition of chloroquine over the cytosine–guanine pair (69).

Perkow (*70*) postulated that a decreased electron density at what he called the *biologically active center* of the drug constitutes a prerequisite for the formation of a bond with the receptor. In fact there are several enzymes that, as a result of their electron-rich regions, can function as electron donors to electron-deficient areas of inhibitors. This would constitute a case analogous to the one studied by Shifrin (*71*), concerning charge transfer, but an *intra-* and not *inter*molecular one, in a nicotinamide derivative series.

Several other examples of complexation by charge transfer can be found elsewhere (*8*), including the hypothetical one that would occur between the C-3 of indole and the pyridine ring, as represented in Figure 7.16.

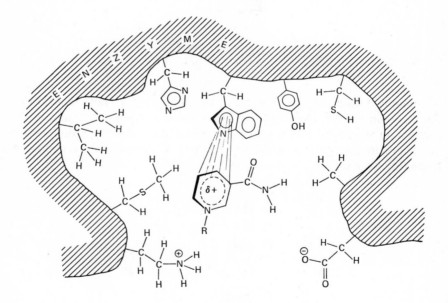

Fig. 7.16. Schematic representation of a hypothetical situation where the nicotinamide moiety of NAD$^+$ is located in the neighborhood of the indole group of a trytophan residue, in such a manner that the electron donation from C-3 of indole to the pyridinium ring may produce a transfer-charge transition. [Adapted from (*72*).]

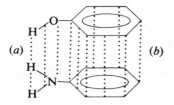

Fig. 7.17. Interaction through charge transfer: (a) localized, between two specific groups; (b) generalized, between the molecule electron clouds (4). (Reproduced by permission of the copyright owner.)

Complexations between electron donors and acceptors, by means of charge transfer, can also occur between a drug and a receptor (4). In fact the former as much as the latter can function at one time as donors and at other times as acceptors, since they often contain either electron-rich or electron-deficient regions. Thus a charge transfer as shown in Figure 7.17 is possible.

Although caution should be exercised in stating that association through charge transfer is biologically significant (8), this complexation among various electron-donor drugs and electron-acceptor compounds seems to furnish clear evidence of the pharmacodynamic activity of several hallucinogens (73), certain psychotomimetic (74) and psychotropic drugs (75), and some indole derivatives (63). These results justify the interest with which workers are studying charge transfer complexes in biological systems (76–78), including those involved in drug-receptor interactions at the submolecular level (76), especially after it was suggested that the tranquilizing activity of chloropromazine could be related to its strong electron-donating capacity (79).

VII. MIXED TYPES OF BONDING

The bond between a drug and a receptor through electrostatic attraction between electron-rich donors and electron-deficient acceptors may also be of a mixed type, involving the three types described above; that is, ionic bonding, hydrogen bonding, and charge transfer, in decreasing bond-energy order. Several examples can be given (32). In o-allylphenol the π-electron cloud of the vinyl group can donate electrons to the electron-deficient hydroxylic hydrogen atom; however, this is an intramolecular linkage.

The carboxylate anion, with a high electron density, can form *inter-molecular* electrostatic bonds through electron donations to (a) a cation, (b) a hydrogen that can participate in hydrogen bonding, and (c) a π-base that can participate in charge transfer. Other combinations of drugs and their receptors are possible, including that which occurs with the intervention of hydrophobic forces (*32*).

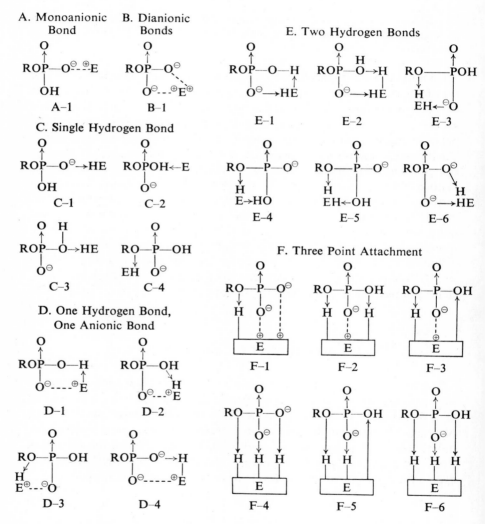

Fig. 7.18. Possible modes of binding of a phosphate ester to an enzyme, E (*80*). (Reproduced by permission of the copyright owner.)

Multifunctional groups, such as peptides and phosphates, can combine with receptors in various ways simultaneously. For instance, in the CONH group the oxygen can be donor and the hydrogen, acceptor: that is, by the way, the bond responsible for the helical portions of proteins. For a phosphate group of a nucleotide 22 different ways can be envisioned for the mode of binding to an enzyme, including by one, two, or three bonds (80). These 22 ways are shown in Figure 7.18.

Heterocyclic rings can establish bonds with receptors in several ways, as shown in Table 7.5. Note that in this table hydrogen bonding is considered

TABLE 7.5   Bonding of Some Monocyclic Heterocycles to Proteins (32)

Heterocycle[b]	Anionic–Cationic	Hydrogen Bond[a]		Charge Transfer[a]		Hydro-phobic Bonding[c]
		Electron Donor	Acceptor	Electron Donor	Acceptor	
Imidazole	Yes	Yes	Yes	Yes	Yes	Poor
Furan	No	Yes	No?	Yes	No?	Yes
Pyrrole	Weak(?)	Yes	No	Yes	No	Yes
Thiophene	No	Yes	Yes?	Yes	Yes?	Yes
Pyrazole	Weak (?)	Yes	No?	Yes	No?	Poor
Triazole	Weak (?)	Yes	Yes	Yes	Yes	No
Pyridine	Weak (?)	Yes	Yes	Yes	Yes	Poor
Pyrimidine	No	Yes	Yes	Yes	Yes	Poor
sym-Triazine	No	Yes	Yes	Yes	Yes	No?

[a] It should be noted that the properties of a heterocycle can be modified by substituting electron-donating or electron-withdrawing groups.
[b] The bonding excludes active hydrogens such as the NH of pyrrole.
[c] Also includes other nonpolar interactions, such as van der Waals forces.

to involve electrons, not protons as in our discussion (Section V of this chapter). For example, pyrimidine can form bonds with a receptor in three different ways:

1. Through hydrophobic interactions, with carbons located at positions 2, 4, 5, and 6.
2. Through acceptance, by the π-electron cloud, of electrons from a donor group of the receptor, forming a charge-transfer complex.
3. Through donation of an electron pair on each nitrogen to an electron-acceptor group of the receptor.

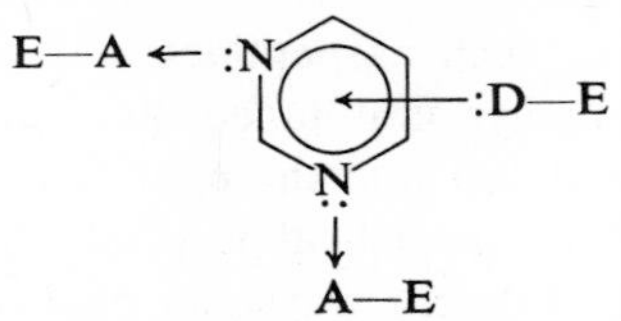

$$E—A \leftarrow :N \bigcirc :D—E$$

$$A—E$$

The introduction into a pyrimidine ring of electron-donor groups modifies radically the properties of the ring. Thus in its tautomeric form, uracil, which is 2,4-dihydroxypyrimidine, can donate electrons to an acceptor group, since the π-electron cloud becomes electron rich and, besides this, its two —CONH— groups can donate electrons from the oxygen and accept electrons for the hydrogen (32).

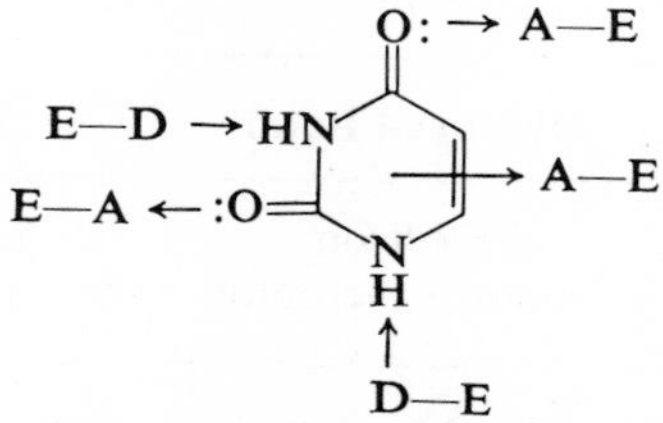

$$O: \rightarrow A—E$$
$$E—D \rightarrow HN$$
$$E—A \leftarrow :O= \rightarrow A—E$$
$$N$$
$$H$$
$$D—E$$

Another pyrimidine derivative, cytosine, besides the bonds already seen in uracil, has two nitrogens that can donate an unshared electron pair and two amine hydrogens that can be acceptors.

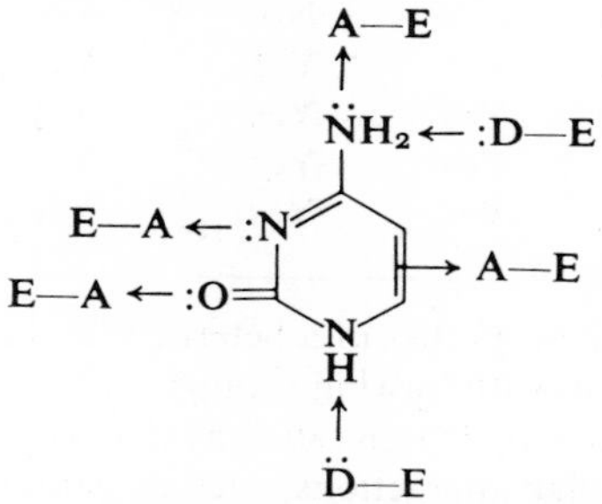

$$A—E$$
$$NH_2 \leftarrow :D—E$$
$$E—A \leftarrow :N$$
$$E—A \leftarrow :O= \rightarrow A—E$$
$$N$$
$$H$$
$$D—E$$

Various amino acid constituents of biological systems, because of the π-framework of their aromatic ring, can function as receptor groups of drugs, establishing mixed bonds. Among others, in a decreasing order of their electron-donating capacity, we have tryptophan > tyrosine > phenylalanine (32).

VIII. HYDROPHOBIC INTERACTION

Water is a solvent with the peculiarity of having its molecules connected by intermolecular hydrogen bonds. In the presence of ions it solvates them, as shown in Figure 7.19.

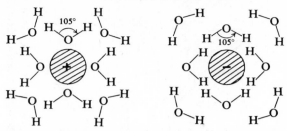

Fig. 7.19. Positive and negative ions solvated by water. [Adapted from (20).]

Hydrocarbons, however, are slightly soluble in water and not solvated by it. Water molecules then, because of the presence of nonpolar regions, arrange themselves in a more orderly manner and are in a higher state of energy than when surrounded entirely by other water molecules. Thus in an internal medium the interaction of two nonpolar chains—for instance, one (*A*) pertaining to a macromolecule of a certain organism and another (*B*) pertaining to a drug that forms a bond with it in order to produce a pharmacological effect—reduces the interface, through the withdrawal of water previously present in the region lying between the two chains. As a consequence the water molecules displaced from their contact with the nonpolar surfaces become disordered (Figure 7.20).

This disorder in the disposition of the water molecules results in an increase of entropy in the system and consequently in a decrease of free energy, which stabilizes the contact between these two nonpolar regions (*15,19,32*). This association, represented in Figure 7.21, is called a *hydrophobic bond* (*81*) or *hydrophobic interaction* (*82,83*). It is a special case of the general phenomenon known as *solvophobic force*, which is greater in water because, among the common inert solvents, it has the greatest surface tension (*84*).

During the process of a hydrophobic interaction, which is highly favorable for complex formation, 0.7 kcal/mole of free energy is liberated for every

$$H_2C \cdots CH_2 \text{ interaction } (83\text{--}86).$$

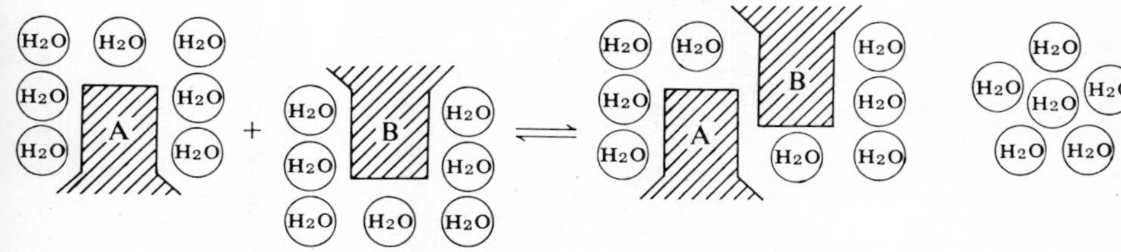

$$n[\text{alkyl chains } (H_2O)_x] \rightleftharpoons (\text{alkyl chains})_n + nx\ H_2O$$

Fig. 7.20. Simplified representation of hydrophobic interaction. [Adapted from (*19*).]

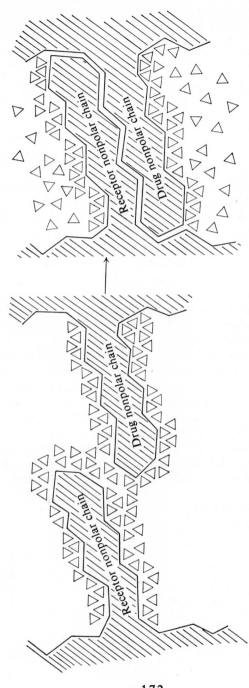

Fig. 7.21. Schematic representation of hydrophobic interaction. The approach of the nonpolar chains one to another results in a more disordered state of some water molecules (represented by triangles) and consequently in an increase of entropy of the system. [Adapted from (19).]

Substituents (90)

Enzyme	Source	Heterocycle	R for Maximum Hydrophobic Bonding	Binding Increment
Dihydrofolic reductase	Pigeon liver	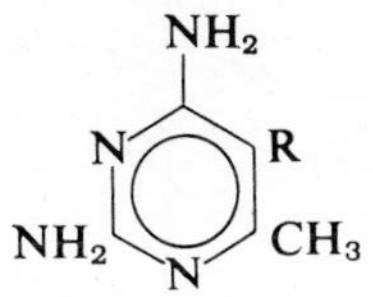	$C_6H_5(CH_2)_4$—	40,000
		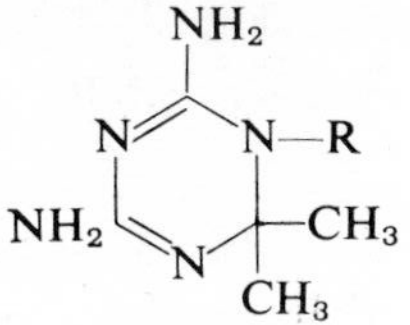	$C_6H_5(CH_2)_4$— C_6H_5— $i\text{-}C_5H_{11}$— $m\text{-}C_6H_4(CH_2)_4C_6H_5$	2,000[a] 700[a] 1,300[a] 20,000
		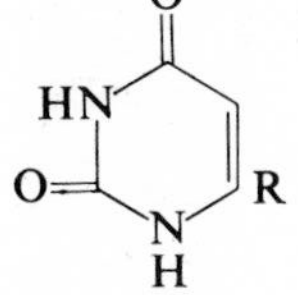	$C_6H_5CH_2$—	18
Thymidine phosphorylase	*Escherichia coli* B	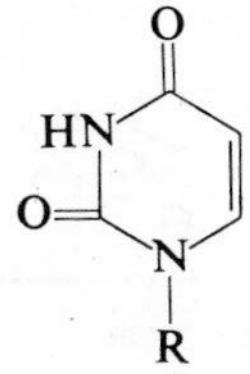	$C_6H_5(CH_2)_5$—	100[b]

[a] Included for comparison.
[b] Higher phenylalkyl analogs not yet investigated, but lower analogs were less effective.

TABLE 7.6 (continued)

Enzyme	Source	Heterocycle	R for Maximum Hydrophobic Bonding	Binding Increment
		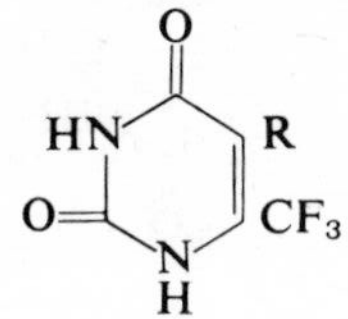	$C_6H_5(CH_2)_4$—	9[b]
Guanase	Rabbit liver	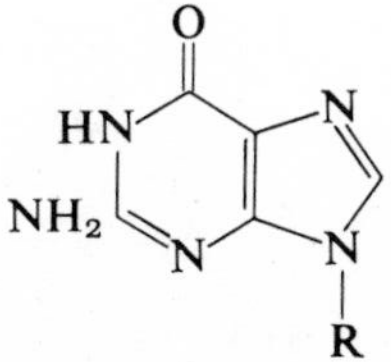	C_6H_5—	28
Xanthine oxidase	Bovine milk	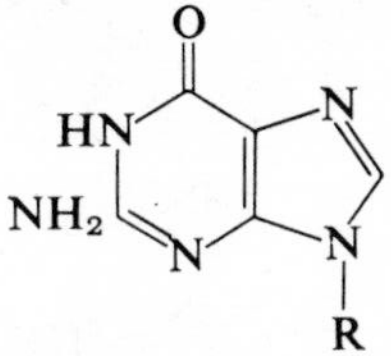	C_6H_5—	100
Succinoadenylate kinosynthetase	Escherichia coli B	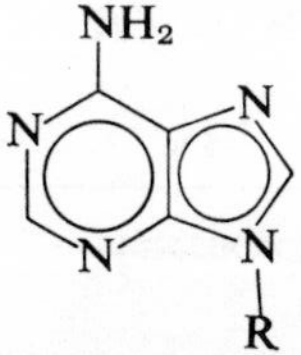	$C_6H_5CH_2$—	11

[b] Higher phenylalkyl analogs not yet investigated, but lower analog are less effective

174

Macromolecules (e.g., enzymes) that interact with drugs have nonpolar chains on their surfaces. Many drugs, equally, possess nonpolar regions in their structures. In both instances these chains can be aryl or alkyl. It is expected, therefore, that in the formation of the macromolecule–drug complex hydrophobic forces intervene, and they can be of quite appreciable magnitude (86,87). Hydrophobic forces also occur in polar groups (88,89) such as in purine and pyrimidine bases (84). This was, in fact, experimentally shown for certain enzymes. Some of the hydrophobic interactions, as well as the increases in bond strength thus obtained, are presented in Table 7.6. Details on hydrophobic interactions may be found elsewhere (83,84,90,91).

IX. VAN DER WAALS FORCES

Also named London's dispersion forces, the van der Waals forces are the most universal form of attraction between atoms (13). They are derived from the polarization induced by two unbonded atoms that approach one another. This polarization causes distortion of the electron cloud surrounding the atoms, and consequently an attraction arises between the electrons of one atom and the positive nucleus of the other. These forces operate in all types of molecules, in polar as well as nonpolar ones (92).

In order for van der Waals forces to appear and to have an appreciable effect it is necessary that distances between interacting atoms be relatively short—namely, from 4 to 6 Å (Figure 7.22). They cannot, however, be much shorter, since the approach of two unlinked atoms is limited by their steric contours. The distance between the atom center and its steric contour is called the *van der Waals radius*, and its value, characteristic for each chemical element, is determined from distances between unlinked atoms in crystals of different substances. Bondi (93) compiled a list of atomic volumes and van der Waals radii. Some of the van der Waals radii values appear in Table 7.7. These contact radii are much longer than covalent bonds.

For the calculation of van der Waals–London forces four contributions are presently considered: E_{el}, electrostatic interaction between net atomic charges; E_{pol}, polarization energy; E_{disp}, dispersion energy; and E_{rep}, repulsion term (94). The value of each of these contributions in a series of compounds, as well as the total value (E_{tot}) and the corrected value (E_{corr}) of this interaction energy, is listed in Table 7.8.

Van der Waals forces have a short duration (10^{-6} sec) and, although weaker than others that act in biological systems, they are of the utmost importance in the stabilization of the protein structure, because their interactions are numerically very superior to the interactions of hydrogen bonds and saline

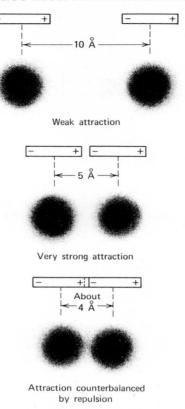

Fig. 7.22. Van der Waals attraction and repulsion forces in relation to electron distribution of monoatomic molecules. [Adapted from (*12*).]

bonds (*95*). Their intensity is given by the following equation:

$$V = \frac{-A}{r^6} + \frac{B}{r^{12}} \tag{IV}$$

where r is the distance that separates the two atomic centers and A and B are constant characteristics of the electronic structure of the atoms (*20*).

Thus the attraction and repulsion forces involved in the drug–receptor interaction by means of van der Waals forces are approximately inversely proportional to the seventh power of the distance between the atoms; that is, by doubling this distance the van der Waals force falls to $\frac{1}{128}$ of its former value (in the same situation a dipole–dipole attraction would be reduced to one-sixteenth and the electrostatic attraction to one-fourth of its initial value) (*13*). In large molecules, such as steroids and fatty acids, the intensity

TABLE 7.7 Van der Waals Radii and Covalent-Bond Radii of Atoms and Groups (*15,20*)

Atom or Group	Van der Waals Radius (Å)	Covalent-Bond Radius (Å)
H	1.2	0.30
O	1.4	0.74[a]
		0.62[b]
S	1.85	—
F	1.35	0.64
Cl	1.80	0.99
Br	1.95	1.14
I	2.15	1.33
C		0.77[a]
		0.67[b]
CH$_3$	2.0	—
P	1.9	1.10
N	1.5	0.74[a]
		0.62[b]
NH$_3$	2.1	
One-half thickness of a benzene ring	1.70	

[a] Single bond.
[b] Double bond.

becomes almost proportional to the fifth power; therefore in these compounds the interaction energy increases substantially. For instance, it was calculated that the interaction energy of two molecules of stearic acid lying parallel to each other and separated by a distance of 4.8 Å is −8 kcal/mole (*96*). Energies of the same magnitude intervene in the complexation between a drug made up of a long hydrocarbon chain or various aromatic rings and a receptor formed by a protein macromolecule (*38*). It is evident, therefore, that van der Waals forces, operating in alkyl chains and aromatic rings, contribute significantly to the drug–receptor bond, reinforcing ionic and dipole interactions, as is indicated by the examples already presented and especially when the drug molecule contains a cavity that is exactly complementary to the salient group on the receptor or vice versa (*12*).

The greater the polarizability of the groups that come close to each other, the greater their interaction, because the maximal forces between the various groups are proportional to the product of their polarizabilities (Table 7.9).

The antiviral activity of some isatin-β-thiosemicarbazone derivatives is related to the van der Waals radii of the substituents in positions 5 and 6 of

TABLE 7.8 Calculated Van der Waals–London Interactions and Experimental Free Energies in Complexes Formed between a Series of Organic Compounds and Tetracyanoethylene (TCNE) (94)

Complex formed with TCNE	Interaction Energy (kcal/mole)						ΔG (kcal/mole)
	E_{el}	E_{pol}	E_{disp}	E_{rep}	E_{tot}	E_{corr}	
Benzene	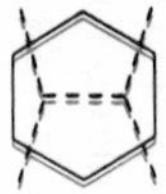 -2.47	-1.35	-3.20	2.23	-4.80	-4.80	$+0.76 \pm 0.12$
Naphthalene	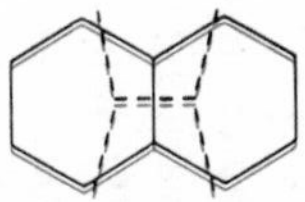 -2.94	-1.76	-4.03	2.70	-6.03	-6.76	-0.02 ± 0.06
Phenanthrene	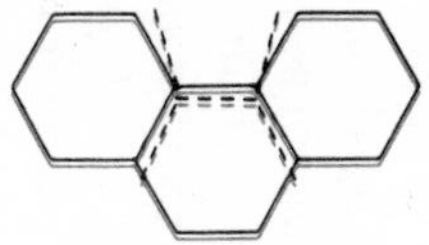 -2.81	-2.18	-4.76	2.98	-6.75	-7.85	-0.46 ± 0.05
Pyrene	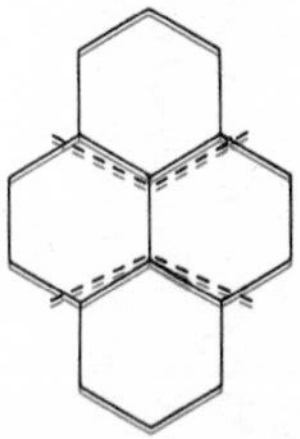 -3.09	-2.45	-5.32	3.62	-7.25	-8.94	-0.61 ± 0.12

Acenaphthalene	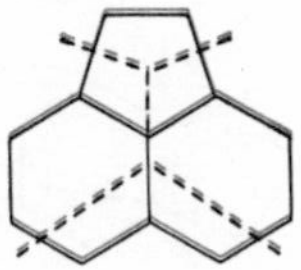 −2.96	−2.07	−4.33	2.96	−6.40	−7.63	−0.62 ± 0.04
Triphenylene	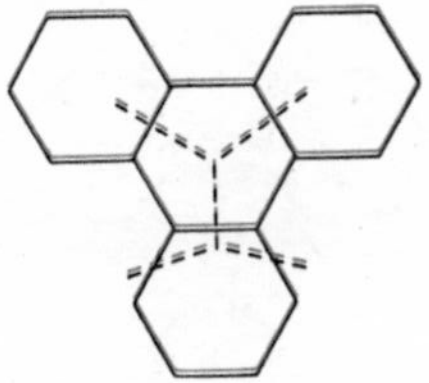 −2.37	−2.80	−5.84	3.55	−7.46	−8.57	−0.75 ± 0.07
Perylene	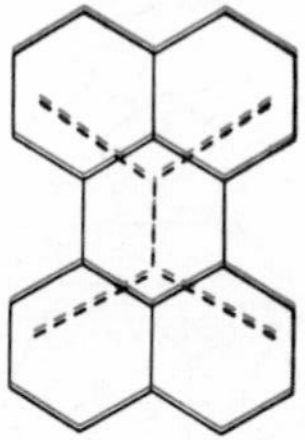 −2.28	−2.71	−5.17	3.49	−6.67	−9.21	−0.83 ± 0.05
3,4-Benzopyrene	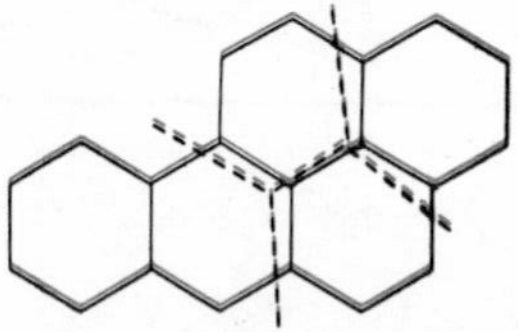 −2.90	−3.03	−6.49	5.28	−7.14	−9.37	−0.97 ± 0.07

TABLE 7.8 (continued)

Complex formed with TCNE		Interaction Energy (kcal/mole)						ΔG (kcal/mole)
		E_{el}	E_{pol}	E_{disp}	E_{rep}	E_{tot}	E_{corr}	
Azulene	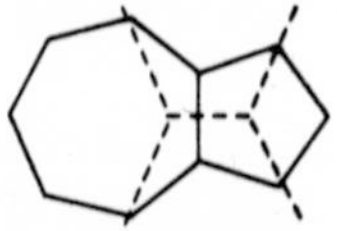	−3.16	−1.80	−3.77	2.90	−5.83	−7.13	−1.59 ± 0.03
Furan	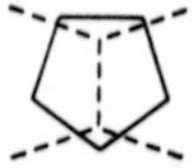	−2.23	−1.29	−2.45	1.73	−4.24	−4.48	0.73 ± 0.02
Thiophene	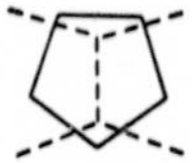	−2.10	−1.91	−3.53	2.24	−5.30	−5.33	0.43 ± 0.02
Dibenzofuran	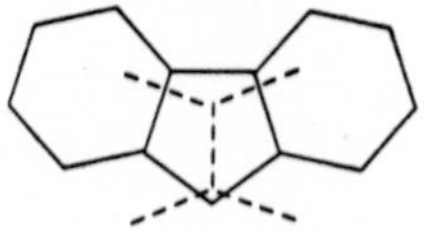	−1.29	−2.00	−4.13	2.64	−4.78	−5.32	−0.03 ± 0.02
Benzofuran	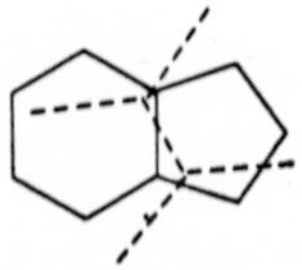	−2.13	−1.76	−3.64	2.48	−5.05	−5.46	−0.04 ± 0.02

Benzothiophene 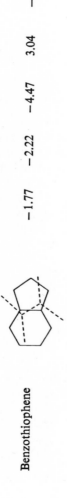	−1.77	−2.22	−4.47	3.04	−5.42	−6.02	−0.04 ± 0.02
Dibenzothiophene	−0.82	−2.61	−5.02	3.21	−5.24	−6.27	−0.17 ± 0.02
Pyrrole	−3.20	−1.71	−2.80	1.87	−5.84	−6.38	—
Indole	−2.65	−2.05	−3.82	2.65	−5.87	−6.70	−0.92 ± 0.03
Carbazole	−2.59	−2.14	−4.33	3.08	−5.98	−6.98	−0.96 ± 0.02

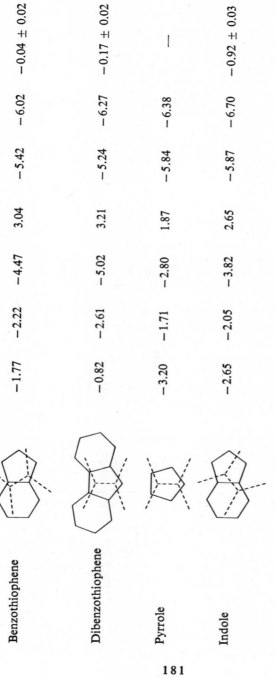

TABLE 7.9 Polarizabilities Relative to Hydrogen for Calculating Relative Van der Waals Forces of the Groups (*15*)

Group	Relative Polarizability
—H	1.0
—F	0.8
—Cl	5.7
—Br	8.5
—I	13.5
—CH$_3$	5.5
—C$_2$H$_5$	10.0
—C$_6$H$_5$	24.8
—C$_{10}$H$_7$	41.7
—C≡N	5.3
—OH	2.5
$\overset{\text{O}}{\underset{\parallel}{—\text{CCH}_3}}$	10.2

the parent molecule. The greater the radius of the substituent element, the smaller will be the biological action of the resultant compound (Table 7.10).

Several other examples might be listed showing that van der Waals forces are present in the interaction of drugs with their receptors (*86,97*).

TABLE 7.10 Relationship of the Van der Waals Radii of Ring-Substituted Isatin-β-thiosemicarbazones to Antivaccinial Activity (*54*)

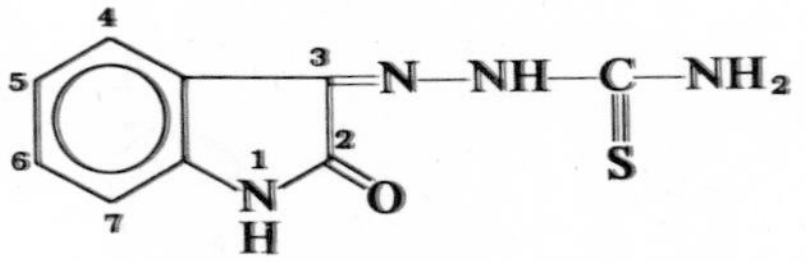

		Relative Activity	
Substituent	Radius (Å)	Position 5	Position 6
—	1.2	100	100
Fluorine	1.35	35.5	43.1
Chlorine	1.80	4.2	11.7
Bromine	1.95	3.1	10.5
Methyl	2.0	0	0.3
Iodine	2.15	0	3.9

Reprinted with permission from the Williams and Wilkins Company

REFERENCES

1. K. J. Brunings, Ed., *Modern Concepts in the Relationships Between Structure and Pharmacological Activity*, Pergamon, Oxford, 1963.
2. J. Büchi, *Grundlagen der Arzneimittelforschung und der synthetischen Arzneimittel*, Birkhauser, Basel, 1963.
3. International Union of Pure and Applied Chemistry and the Italian Society of Pharmaceutical Sciences, *Pharmaceutical Chemistry*, Butterworths, London, 1963.
4. R. S. Schnaare and A. N. Martin, *J. Pharm. Sci.*, **54**, 1707 (1965).
5. L. Pauling, *The Nature of the Chemical Bond*, Cornell University Press, Ithaca, N.Y., 1960.
6. J. O. Hirschfelder, Ed., *Advan. Chem. Phys.*, **12**, 1–630 (1967).
7. Pontificiae Academiae Scientiarum Scripta Varia, *Study Week on Molecular Forces*, North-Holland, Amsterdam, and Wiley, New York, 1967.
8. B. Pullman, Ed., *Molecular Associations in Biology*, Academic, New York, 1968.
9. C. B. Anfinsen, *The Molecular Basis of Evolution*, Wiley, New York, 1959.
10. W. Kauzmann, *Advan. Protein Chem.*, **14**, 1 (1959).
11. G. Némethy, *Ann. N.Y. Acad. Sci.*, **155**, 492 (1969).
12. J. D. Watson, *Molecular Biology of the Gene*, Benjamin, New York, 1965.
13. A. Albert, *Selective Toxicity*, 3rd ed., Wiley, New York, 1965.
14. A. L. Lehninger, *Bioenergetics*, Benjamin, New York, 1965.
15. D. Pressman and A. L. Grossberg, *The Structural Basis of Antibody Specificity*, Benjamin, New York, 1968.
16. O. Reutov, *Theoretical Principles of Organic Chemistry*, Mir Publishers, Moscow, 1967.
17. D. F. Heath, *Organophosphorus Poisons*, Pergamon, New York, 1961.
18. J. M. van Rossum, "Receptor Theory in Enzymology," in E. J. Ariëns, Ed., *Molecular Pharmacology*, Vol. II, Academic, New York, 1964, pp. 199–255.
19. K. D. Kopple, *Peptides and Amino Acids*, Benjamin, New York, 1966.
20. S. A. Bernhard, *The Structure and Function of Enzymes*, Benjamin, New York, 1968.
21. J. M. van Rossum, *Advan. Drug Res.*, **3**, 189 (1966).
22. O. Gisvold, "Cholinergic Agents and Related Drugs," in C. O. Wilson, O. Gisvold, and R. F. Doerge, Eds., *Textbook of Organic Medicinal and Pharmaceutical Chemistry*, 5th ed., Lippincott, Philadelphia, 1966, pp. 453–467.
23. J. M. Sprague, *Topics Med. Chem.*, **2**, 1 (1968).
24. H. P. Burchfield and E. E. Storrs, "Electronic and Steric Aspects of Fungicidal Action," in D. C. Torgeson, Ed., *Fungicides*, Vol. II, Academic, New York, 1969, pp. 61–100.
25. J. L. Strominger and D. J. Tipper, *Am. J. Med.*, **39**, 708 (1965).
26. E. Rauenbusch, *Antibiot. Chemother.*, *(Basel)*, **14**, 95 (1968).
27. G. P. Warwick, *Rev. Pure Appl. Chem.*, **18**, 245 (1968).
28. V. N. Iyer and W. Szybalski, *Science*, **145**, 55 (1964).
29. P. D. Bartlett, S. D. Ross, and C. G. Swain, *J. Am. Chem. Soc.*, **69**, 2971 (1947); *ibid.*, **71**, 1415 (1949).
30. N. B. Chapman and D. J. Triggle, *J. Chem. Soc.*, 1385 (1963).
31. B. Belleau, *J. Med. Pharm. Chem.*, **1**, 327 (1959).

32. B. R. Baker, *Design of Active-Site-Directed Irreversible Enzyme Inhibitors*, Wiley, New York, 1967.
33. B. R. Baker, *J. Pharm. Sci.*, **53**, 347 (1964).
34. B. R. Baker, *Biochem. Pharmacol.*, **11**, 1155 (1962).
35. B. R. Baker, G. J. Lourens, R. B. Meyer, Jr. et al., *J. Med. Chem.*, **11**, 26, 34, 38, 475, 483, 486, 489, 495, 666, 672, 677 (1968); *ibid.*, **12**, 224, 668, 672, 680, 684 (1969).
36. B. R. Baker and J. A. Hurlbut, *J. Med. Chem.*, **11**, 233, 241 (1968).
37. B. R. Baker, W. F. Wood, and J. A. Kozma, *J. Med. Chem.*, **11**, 644, 650, 652, 656, 661 (1968); *ibid.*, **12**, 211, 214 (1969).
38. E. W. Gill, *Progr. Med. Chem.*, **4**, 39 (1965).
39. J. Büchi and X. Perlia, *Arzneimittel-Forsch.*, **10**, 1 (1960).
40. J. Büchi and X. Perlia, *Farmaco, (Pavia), Ed. Sci.*, **18**, 197 (1963).
41. J. M. Ritchie and P. Greengard, *Ann. Rev. Pharmacol.*, **6**, 405 (1966).
42. J. Büchi, K. Müller, X. Perlia, and M. A. Preiswerk, *Arzneimittel-Forsch.*, **16**, 1263 (1966).
43. W. C. Bowman, H. J. Rand, and G. B. West, *Textbook of Pharmacology*, Blackwell, Oxford, 1968.
44. G. C. Pimentel and A. L. McClellan, *The Hydrogen Bond*, Freeman, San Francisco, 1960.
45. N. D. Sokolov, *Ann. Chim.*, **10**, 497 (1965).
46. W. C. Hamilton and J. A. Ibers, *Hydrogen Bonding in Solids*, Benjamin, New York, 1968.
47. R. Srinivasan and K. K. Chacko, "Hydrogen Bonds Involving Sulphur," in G. N. Ramachandran, Ed., *Conformation of Biopolymers*, Vol. II, Academic, New York, 1967, pp. 607–615.
48. G. A. Sim, *Ann. Rev. Phys. Chem.*, **18**, 57 (1967).
49. W. C. Hamilton, "On Hydrogen Bonding in Inorganic Crystals: Some Generalizations, Some Recent Results, and Some New Techniques," in A. Rich and N. Davidson, Eds., *Structural Chemistry and Molecular Biology*, Freeman, San Francisco, 1968, pp. 466–483.
50. J. Donohue, "Selected Topics in Hydrogen Bonding," in A. Rich and N. Davidson, Eds., *Structural Chemistry and Molecular Biology*, Freeman, San Francisco, 1968, pp. 443–465.
51. B. M. Craven and W. J. Takei, *Acta Cryst.*, **17**, 415 (1964).
52. J. Gaultier and C. Hauw, *Acta Cryst.*, **B25**, 546 (1969).
53. T. C. Daniels and E. C. Jorgensen, "Physicochemical Properties in Relation to Biologic Action," in C. O. Wilson, O. Gisvold, and R. F. Doerge, Eds., *Textbook of Organic Medicinal and Pharmaceutical Chemistry*, 5th ed., Lippincott, Philadelphia, 1966, pp. 4–62.
54. P. W. Sadler, *Pharmacol. Rev.*, **15**, 407 (1963).
55. M. Sax and J. Pletcher, *Science*, **166**, 1546 (1969).
56. A. Cammarata and R. L. Stein, *J. Med. Chem.*, **11**, 829 (1968).
57. C. H. Jarboe, L. A. Porter, and R. T. Buckler, *J. Med. Chem.*, **11**, 729 (1968).
58. L. J. Andrews and R. M. Keefer, *Molecular Complexes in Organic Chemistry*, Holden-Day, San Francisco, 1964.
59. J. Rose, *Molecular Complexes*, Pergamon, Oxford, 1967.

60. E. N. Gur'yanova, *Russian Chem. Rev.* (Engl. Trans.), **37**, 863 (1968).

61. E. M. Kosower, *Molecular Biochemistry*, McGraw-Hill, New York, 1962.

62. T. C. Bruice and S. J. Benkovic, *Bioorganic Mechanisms*, Vol. II, Benjamin, New York, 1966.

63. P. Millié, J. P. Malrieu, J. Benaim, J. Y. Lallemand, and M. Julia, *J. Med. Chem.*, **11**, 207 (1968).

64. G. Cilento and K. Zinner, *Biochim. Biophys. Acta*, **120**, 84 (1966); **143**, 88 (1967).

65. G. Cilento and K. Zinner, *Biochim. Biophys. Acta*, **143**, 93 (1967).

66. G. Cilento and K. Zinner, *Arch. Biochem. Biophys.*, **120**, 244 (1967).

67. G. Cilento and D. L. Sanioto, *Arch. Biochem. Biophys.*, **110**, 133 (1965).

68. G. Cilento and D. L. Sanioto, *Ber. Bunsenges. Phys. Chem.*, **67**, 426 (1963).

69. F. E. Hahn, R. L. O'Brien, J. Ciak, J. L. Allison, and J. G. Olenick, *Mil. Med.*, Suppl. 9, **131**, 1071 (1966). For corroboration see also recent papers: K. Van Dyke, C. Szustkiewicz, C. H. Lantz, and L. H. Saxe, *Biochem. Pharmacol.*, **18**, 1417 (1969); H. Sternglanz, K. L. Yielding, and K. M. Pruitt, *Mol. Pharmacol.*, **5**, 376 (1969).

70. W. Perkow, *Arzneimittel-Forsch.*, **16**, 1287 (1966).

71. S. Shifrin, *Biochemistry*, **3**, 829 (1964).

72. S. Shifrin, "Charge-Transfer Complexes in Enzyme-Coenzyme Models," in B. Pullman, Ed., *Molecular Associations in Biology*, Academic, New York, 1968, pp. 323–341.

73. S. H. Snyder and C. R. Merril, *Proc. Natl. Acad. Sci., U.S.*, **54**, 258 (1965).

74. N. W. Gabel and L. G. Abood, *J. Med. Chem.*, **8**, 616 (1965).

75. T. Nogrady and A. A. Algieri, *J. Med. Chem.*, **11**, 212 (1968).

76. A. G. Szent-Györgyi, *Introduction to a Submolecular Biology*, Academic, New York, 1960.

77. E. M. Kosower, *Progr. Phys. Org. Chem.*, **3**, 81 (1965).

78. F. J. Bullock, "Charge Transfer in Biology," in M. Florkin and E. H. Stotz, Eds., *Comprehensive Biochemistry*, Vol. 22, Elsevier, Amsterdam, 1967, pp. 81–165.

79. G. Karreman, I. Isenberg, and A. Szent-Györgyi, *Science*, **130**, 1191 (1959).

80. B. R. Baker, P. M. Tanna, and G. D. F. Jackson, *J. Pharm. Sci.*, **54**, 987 (1965).

81. H. S. Frank and M. W. Evans, *J. Chem. Phys.*, **13**, 507 (1945).

82. R. Breslow, *Organic Reaction Mechanisms*, 2nd ed., Benjamin, New York, 1969.

83. G. Némethy, *Angew. Chem., Intern. Ed.*, **6**, 195 (1967).

84. O. Sinanoğlu, "Solvent Effects on Molecular Associations," in B. Pullman, Ed., *Molecular Associations in Biology*, Academic, New York, 1968, pp. 427–445.

85. G. Némethy and H. A. Scheraga, *J. Phys. Chem.*, **66**, 1773 (1962); *ibid.*, **67**, 2888 (1963).

86. B. Belleau and G. Lacasse, *J. Med. Chem.*, **7**, 768 (1964).

87. B. Belleau, *Advan. Drug Res.*, **2**, 89 (1965).

88. H. A. Scheraga, R. A. Scott, G. Vanderkooi, S. J. Leach, K. D. Gibson, T. Ooi, and G. Némethy, "Calculations of Polypeptide Structures from Amino Acid Sequence," in G. N. Ramachandran, Ed., *Conformation of Biopolymers*, Vol. I, Academic, New York, 1967, pp. 43–60.

89. K. D. Gibson and H. A. Scheraga, *Proc. Natl. Acad. Sci. U.S.*, **58**, 420 (1967).

90. B. R. Baker, *J. Chem. Educ.*, **44**, 610 (1967).

91. B. R. Baker, *J. Pharm. Sci.*, **56**, 959 (1967).

92. L. Pauling, *General Chemistry*, Freeman, San Francisco, 1947.
93. A. Bondi, *J. Phys. Chem.*, **68**, 441 (1964).
94. M. J. Mantione, "Les forces de van der Waals-London dans les complexes dits de transfert de charge," in B. Pullman, Ed., *Molecular Associations in Biology*, Academic, New York, 1968, pp. 411–426.
95. H. G. Mautner, *Pharmacol. Rev.*, **19**, 107 (1967).
96. L. Salem, *Nature*, **193**, 476 (1962).
97. P. Claverie, B. Pullman, and J. Caillet, *J. Theoret. Biol.*, **12**, 419 (1966).

CHAPTER

8

TOPOGRAPHY OF
RECEPTORS

Although it is possible to interpret the actions of drugs at receptors without considering these as more than hypothetical structures, it is natural to consider what such structures may be and what they may do, especially as any information about this should lead to a fuller understanding of the mode of action of drugs.

R. B. Barlow

I. ATTEMPTS TO DETERMINE RECEPTOR TOPOGRAPHY

In order to facilitate the understanding of ways in which drug–receptor interactions occur constant attempts are being made to determine the topography of certain receptors (*1–8*). Among the methods used, the outstanding ones are covalent labeling (*6,7,9–12*), the use of antimetabolites (*13*), and experiments with substances of rigid structure shaped so that they will fit well into the hypothetical receptor sites (*13–17*). The purpose of these researches is either to identify and isolate directly the receptor or deduce indirectly its topography from biological effects produced by drugs; that is, based on the relationship between structure and mode of action (*5,7*).

Analogous attempts have been made with the aim of identifying the active site and the mechanism of action of some enzymes (*18–20*) through the application of several techniques, including the use of nuclear-magnetic-resonance spectroscopy, which is also employed in studies of drug binding sites (*21–25*).

Obviously the maps obtained in this way—with their surface contour, charge distribution, and, in some cases, even the presence of certain chemical groups—are only hypothetical and subject to periodic alteration as new knowledge is acquired on this very complex and as yet insufficiently studied area (*7,26*).

For illustration this chapter presents some examples of receptor maps, without going into details, which can be found in the cited literature.

II. RECEPTORS OF ANALGETICS

Taking into consideration that analgetics derived from, or analogous to, morphine have in common the N-methyl-γ-phenylpiperidino moiety, Beckett

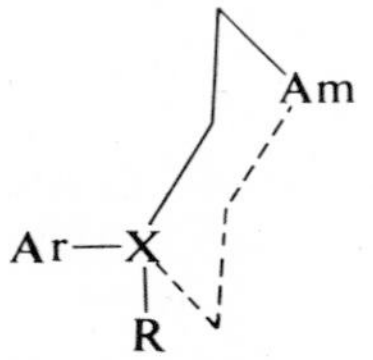

and Casy (*27–30*) proposed the receptor topography shown in Figure 8.1. There three sites are essential:

1. A flat structure that allows a linkage with the aromatic ring of the drug through van der Waals–type forces.

2. An anionic site able to associate with the positively charged basic center of the drug.

3. A suitably oriented cavity in order to accommodate the —CH_2CH_2— portion (relative to carbons 15 and 16) projecting from the piperidine ring that lies in front of the plane containing the aromatic ring and the basic center (*28*).

It was found that the configuration of morphine arbitrarily chosen as the basis for an original receptor diagram actually represents (+)-morphine and not (−)-morphine (*29,30*), which is the natural isomer. The absolute configuration of (−)-morphine has been recently elucidated (Figure 8.2).

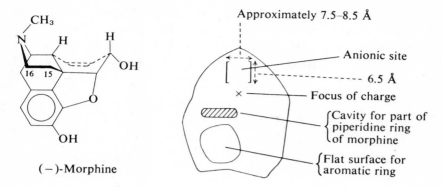

Approximately 7.5–8.5 Å

Anionic site

6.5 Å

Focus of charge

Cavity for part of piperidine ring of morphine

Flat surface for aromatic ring

(−)-Morphine

Fig. 8.1. Receptor site of analgetics derived from, and analogous to, morphine (*30*). (Reprinted with permission of the Editor.)

Synthetic analgetics that are analogous in action to morphine have a much simpler structure (*32–37*). Their general structure can be represented by the formula

$$Am—C_nH_{2n}—X—Ar$$
$$\underset{R}{|}$$

where the basic amine function (Am), usually tertiary, is linked to a central highly substituted atom (X) through a hydrocarbon chain, generally consisting of two carbon atoms (*38*). Several synthetic analgetics have in common the N-methyl-γ-phenylpiperidino moiety. Others which do not contain it are capable of assuming a conformation in which a part of the molecule resembles that moiety. Synthetic analgetics are found among derivatives of 4-phenylpiperidine (families of meperidine, prodine, ethoptazine, prodilidine, and others), of diphenylpropylamine (families of methadone, dimepheptanol, dextromoramide, and others), of dithienylbutenylamine

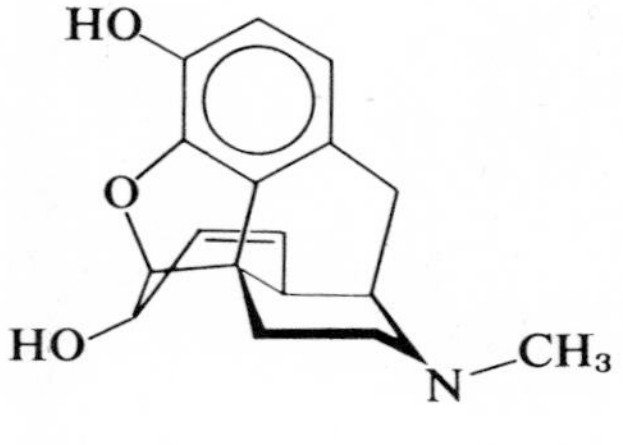

HO

O

HO   N—CH₃

Fig. 8.2. Absolute configuration of (−)-morphine (*31*).

(family of thiambutene), of 3-phenyl-3-acyloxybutylamine (propoxyphene type), and analogous nitrogenous derivatives (phenampromid type). Morphine's opioid antagonists have the same general structure (*39*):

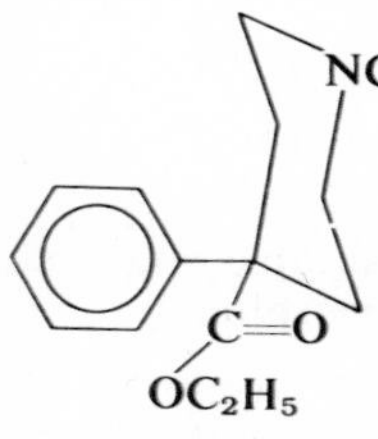

Meperidine 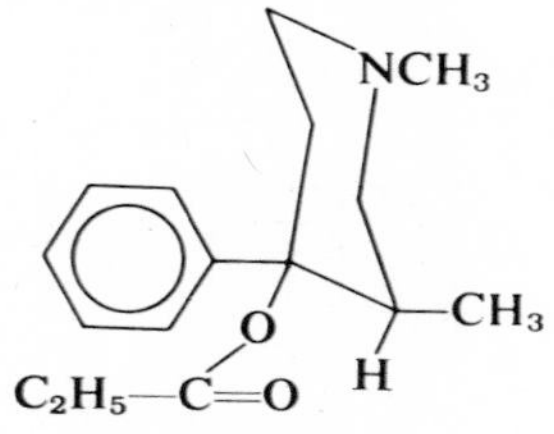   Prodine 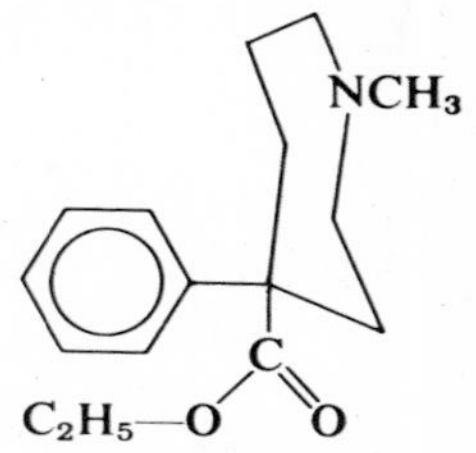   Ethoheptazine

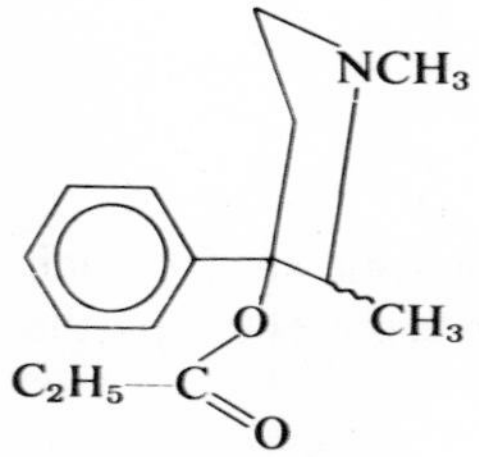

Prodilidine 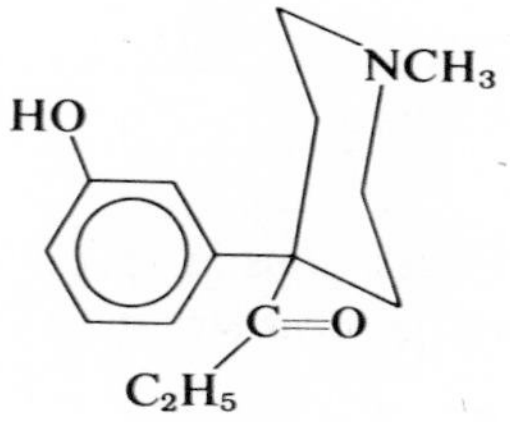   Ketobemidone 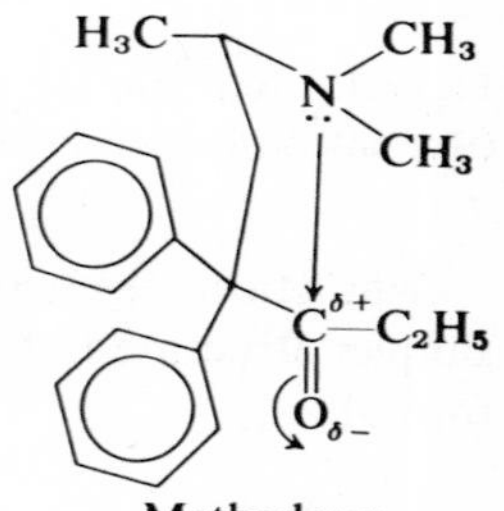   Methadone

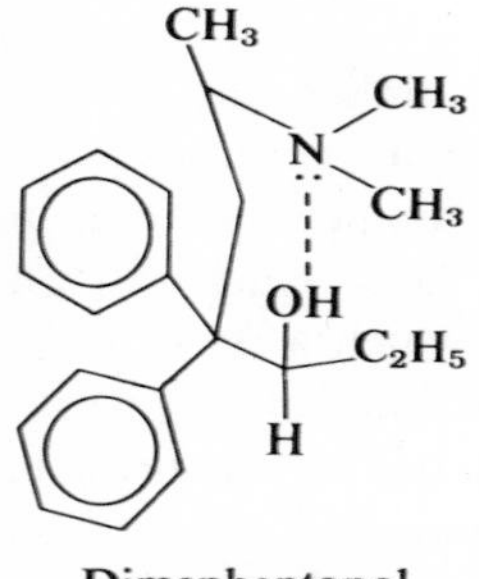

Dimepheptanol 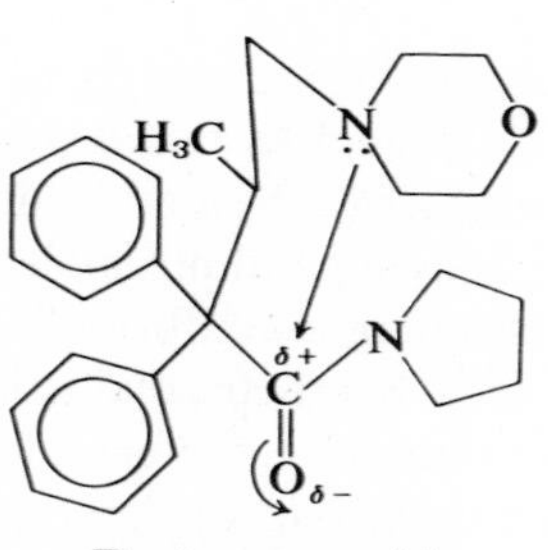   Dextromoramide 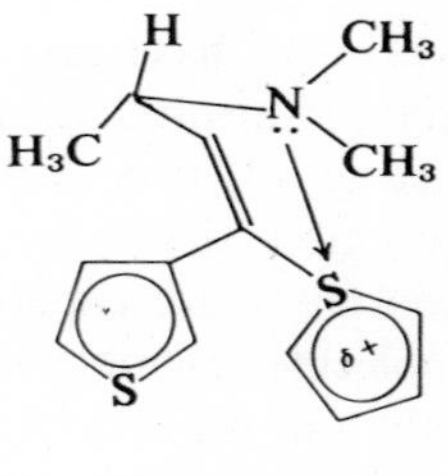   Dimethylthiambutene

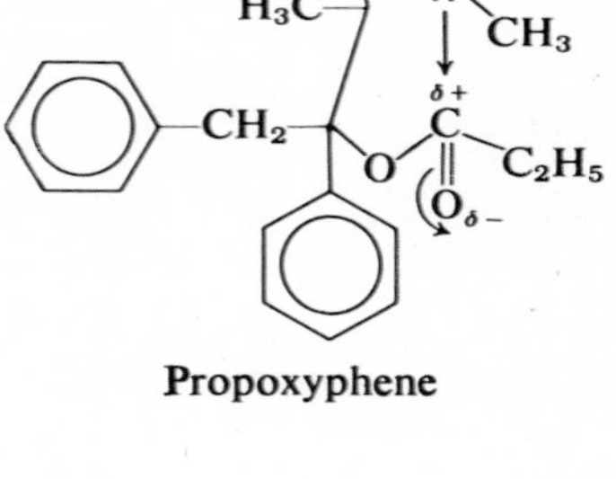

Propoxyphene 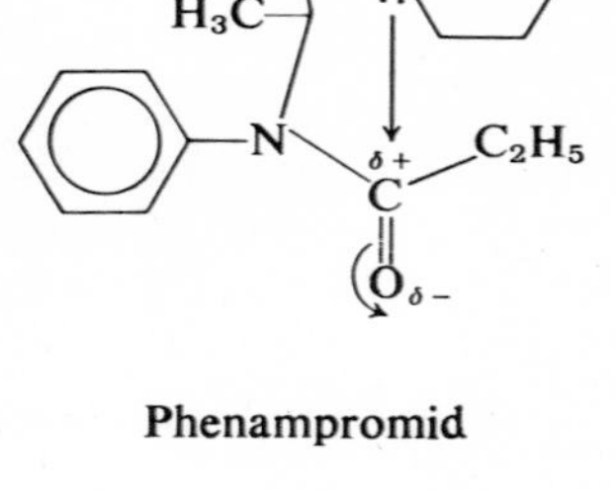   Phenampromid

Following research on methadone asymmetry (40) and methadol stereochemistry (41,42) done by other authors, Casy and Hassan (43) produced evidence for hydrogen-bond formation in some tertiary amino alcohols related to methadone, which would compel them to adopt the conformation of the characteristic general structure of analgetics.

First, it was suggested that for obtaining analgetic action in these morphine-like compounds the preferred conformation of the phenyl group was axial (28). However, later on, in structurally related isomers it was observed that analgetic activity was the same whether the phenyl position was axial or equatorial (44), and that some of them may even exist in both conformations, as is the case of trimeperidine. In fact it was shown that no definite conformation of the phenyl group is necessary for analgetic action (34,45, 46).

The attractive hypothesis of Beckett and Casy, which admits an essentially inflexible receptor site, had to be modified when it was found that certain analgetics, although possessing high activity, did not present an exactly complementary structure to the proposed receptor area. For this and other reasons and on the basis of the fact that macromolecules may undergo conformational changes (47–53), Portoghese (54,55) postulated that the formation of different complexes of narcotic analgetics with receptors can, in many cases, involve different modes of interaction instead of only one type of drug–receptor complexation.

The same author acknowledged also the possibility of an induced fit, a theory proposed by Koshland (47,56), which is discussed in Chapter 9, as a contributing factor to the binding of the receptor to different analgetics. In summary, he assumed that there may exist three different interactions between receptor and analgetic:

1. Interaction of different analgetics with a single species of receptors: (a) identical interaction; (b) differing interaction.

2. Interaction of different analgetics with two or more species of receptors common to the different analgetics: (a) identical partitioning on the receptors by different analgetics; (b) dissimilar partitioning on the receptors by different analgetics.

3. Interaction of different analgetics with two or more species of receptors not common to the different analgetics.

It is quite possible, according to Portoghese, that cases 1 and 2 are the predominant types of interaction. Case 1(b) is represented in Figure 8.3. However, the lack of consistency in analgetic activity–structure relationship did not permit the determination of the exact topography of analgetic receptors (54).

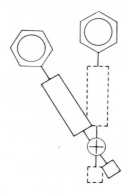

Fig. 8.3. The protonated amine nitrogen is represented by ⊕, the square denotes an *N*-substituent, and the rectangle depicts another portion of the molecule. The different positions of molecular binding are shown by the heavy and dashed lines (*54*). (Reprinted by permission of the American Chemical Society and of the author.)

However, after considering that the more active enantiomers of the methadone family have a configuration opposite to that which would fit better into the hypothetical receptor envisioned by Beckett and Casy, Portoghese postulated that the interaction of analgetics with receptors would occur as represented schematically in Figure 8.4. The dipoles that these narcotics develop may attach to the receptor by hydrogen bonding, either donating a proton (*X*) or accepting one (*Y*).

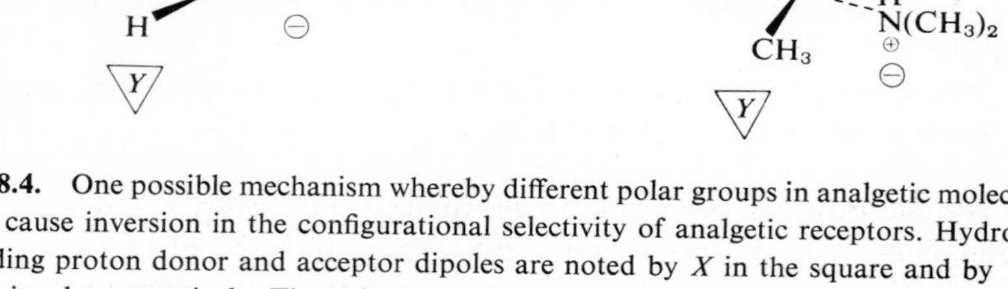

Fig. 8.4. One possible mechanism whereby different polar groups in analgetic molecules may cause inversion in the configurational selectivity of analgetic receptors. Hydrogen bonding proton donor and acceptor dipoles are noted by *X* in the square and by *Y* in the triangle, respectively. The anionic site is represented by ⊖. Left: 3S : 6S-methadol; right: R-methadone (*54*). (Reprinted by permission of the American Chemical Society and of the author.)

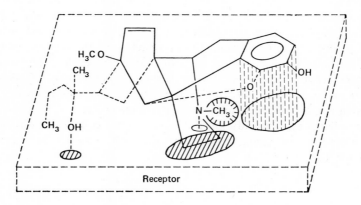

Studies by Bentley and co-workers (57) with the 6,14-endoethenotetra-hydrothebaine series, which is analogous to oripavine, indicate that in general, by maintaining R and R″ constant, the analgetic activity increases progressively when the side chain R′ increases in the following order: H, CH_3, C_2H_5, C_3H_7. The compound in which R is H, R′ is n-Pr, and R″ is CH_3 and in which the double bond C_{17}—C_{18} has been saturated, is 12,000 times more active than morphine. The substitution on nitrogen by groups usually associated with narcotic antagonism (allyl, cyclopropylmethyl) results in compounds with antagonistic activity only where R′ is H, CH_3, or C_2H_5. The most potent analgetic antagonists are found in the phenol series; that is, when R is H. Reduction of the 6,14-ethene bridge brings about only slight alterations in their activity, may it be analgetic or antagonistic. A reversal of the stereochemistry at C-19, even though not thoroughly studied, showed that a variation of the alkyl group R′ does not affect analgetic action; the absence of the alcoholic group, however, decreases it strongly. It may be inferred therefore that the alcoholic group is also involved in the attachment between the analgetic substance and the receptor surface (58). Based on these studies Bentley and his colleagues concluded that several of their compounds, although possessing a much greater analgetic action than morphine,

Fig. 8.5. A more general hypothetical receptor region of analgetics (58).

would not be more acceptable than morphine at the receptor surface represented by Beckett and Casy. One very attractive hypothesis advanced to explain the high activity of these compounds is that they would have additional bond sites with the receptor surface. By analogy to what is admitted to happen with epinephrine and similar compounds, an additional bond could form with the alcoholic hydroxyl at C-19. The receptor site that, according to Harris and Dewey (58), would accommodate practically all known analgetics, is represented in Figure 8.5.

In experiments carried out with two isomers of 2-methyl-5-phenyl-5-carbethoxy-2-azabicyclo[2.2.1]heptane, diastereomers analogous to meperidine but of rigid conformation, Portoghese and co-workers (34) showed that the *endo* isomer is about 3.7 times more active than the *exo* isomer, and they found a direct relationship between the concentration level of these two compounds in the brain and their liposolubility.

2-Methyl-5-*exo*-phenyl-5-
carbethoxy-2-azabicyclo-
[2.2.1]heptane

2-Methyl-5-*endo*-phenyl-5-
carbethoxy-2-azabicyclo-
[2.2.1]heptane

They came to the conclusion that in analgetics analogous to meperidine the conformational requirement is low, which might be due to different modes of interaction with receptors of analgetics. The apparent lack of conformational specificity in these two compounds studied—which might not be narcotic analgetics—does not necessarily imply that the same happens with highly potent analgetics. In fact the most active of the 4-phenylpiperidino derivatives are the ones in which the aromatic and piperidine rings approach coplanarity (35). Portoghese's studies stressed the importance of taking into account not only *structural features* but also *physical characteristics* in the interpretation of biological activities of diastereoisomers.

From all the facts already known about analgetics it seems obvious that the concept of an analgetic receptor site will have to be reevaluated completely (8).

III. RECEPTORS OF ANTI-INFLAMMATORY AGENTS

Among the various anti-inflammatory agents used in therapeutics (59) indomethacin is one of the most modern and efficient ones. This is the reason why it has been so thoroughly studied, even to the extent of establishing the relationship between its chemical structure and biological activity. Attempts were also made to determine the topography of its hypothetical receptor site. With this objective in mind researchers have tried to establish the configuration and preferred conformation of indomethacin and its derivatives. Of all α-methyl analogs of indomethacin studied, only the dextrorotatory enantiomers showed anti-inflammatory and antipyretic actions. Further, it seems that the preferred conformation of the *p*-chlorophenyl moiety is the *cis* position in relation to the methoxyphenyl moiety of the indole ring.

The study of the stereochemistry of indenylic isosteres of indomethacin provided new elements to postulate a receptor-surface topography. Thus, by resorting to physical analyses—such as nuclear magnetic resonance, X-ray diffraction, ultraviolet absorption—, confirmed by isomerization experiments, it was concluded that, of the geometrical isomers of 1-*p*-chlorobenzylidene-5-methoxy-2-methyl-3-indenylacetic acid the one that showed greater activity had a *p*-chlorobenzylidine moiety in the *cis* position in relation to the methoxyphenyl moiety. Likewise, due to steric hindrance by the proton at C-7 of the indene ring, the *p*-chlorophenyl moiety is compelled to project itself out of the plane.

Thus, by taking into account the conformation of indomethacin and its derivatives, for analogs of this anti-inflammatory drug Shen (60) proposed the receptor site shown in Figure 8.6.

On the other hand, on the basis of the interatomic distances of some anti-inflammatory agents and inflammagenic amines, it was recently postulated that both groups of drugs might act on common receptors (see Section XII in this chapter).

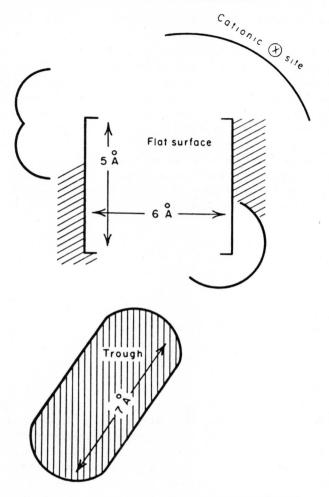

Fig. 8.6. Receptor-site contour for indomethacin analogs (60).

IV. RECEPTORS OF LOCAL ANESTHETICS

With reference to this type of receptor, comments and some illustrations can be found in Chapter 5, Section IV, and Chapter 7, Section III.

Based on recent experiments, Thyrum and co-workers (*61*) advanced the hypothesis that local anesthesia results from an interaction between local anesthetics and thiamine. Thus, according to these authors, procaine interacts with thiamine pyrophosphate (TPP) to form a complex, as represented below:

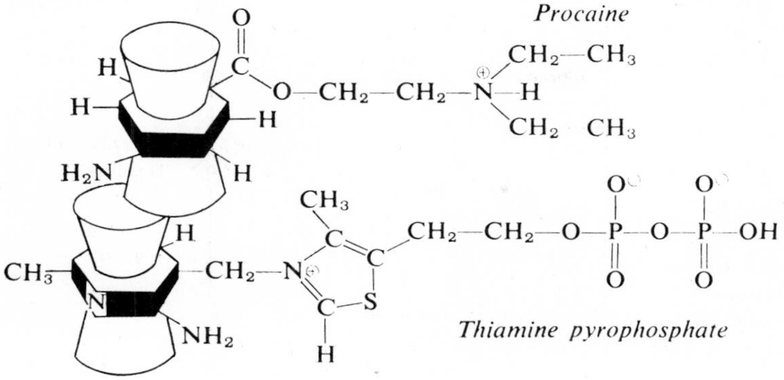

By interacting with membrane macromolecules, the procaine–TPP complex causes alterations in cell-membrane diffusion properties leading to local anesthesia.

For details on mechanism of action of local anesthetics the reader is referred elsewhere (*62,63*).

V. CHOLINERGIC RECEPTORS

For a better understanding of the sections dealing with cholinergic and adrenergic receptors, it is necessary to review briefly what occurs in the autonomic nervous system (*64*). This system regulates the visceral functions of the organism and has central and peripheral parts. The peripheral portion, in which we are interested, is represented in Figure 8.7. The two portions of the autonomic nervous system, known as sympathetic and parasympathetic, are different anatomically, physiologically, and pharmacologically. When stimulated, they liberate at their synapses the so-called chemical mediators. Owing to their endogenous origin and chemical structure, these mediators are called biogenic amines: acetylcholine is liberated by the cholinergic nerves, and epinephrine and norepinephrine by the adrenergic nerves. The effects they produce may be parallel or opposite (Table 8.1).

Drugs that mimic the action of acetylcholine are called parasympathomimetics. Drugs that mimic the action of epinephrine and norepinephrine are called sympathomimetics. Inhibitors of the actions of biogenic amines receive the names of cholinergic blocking agents and adrenergic blocking agents, respectively.

The transmission of the nervous impulse occurs with a variation of the

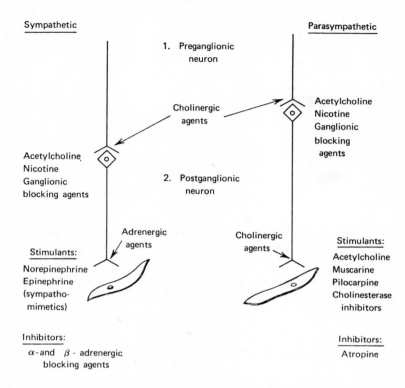

Fig. 8.7. Schematic representation of peripheral efferent vegetative system, with synapses, chemical mediators, and stimulant and inhibitory drugs (65).

TABLE 8.1   Actions of the Autonomic Nerves on Various Effectors (3)

Effector	Response to Sympathetic Nerves	Response to Parasympathetic Nerves	Nature of Responses
Eye:			
Pupil	Dilation	Constriction	Opposed
Iris:			
Radial muscles	Contraction		
Circular muscles		Contraction	
Accommodation		Near vision	
Ciliary muscle		Contraction	

TABLE 8.1 *(continued)*

Tarsal muscle	Contraction		
Orbital muscle	Contraction		
Nictitating membrane (cat, etc.)	Contraction		
Glands:			
Sweat	Secretion[a]		
Salivary	Secretion	Secretion	Parallel
Lacrimal		Secretion	
Respiratory tract		Secretion	
Gastrointestinal tract		Secretion	
Piloerectors	Contraction		
Bronchioles	Relaxation	Contraction	Opposed
Heart:			
Sinus nodal rhythm	Acceleration	Slowing	Opposed
AV node refractory period	Reduced	Increased	Opposed
Atrial conduction rate	Increased	Increased	Parallel
Atrial contraction force	Increased	Decreased	Opposed
Ventricular contraction force	Increased	Decreased (?)	Opposed
Blood vessels:			
Muscle	Dilation		
Coronary	Dilation	Constriction	Opposed
Skin	Constriction		
Viscera	Constriction		
Salivary gland	Constriction	Dilation	Opposed
Erectile tissue	Constriction	Dilation	Opposed
Gastrointestinal tract:			
Muscle wall	Relaxation	Contraction	Opposed
Sphincters:	Contraction	Relaxation	Opposed
Cardiac		Relaxation[b]	
Ileocecal	Contraction		
Spleen	Contraction		
Urinary bladder:			
Fundus	Relaxation	Contraction	Opposed
Trigone and sphincter	Contraction	Relaxation	Opposed
Uterus:			
Nonpregnant			
Cat	Relaxation		
Human	Contraction		
Pregnant	Contraction		
Liver	Glycogenolysis		

[a] Cholinergic fibers.
[b] Adrenergic fibers.

Reproduced by permission of McGraw-Hill Book Company.

action potential—that is, alteration of electric charge—which can be recorded by means of suitable instruments. This action potential derives from the movement of ions in and out of the interior of the nerve-fiber membrane.

In the resting state the membrane has a much greater permeability to potassium and chloride ions than to sodium ions. When the distribution of ions inside and outside the membrane is unequal, the membrane is said to be polarized. Its action potential, which then has a negative value, depends on the extracellular concentration of potassium and chloride ions. In this state the chemical mediators are liberated in the synapses slowly but continuously, in general in an amount insufficient to cause initiation of a propagated impulse (Figure 8.8).

During the rising phase of the action potential, the membrane becomes more permeable to sodium ions than to potassium ions. With the entry of sodium ions the nerve-fiber membrane becomes positively charged in relation to the environment—the membrane is then said to be depolarized. This depolarization is a consequence of the sudden liberation of a great quantity of chemical mediators in the synapses.

At the falling phase of the action potential the membrane has a greater

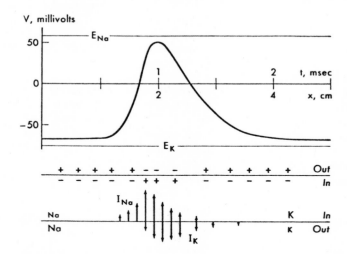

Fig. 8.8. Descriptions of an impulse in a squid axon propagating to the left as a function of time t at one point or distance x at one time. At rest (left) the potential (top) is near the potassium potential E_K, there is a deficit of positive charges inside the axon (center) and the ion currents (bottom) are negligible. The increase in potential as the impulse approaches allows an inward sodium current I_{Na}, which further increases V and I_{Na}. As the potential approaches E_{Na}, I_{Na} decreases, I_K increases until, after the peak of the spike, the outward I_K dominates to return V to the rest potential (66). (Reprinted by permission of the Regents of the University of California.)

permeability to potassium ions and lesser permeability to sodium ions. The membrane returns to the polarized state and assumes again a negative value. The chemical mediators are again liberated, slowly but continuously.

The various phases of movements of ions across the membrane of the nerve fiber are represented in Figure 8.9.

Cholinergic agents are drugs that act on the effector cells, producing effects

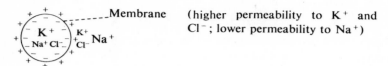 _____Membrane   (higher permeability to K^+ and Cl^-; lower permeability to Na^+)

Resting phase

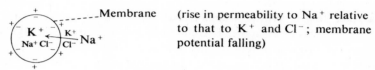 _____Membrane   (rise in permeability to Na^+ relative to that to K^+ and Cl^-; membrane potential falling)

Early rising phase of nerve action potential

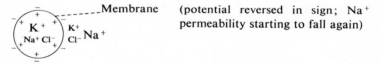 _____Membrane   (potential reversed in sign; Na^+ permeability starting to fall again)

Peak of action potential

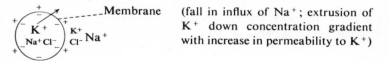 _____Membrane   (fall in influx of Na^+; extrusion of K^+ down concentration gradient with increase in permeability to K^+)

Decline of action potential

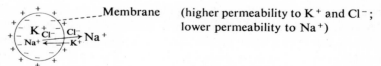 _____Membrane   (higher permeability to K^+ and Cl^-; lower permeability to Na^+)

Completion of return to resting phase (refractory)

Fig. 8.9. The movement of ions across the nerve-fiber membrane during the passage of a nerve impulse. The extracellular concentration of sodium is greater than that in the cells; the converse is true for potassium (67).

similar to those brought about by acetylcholine. According to their mode of action, they can be classified as follows:

1. Direct cholinergic agents—those that, due to their structural similarity with acetylcholine, exert an analogous action to that of this chemical mediator.

2. Indirect cholinergic agents—those that inhibit the action of cholinesterase; in this way they prevent this enzyme from hydrolyzing acetylcholine, which as a consequence will accumulate.

More details on this matter can be found elsewhere (68–70).

Acetylcholine produces two types of effects: nicotinic and muscarinic. The nicotinic effects are analogous to those produced by nicotine; that is, on ganglia and the motor plate. These effects are blocked by tetraethylammonium ions. The muscarinic effects are similar to those produced by muscarine and pilocarpine—that is, on the postganglionic parasympathetic receptors. Such effects are blocked by atropine. Therefore it is assumed that for acetylcholine there are two types of receptor: nicotinic and muscarinic. These receptors show differences, at least in the spatial disposition of their active sites. Besides interacting with those receptors, acetylcholine combines with acetylcholinesterase, in the process of its hydrolysis. In a recent review Durell et al. (71) examined the biochemical aspects of acetylcholine action.

As a result of many studies on this subject several attempts have been made to determine with precision the topography and conformational requirements of the receptor sites of cholinergic agents, especially on the basis of the conformation of acetylcholine and analogous substances, using structurally rigid compounds (16,50,72–75). However, in spite of all these efforts, doubts on the nature of cholinergic receptors still persist (76). It is assumed, however, that the active site of the acetylcholine receptor cannot be identical to that of the acetylcholinesterase because, besides other important differences (77), the former, conversely to what happens with the latter, does not hydrolyze acetylcholine.

As far as the diversity of effects produced by acetylcholine is concerned, a hypothesis that has been advanced states that all these effects result from the different conformations of the molecule of this chemical mediator, but so far no agreement has been reached as to which conformation is responsible for the nicotinic action and which for the muscarinic action (78). The conformations usually invoked in these studies are the ones shown in Figure 8.10. At first it was suggested that conformation II was responsible for the muscarinic action, and conformation I, for the nicotinic action. Further studies, however, seem to favor the opposite (74); that is, conformation II is responsible for the nicotinic action, and conformation I, for the muscarinic action. In effect the structure of the muscarine molecule determined in crystalline muscarine

I

II

Muscarine Nicotine

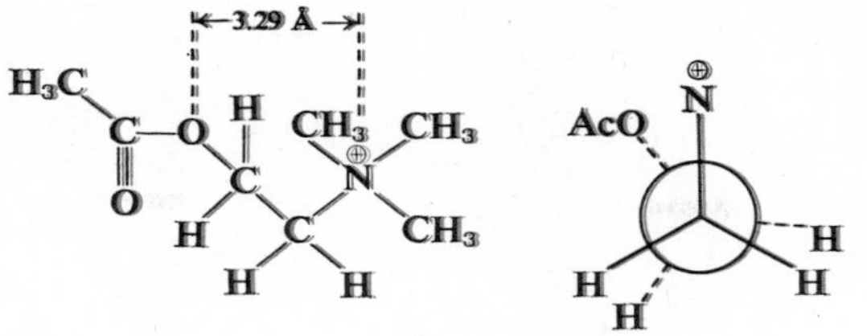

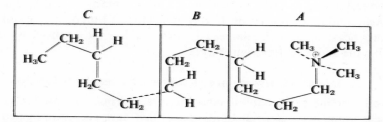

Fig. 8.10. Conformation of cholinergic agents.

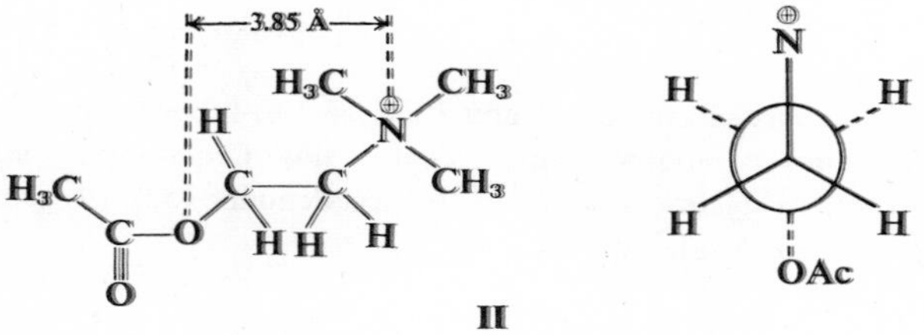

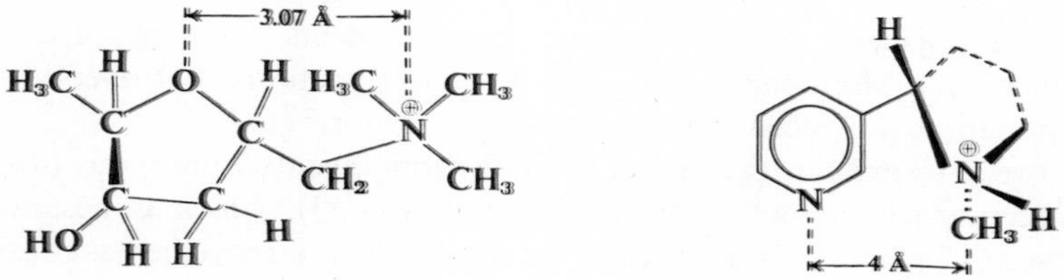

iodide has a great similarity to conformation I, which supports the latter hypothesis (*79*). It was also seen that, whereas the nicotinic receptor does not show a steric specificity, the muscarinic receptor is highly stereoselective (*16*).

In 1965 Belleau (*80*) advanced the hypothesis that the cholinergic receptor would be comprised of the three compartments represented in Figure 8.11. The muscarinic receptor would encompass three nonpolar compartments,

Fig. 8.11. Schematic representation of the cholinergic receptor. Muscarinic receptor: *A*, *B*, and *C* are nonpolar. Nicotinic receptor: *B* is semipolar or polar (*80*).

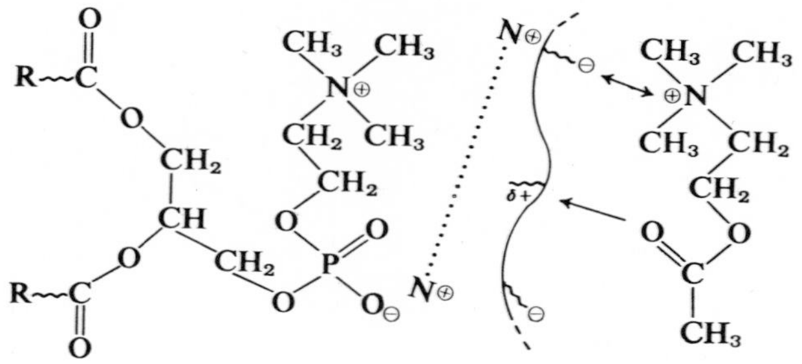

Fig. 8.12. Proposed mechanism of combination of (+)-tubocurarine or other bis-quaternary ammonium compound with receptor site. Cross-linking stabilizes the protein–lecithin complex against dissociation by acetylcholine (*82*). (Reprinted by permission of the New York Academy of Sciences.) S. Ehrenpreis, " Possible Nature of the Cholinergic Receptor "

whereas the nicotinic one would be formed by one polar or semipolar compartment adjacent to two nonpolar compartments. This hypothesis was modified in a later paper (see part A of this section), but even the new interpretation was recently questioned by Ehrenpreis (*81*).

In order to explain the action of cholinergic agents Ehrenpreis (*82*) used the receptor-site model proposed by Watkins (*83*), which is described in Chapter 6, Section I. This site, which controls the ion movements, consists of a protein–lecithin complex, located within the postsynaptic membrane. As a result of the action of acetylcholinesterase this complex dissociates, causing the membrane to open and increasing its permeability to ions. A potent cholinergic agent therefore would be one that is highly efficient in dissociating the complex. A great intensity of pharmacodynamic action does not necessarily derive from a strong binding, that is, high affinity. The determinant factor of the specificity of interaction would be the complementarity between the protein surface and the cholinergic agent. Depending on the tissue, either true- or pseudo-cholinesterase could participate as the receptor. This would explain why either acetylcholine or butyrylcholine is the more potent agonist on several tissues and why the action of a muscarinic agent is different from the action of a nicotinic agent. In this model the (+)-tubocurarine can bind to two negative sites simultaneously and stabilize the complex by cross-linking the active center (Figure 8.12).

efficacy ←

A. Interaction between Acetylcholinesterase and Its Substrates

Acetylcholine is the natural substrate of acetylcholinesterase, an enzyme present in the nervous tissue of all species that have been investigated (*84*). Leuzinger and co-workers recently not only obtained acetylcholinesterase in large amount in crystaline form (*85,86*) but also showed that it has a dimeric hybrid structure with only two active sites (*87*). Through the catalyzing action of acetylcholinesterase, acetylcholine is hydrolyzed to produce acetate and choline (*63*):

$$(CH_3)_3\overset{\oplus}{N} \overset{CH_2}{\underset{CH_2}{\diagdown}} \overset{O}{\underset{\overset{\|}{O}}{\underset{OH}{\diagup}}} \overset{CH_3}{C} + H_2O \rightleftharpoons (CH_3)_3\overset{\oplus}{N} \overset{CH_2}{\underset{CH_2}{\diagdown}} \overset{OH}{\diagup} + \underset{\overset{\|}{O}}{O-C-CH_3}$$

<table>
<tr><td>Anionic site</td><td>Esteratic site</td><td>Anionic site</td><td>Esteratic site</td></tr>
<tr><td colspan="2" align="center">Acetylcholinesterase</td><td colspan="2" align="center">Acetylcholinesterase</td></tr>
</table>

Another representation can be seen in Figure 8.13. Here the nucleophilic group of the enzyme is comprised of the oxygen atom belonging to serine; the nucleophilicity of this group is enhanced by the formation of hydrogen bonding between hydroxy group and the imidazole ring (of histidine) which functions as a general catalyst of bases (*88–90*).

A more modern and more detailed representation of the interaction between acetylcholine and acetylcholinesterase is shown in Figure 8.14. It is assumed that the esteratic site of acetylcholinesterase contains a histidine residue adjacent to a hydroxy group in a serine residue. Russian authors (*14*) prefer to call the esteratic center simply the esterophilic point, since it has affinity for the ester group of acetylcholine.

It seems, therefore, that in the interaction of acetylcholine with acetyl-cholinesterase four groups in two sites of the enzyme are involved: at the anionic site the interaction is between a phosphate group of the enzyme and the trimethylammonium group of acetylcholine; at the esteratic site the imidazole nucleus of the enzyme interacts with the acetyl group of acetyl-choline by establishing a covalent bond with the carboxylic carbon, an unidentified bond with the carboxylic oxygen, and dipolar forces in the ester oxygen atom (*91*).

Although it was suggested some years ago that acetylcholinesterase and the

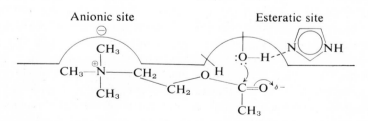

Fig. 8.13. Hydrolysis of acetylcholine through the catalytic action of acetylcholin-esterase.

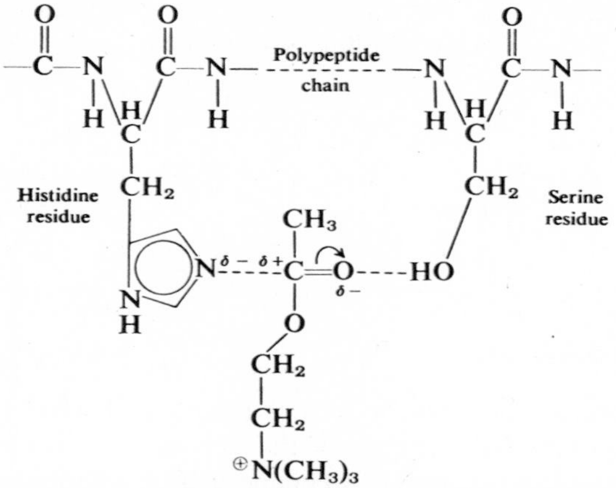

Fig. 8.14. Hypothetical adsorption of acetylcholine at the esteratic site of acetyl-cholinesterase (*1*).

acetylcholine receptor of excitable membranes were identical, comparative studies have shown quite conclusively that this is not so (*8*).

In the interaction of acetylcholine with its receptor site it is assumed that the ester oxygen has a partial positive charge ($\delta+$). Calculations relative to the electron distribution in the acetylcholine molecule, but in which only the π-electron system was considered, have confirmed that this really occurs:

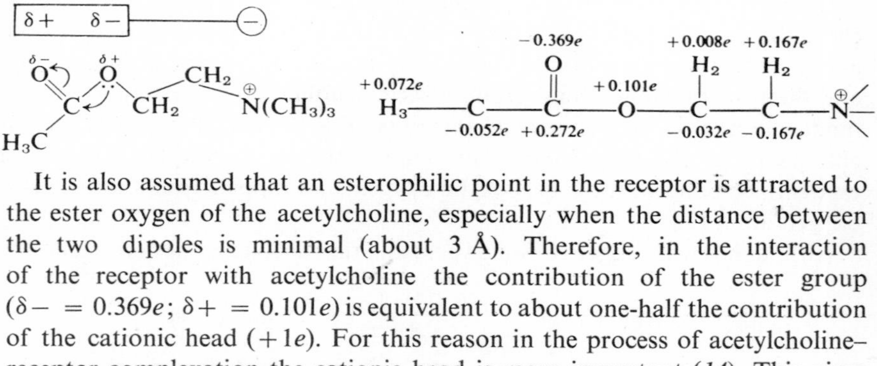

It is also assumed that an esterophilic point in the receptor is attracted to the ester oxygen of the acetylcholine, especially when the distance between the two dipoles is minimal (about 3 Å). Therefore, in the interaction of the receptor with acetylcholine the contribution of the ester group ($\delta- = 0.369e$; $\delta+ = 0.101e$) is equivalent to about one-half the contribution of the cationic head ($+1e$). For this reason in the process of acetylcholine–receptor complexation the cationic head is more important (*14*). This gives support to Cavallito's hypothesis (*92*), which is discussed later on.

The hydrolysis of acetylcholine seems to proceed in accordance with the mechanism proposed by Cunningham (*93*), represented in Figure 8.15.

Taking into consideration the stereoselectivity of acetylcholine-type compounds and of the inhibitors of acetylcholinesterase, Krupka and Laidler (*94*) postulated that the active site of this enzyme would be three-dimensional, and they represented it accordingly. Though quite suggestive, the representation

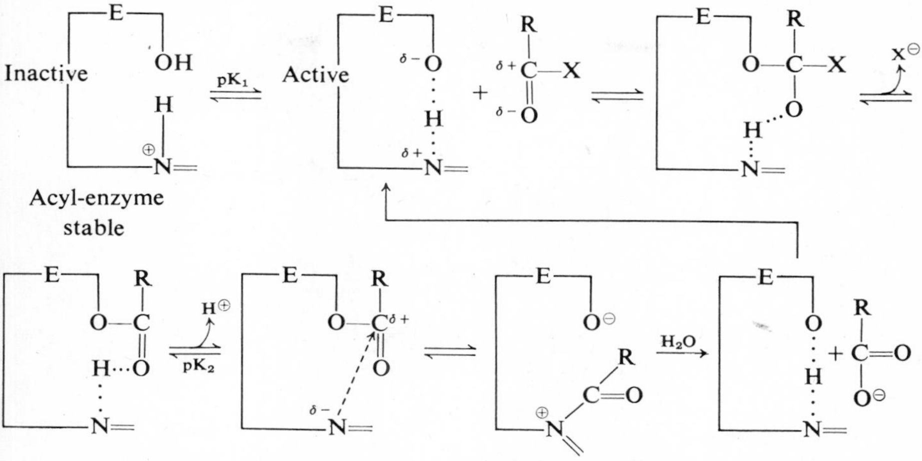

Fig. 8.15. Mechanism of enzymic hydrolysis. The active site involves two hydrogen bonds between a hydroxy group of serine and an uncharged imidazole nucleus. Nucleophilic oxygen of the hydroxy group attacks the carbonyl function of the substrate. With expulsion of the ester alcoholic portion the acylated enzyme is formed. Afterward the nucleophilic attack of imidazole nitrogen on the newly formed ester linkage in the acylated enzyme results in acylimidazole, which is rapidly hydrolyzed, producing the acid and the active enzyme (*93*).

proposed by them cannot be completely correct, because they considered acetylcholine as having an *anti* conformation, whereas all known choline esters have a *gauche* conformation (*91*). For this reason the hypothetical topography of the active center of acetylcholinesterase was modified by Beckett (*76*), who has represented it as shown in Figure 8.16. By tautomeric changes, the *same* nitrogen atom of the imidazole residue present in this structure could form a hydrogen bond, either donating or accepting a proton. In the first case it could attach itself to the hydroxy group of muscarine, and in the second case, to the carboxylic oxygen of muscarone or to the ether oxygen of the dioxolanes (*76*):

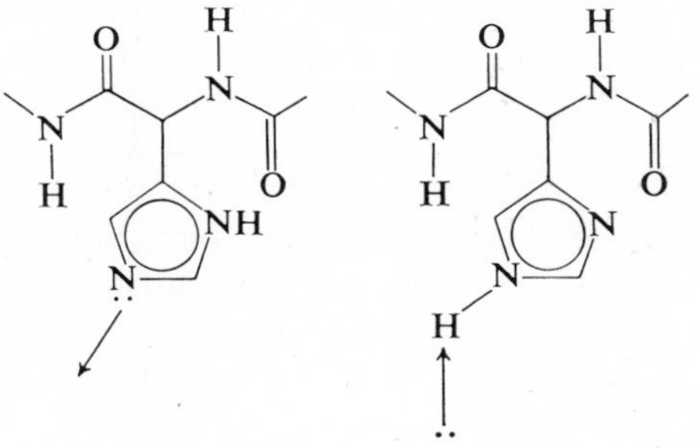

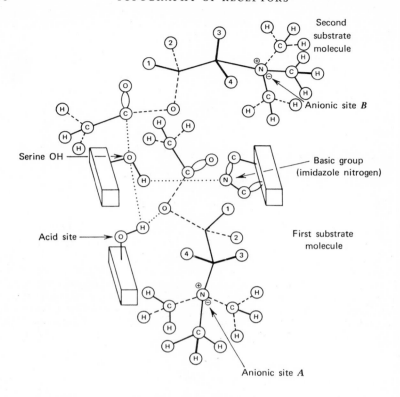

Fig. 8.16. Acetylcholine molecules at the proposed active site of acetylcholinesterase (76). (Reprinted by permission of the New York Academy of Sciences.)

Considering that in the solid state of acetylcholine bromide the N^+ cation is surrounded by four Br^- anionic charges, Canepa (95) suggested that the cholinergic membrane receptor contains in its structure four partially mobile anionic charges whose tetrahedral distribution forms the receptor's cavity. Each anionic charge constitutes a component of the receptor unit. The centers of three of the anionic components lie on the surface of the receptor membrane; the distances between them on the resting membrane are at least 9 to 10 Å, in order to allow for partial penetration of the cationic head of acetylcholine; the remaining anionic component is be about 6 Å below the surface. The limited mobility of the three anionic components of the tetrahedral receptors, and hence the variation of the interunit receptor distances, would explain the increase or decrease in membrane permeability to cations (Figure 8.17).

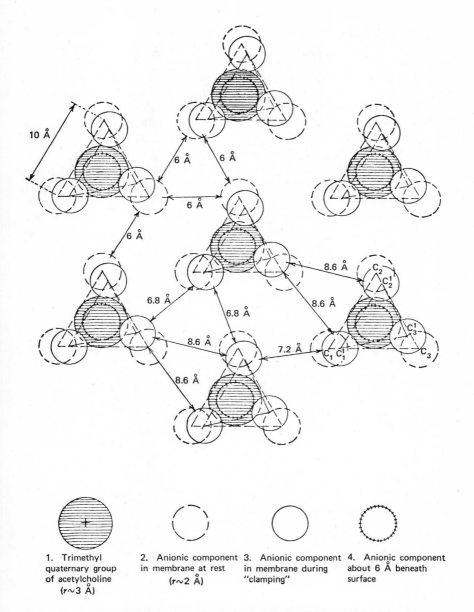

Fig. 8.17. Preferred orientation distribution of simplified nicotine-like receptors. Intercomponent external distances are 6 Å at rest and 6.8 to 8.6 Å when clamping occurs (95). (Reprinted by permission of the New York Academy of Sciences.)

Based on speculated minimal features of acetylcholine receptors, Cavallito (*92*) postulated that the anionic site of the cholinergic receptor could be constituted by the phosphate group, present in many biological compounds and a center of high electron density. Such a receptor region could accommodate multiple-point and secondary bonding electrostatic interactions with acetylcholine. The action of this compound results either in conformational modifications, if the receptor is located in flexible molecules, or in conformational adaptability, when the receptor is a part of more rigid molecules. The conformational changes induced in the receptor would also alter the structure of contiguous water molecules. Thus a phosphate polyanionic grid as a component of the receptor (Figure 8.18), through the action of different cations, would undergo a considerable conformational and electrostatic change, depending on the presence or absence of cations and their position. Such an accommodating anionic receptor structure would allow binding with agonists

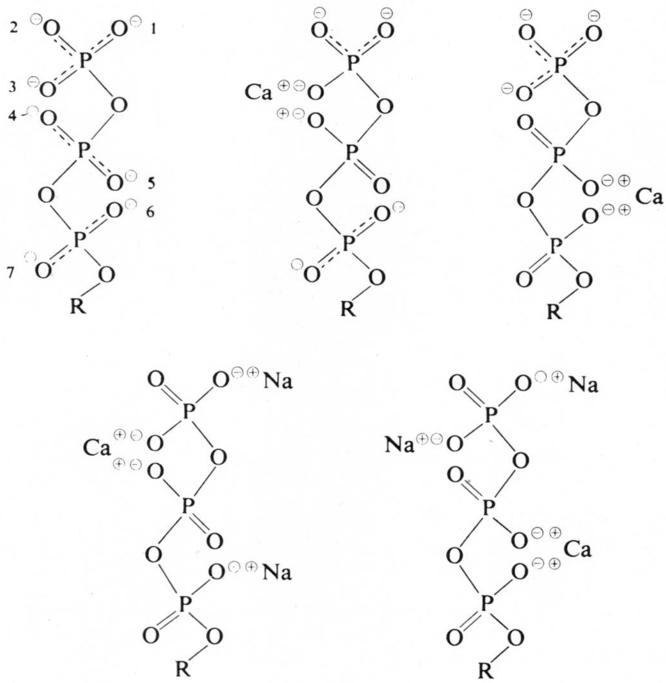

Fig. 8.18. Cholinergic-receptor anionic site proposed by Cavallito. As part of a polyanionic structure, it can undergo considerable conformational and electrostatic change induced by different cation species. Furthermore the different configurational variants can have correspondingly different structures among the hydrogen-bonded associated water molecules (*92*). (Reprinted by permission of the New York Academy of Sciences.)

or antagonists and would produce modifications in the characteristics of the structure of water molecules in the neighborhood of the receptor or alterations to cation permeability in the interface.

Some authors (*90,96*) suggested that acetylcholinesterase can undergo reversible changes in conformation, since it is an allosteric enzyme (*97*). Recent experimental data indicate that acetylcholinesterase does undergo conformational changes. For instance, having used the optical-rotatory-dispersion technique, Kitz and Kremzner (*98*) reported conformational changes induced in highly purified acetylcholinesterase by heat, strong base, a substrate, and anticholinesterase agents. Podleski (*77*) advanced the idea that receptor activation very likely involves conformation modifications, but that the active site of the acetylcholine receptor differs from that of acetylcholinesterase. By following a similar line of reasoning, from evidence obtained in their experiments with the electroplax of the electric eel (*99*), Karlin and co-workers postulated that the acetylcholine receptor contains both sulfhydryl and disulfide groups (*100,101*) and that its active site, at least after a disulfide bond has been reduced, is sufficiently flexible to permit competition between a free inhibitor and a covalently attached activator, assuming that they bind to the same site (*12*). Having found a similar inhibitory potency of acetylcholinesterase in the choline esters of *cis*- and *trans*-4-*tert*-butylcyclo-hexanecarboxylic acid, Kay and Robinson (*102*) assumed that the *cis* isomer binds to the active site in a thermodynamically unstable conformation. To explain the inhibition of acetylcholinesterase by β-trimethylammoniopropionate esters of *cis*- and *trans*-4-*tert*-butylcyclohexanol, they suggested that the "reverse esters" and acetylcholine derivatives attach to the enzyme-receptor area in different ways. On the other side, Cammarata and Stein (*103*), by using the multiple-regression technique where possible, made attempts to determine how the interaction of the 3-hydroxyphenyltrimethyl-ammonium derivatives with acetylcholinesterase would occur. They calculated some σ and π properties of these compounds and concluded that position 1 interacts with a negative group of acetylcholinesterase and position 3, with an electrophilic species through hydrogen bonding.

$$X = H,\ 4\text{-}CH_3,\ 5\text{-}CH_3,\ 6\text{-}CH_3,\ 4\text{-}OCH_3,\ 6\text{-}OCH_3$$

In order to explain the interaction of certain cholinergics with acetyl-cholinesterase, Belleau (*104*) applied his macromolecular perturbation theory (*50*) and calculated various thermodynamic parameters, such as free energies, enthalpies, and entropies of binding of $C_nH_{2n+1}\overset{\oplus}{N}(CH_3)_3$ on acetylcholinesterase (105), shown in Table 9.1 (Chapter 9). He assumed that the tetramethylammonium moiety and the alkyl chains bind to acetylcholinesterase independently. Therefore, by subtracting the contribution of the tetramethylammonium ion from the individual values of ΔH and ΔS listed in Table 9.1, he calculated the thermodynamic parameters that characterize the binding of the alkyl chains (Table 8.2). He deduced that the binding of all the hydrocar-

TABLE 8.2 Enthalpies and Entropies of Binding of $C_nH_{2n+1}\overset{\oplus}{N}(CH_3)_3$ *minus* the contribution of $\overset{\oplus}{N}(CH_3)_4$ (104)

n	$\delta\Delta H$ (cal/mole)	$\delta\Delta S$ (e.u.)
1	–	–
2	150	1.2
3	280	2.0
4	1380	6.7
5	1200	4.6
6	2050	7.7
7	2100	8.7
8	2200	9.9
9	2200	10.5
10	2340	12.5
11	3840	19.2
12	3850	20.5

Reprinted by permission of the New York Academy of Sciences and of the author.

bon residues, regardless of chain length, is basically unfavorable (since it is an endothermic process), so that the driving force for adsorption is exclusively entropic in origin. For this reason he ascribed to the water structure of the internal environment the determinant role in the complexation between drug and enzyme, proposing that this occurs as shown in Figure 8.19.

The direct cholinergics manifest the same action as acetylcholine because of their similarities in chemical structure, such as distance between polar groups and charge distribution (62,65). All of them have a chain of five atoms, which is a feature of direct cholinergics known as the *five-atom-chain rule*. It should be noted that the distances indicated in Figure 8.20 correspond approximately to the ones found between certain positions of protein groups, as was shown in Chapter 5, Section III.

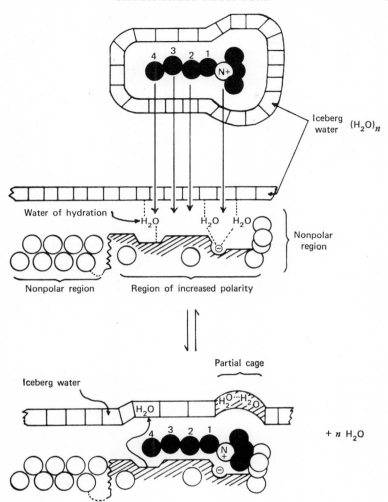

Fig. 8.19. Schematic representation of the physical interaction mechanism of butyl-trimethylammonium with the acetylcholinesterase surface. Note that the fourth carbon atom causes the loss of one water molecule of hydration. Filled circles = CH_2 groups; open circles = nonpolar residues (*104*). (Reprinted by permission of the New York Academy of Sciences.)

Recently some attempts were made to isolate and identify the receptor substance of acetylcholine in solution, but without any decisive results (*7,82*). Since acetylcholinesterase has been obtained in the pure crystalline state (*85–87*), researches aiming at the determination of acetylcholine-receptor topography, and therefore of cholinergic and cholinergic blocking agents,

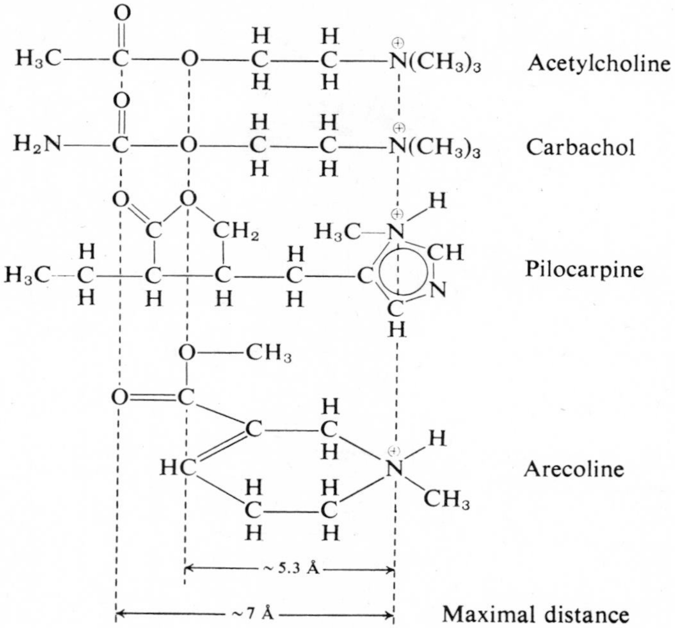

$$H_3C\!-\!\overset{\displaystyle O}{\overset{\|}{C}}\!-\!O\!-\!\overset{H}{\underset{H}{C}}\!-\!\overset{H}{\underset{H}{C}}\!-\!\overset{\oplus}{N}(CH_3)_3 \quad \text{Acetylcholine}$$

$$H_2N\!-\!\overset{\displaystyle O}{\overset{\|}{C}}\!-\!O\!-\!\overset{H}{\underset{H}{C}}\!-\!\overset{H}{\underset{H}{C}}\!-\!\overset{\oplus}{N}(CH_3)_3 \quad \text{Carbachol}$$

Pilocarpine

Arecoline

~5.3 Å

~7 Å   Maximal distance

Fig. 8.20. Similarities in cholinergic agents (*65*).

will be facilitated. At present the only certain thing is that the receptor site in acetylcholinesterase is composed at least of one anionic group—the nature of which has not yet been proved—which is easily accessible (*106*).

B. Muscarinic Receptors

Studies carried out with several isomers of muscarine, muscarone, dioxolane, and acetylmethylcholine have led to the postulation of the existence of

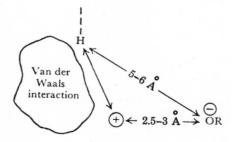

Fig. 8.21. Proposed structure of muscarinic receptor (*107*).

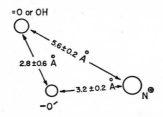

Fig. 8.22. Model of forces representing muscarinic receptor. These forces coincide with the three principal atoms of acetylcholine, muscarine, and muscarone molecules (*108*).

a common muscarinic receptor that possesses (a) an anionic site that associates with a charged cationic head of these molecules, and (b) a chemical grouping that is able to react with an alcoholic hydroxyl, a ketone, an ether oxygen, and the carbonyl group of an ester (*76*). The dimensions and the interaction forces in this complexation are represented in Figure 8.21.

Through molecular-orbital calculations Kier (*108*) determined the preferred conformations of acetylcholine, L-(+)-muscarine and D-(−)-muscarone, and suggested a model for the muscarinic receptor (Figure 8.22). Data gathered in research with conformationally rigid analogs of acetylcholine led Cannon and co-workers (*16*) to suggest that attachment of acetylcholine to the muscarinic receptor involves its *trans* conformation.

The interaction of acetylcholine with a muscarinic receptor is usually represented as shown in Figure 8.23. The complexation of (+)-2S:3R:5S-muscarine with the same receptor is depicted in a very similar manner (Figure 8.24).

Experiments carried out with compounds of a structure analogous to that of acetylcholine—where molecular dimensions, conformation, and charge distribution have been taken into consideration—induced researchers to propose for S-(−)-hyoscyamine, a potent and specific antagonist of the muscarinic effects of acetylcholine, the receptor shown in Figure 7.7 (Chapter 7, Section III).

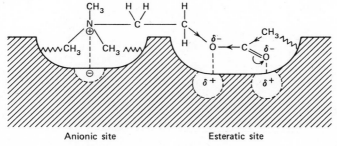

Fig. 8.23. Complexation of acetylcholine with the muscarinic receptor through electrostatic, dipolar, and hydrophobic interactions (*109*).

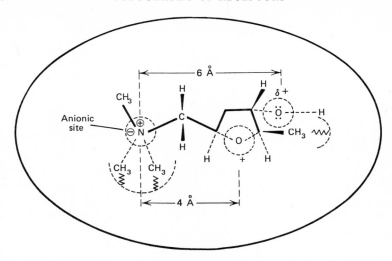

Fig. 8.24. Interaction of (+)-muscarine with its hypothetical receptor (*109*).

Kuznetsov and Golikov (*110*) suggested that the active part of the receptor in a cellular membrane consists of two parallel protein chains linked by ionic and hydrogen bonds. The depolarizing action of acetylcholine results from the rupture of the hydrogen bonding caused by its interaction with one of these chains and the consequent passage of ions. Antagonists, such as benzilonium, also cross the protein chains but interact with *both*; this keeps them attached and prevents the flow of ions. This interpretation is schematically represented in Figure 8.25.

For cholinergic blocking agents Ariëns (*111*) proposed a more sophisticated receptor. It includes an additional acceptor area, to which the haptophoric part of the drug is attached. The haptophore acts as a selecting carrier for the

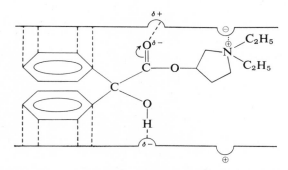

Fig. 8.25. Interaction of benzilonium with the muscarinic receptor (*110*).

fixing groups. This occurs, for instance, in the interaction of benzilylcholine mustard, the fixing groups of which are alkylating.

Acetylcholine receptor

Reversible blockade

Acetylcholine receptor

Reversible phase

Irreversible blockade

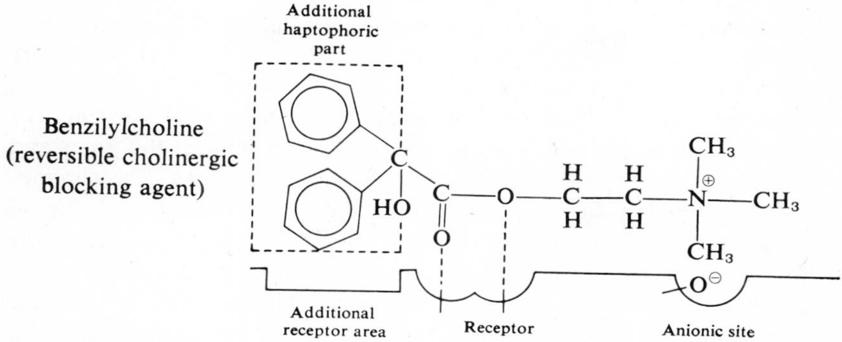

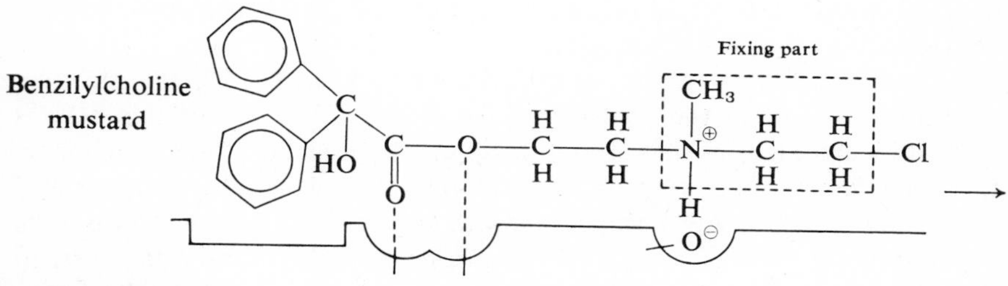

C. Nicotinic Receptors

The measure of the nicotinic activity of nicotine enantiomers and analogous compounds indicates that the interaction of acetylcholine with the nicotinic receptor does not involve binding through more than two points.

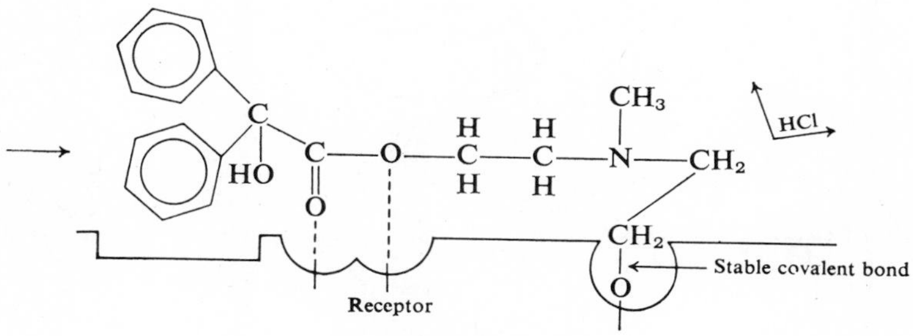

This suggests that in the nicotinic sites optical isomerism is of little importance (*78*).

On the basis of results obtained with autoradiographic fixation methods of radioactive curariform or cholinergic molecules in the end plates of mice diaphragms, Waser (*112,113*) proposed a hypothetical model of a very suggestive cholinergic receptor (Figure 8.26). According to his hypothesis, acetylcholine and other cholinergic compounds, when depolarizing the synaptic membrane of a motor plate, produce an opening of the pores and the consequent exchange through them of K^+ and Na^+ ions. The cholinolytics, and still better the cholinergic blocking agents, being made up of bulky molecules and having great chemical affinity for specific groups of the receptor, to which they are attracted by electrostatic forces, close the pore and thus prevent the aforementioned ion exchange (Figure 8.27). Cholinergic blocking agents can be removed from their binding to the receptor site, but this demands a high concentration of cholinergics. Likewise, from his experiments Waser (*114*) concluded that three types of receptors exist in the terminal motor plate: curarimimetic receptors, cholinergic receptors, and the active centers of specific cholinesterase.

In accordance with Waser, and as shown in Figure 8.27, the nicotinic receptor is a pore in the postsynaptic membrane. The rim of this pore is formed by anionic sites that attract the quaternary nitrogen of acetylcholine. Inside the lumen of the pore are the esteratic sites at which the ester group of acetylcholine is attached. Compounds with groups bulky enough to close the opening of the pore, such as (+)-tubocurarine, would act as antagonists to the actions of acetylcholine at the neuromuscular synapses in skeletal muscles, because they would prevent not only the access of acetylcholine but also the

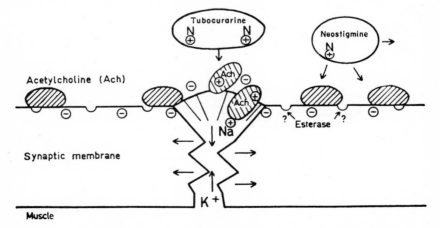

Fig. 8.26.   Schematic representation of the cholinergic receptor area of end plates (*112*).

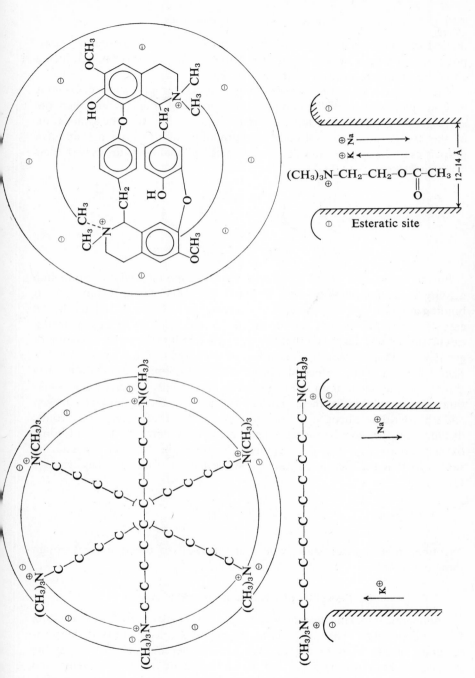

Fig. 8.27. Nicotinic receptor, according to Waser (*114*).

inward and outward flow of ions. In the specific case of bisquaternary compounds, they might bridge the orifice of the pore and deform it, producing
agonistic or antagonistic effects (*112,113*).

The hypothesis of Waser, by admitting a nonflat receptor surface, explains
why nonplanar tetrahydroquinoline compounds are more potent than the
corresponding quinolinium ions. It supports also the idea that the localization
of the charge and the molecular conformation of the drug are additive
properties in the complexation of cholinergics and analogous drugs with their
respective receptors (*115*).

Furthermore, as a common characteristic compounds with nicotine-like
activity have an onium head as an essential part. Other features contribute to
binding at a nearby site to increase or decrease the intensity of activity. In the
case of substituted phenyl choline ethers, on the basis of molecular-orbital
calculations it was suggested that the aromatic ring interacts with a secondary
group(s) in the receptor by formation of a charge-transfer complex (*116*).
Kier (*117*), by using extended Hückel theory in similar calculations, has
shown that the nicotinium ion can exist in two equally preferred conformations. But in only one of these are there two atoms—the quaternary nitrogen
and the pyridine nitrogen atom—of comparable charge and interatomic
distance to the corresponding ones—quaternary nitrogen and carbonyl
oxygen atoms—found in acetylcholine (*108*). On the basis of his data, he
suggested that the nicotinic-acting molecule has the following key features
(*117*):

$$\overset{\ominus\delta}{X} \xleftarrow{\quad 4.85 \pm 0.1 \text{ Å} \quad} \overset{\oplus}{N}{-}$$

Nicotine, in its ionized state, would attach itself to the receptor through
these two points.

D. Receptors of Cholinergic Blocking Agents

Cholinergic blocking agents are drugs that block the activity resulting
from acetylcholine. They may act at different sites, such as (a) at the post-
ganglion terminations of the parasympathetic nervous system; (b) at the
ganglia of both sympathetic and parasympathetic nervous system; and
(c) at the neuromuscular junctions of the voluntary nervous system (*118,119*).

The first group, known as cholinolytics, parasympatholytics, or anticholinergics, are antimuscarinics, because they produce the following effects: mydriatic, cycloplegic, antispasmodic, and antisecretory (*118*). It is admitted that they compete for the receptor sites of acetylcholine by preventing it from attaching itself to these sites and thus interrupting the transmission of the nervous impulse (*120*). They belong to different chemical classes—amino alcohols, derivatives of amino alcohols (esters, ethers, carbamates), amines, diamines, amino amides, and other groups—but in general they have a cationic head, an alcoholic hydroxyl, an ester group, and a cyclic substituent, usually aromatic. The conformation is also important, because the receptor is quite stereoselective. A typical example of a cholinolytic compound is S-(−)-hyoscyamine. Its interaction with the receptor is represented in Figure 7.7 (Chapter 7, Section III).

Another hypothesis on the mode of complexation of these cholinolytics was advanced by Kuznetsov and Golikov (*110*) and is explained in Section V.B of this chapter (Figure 8.25).

The cholinergic blocking agents that act at the ganglionic synapses of both the sympathetic and parasympathetic nervous systems are generally called ganglionic blocking agents or ganglioplegics, owing to their ability to block the transmission of impulses through the autonomic ganglia. Several of these drugs possess two quaternary nitrogens separated by a chain of six atoms; hence this chain is called the *ganglioplegic distance*. As to the mode of action, they are divided into three groups (*121*):

1. Depolarizing ganglionic blocking agents. Actually they are ganglionic stimulants, producing a nicotinic effect, but are not used clinically.

2. Nondepolarizing competitive ganglionic blocking agents. They compete with acetylcholine for the receptor sites, but do not produce transmission of nervous impulses. Examples are tetraethylammonium salts, hexamethonium, azamethonium, trimethaphan, and mecamylamine (which, besides possessing a competitive action, has also a noncompetitive one—it is a dual antagonist).

3. Nondepolarizing noncompetitive ganglionic blocking agents. The effect they produce does not result from interaction with the receptor site of acetylcholine but with the noncompetitive receptors of the ganglia. Examples are chlorisondamine and trimethidinium (*118*).

Taking into account the experimental data of other authors, Goldstein and co-workers (*5*) proposed that there are two different receptors for acetylcholine: one in the ganglion cell and the other in the muscle end plate. These receptors differ essentially in the distance between anionic sites. The ganglionic site interacts strongly with hexamethonium; hence this drug is a ganglionic blocker, because it prevents the receptor from responding to acetylcholine. Decamethonium, however, is too long to fit the ganglionic receptor; it acts as a neuromuscular blocking agent by preventing complexation of acetylcholine with the muscle end plate receptor (Figure 8.28).

According to Barlow (*1*), bisonium salts bind to their receptors at two points, so that the interaction of a ganglionic blocker with its receptor is as shown in Figure 8.29.

The cholinergic blocking agents at the neuromuscular junction are drugs that bring about voluntary-muscle relaxation and have some points in common with some ganglionic blockers. Since their activity is similar to that of curare, they are also called curariform or curarimimetic drugs. According

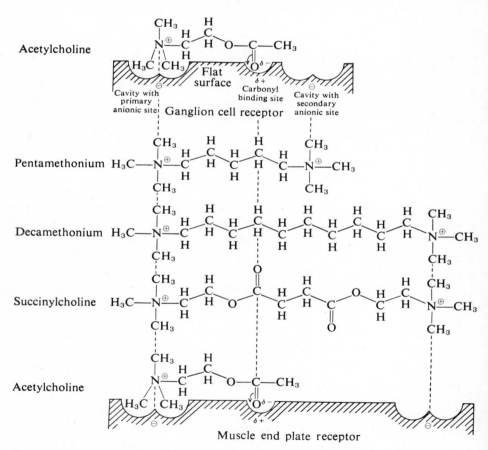

Fig. 8.28. Hypothetical acetylcholine receptors: in ganglion cell (above) and in muscle end plate (below). [Adapted from (*5*).]

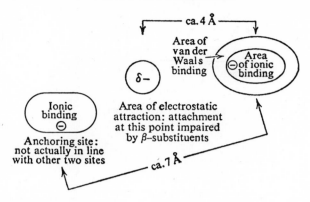

Fig. 8.29.   Representation of a hypothetical ganglionic receptor (*1*).

to their mode of action, these drugs are classified (*118*) into three types:

1. Depolarizing blocking agents. They cause depolarization of the membrane of the muscle end plate, similar to that produced by acetylcholine itself —owing to its nicotinic effect—at ganglia and neuromuscular junctions; examples are decamethonium and succinylcholine.

2. Competitive blocking agents. It is thought that they compete with acetylcholine for the receptor sites but are unable to effect the depolarization characteristic of the natural neuroeffector; examples are tubocurarine and gallamine.

3. Mixed blocking agents. These act by both of the aforementioned mechanisms; examples are decamethonium and succinylcholine, which, although usually considered as depolarizing agents, act also through a competitive mechanism.

As to the way in which these bisquaternary compounds interact with the molecule of cholinesterase, there are four possibilities, which are schematically represented in Figure 8.30.

Considering that many of the compounds that manifest curarizing activity are characterized by a chain of 10 atoms between the two quaternary nitrogens, as in the case of (+)-tubocurarine, succinylcholine, and decamethonium, this chain is known as the *curarizing distance* ("C-10 structure") and is equivalent to about 14 Å.

To this class of agents belong also some bisonium salts, which have only six carbons between the quaternary nitrogens. Actually, however, the separation between positive charges is about 14 Å, which corresponds to the C-10 structure. Derivatives of hexamethonium, listed in Table 8.3, are an example. As result of the $+I$ inductive effect of the aromatic ring, the

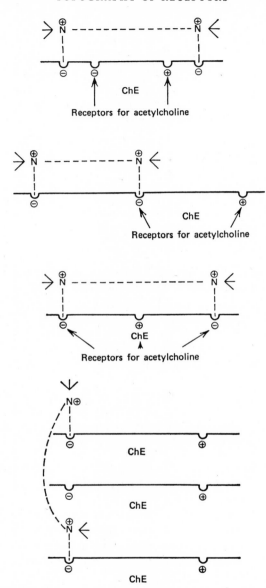

Fig. 8.30. Interaction of bisquaternary compounds with cholinesterase (ChE) (*122*).

positive charge of the nitrogen decreases, and a partial positive charge appears in the phenyl group. Hence, in comparison with hexamethonium, as a ganglionic blocker compound **II** is much less active, but as a muscle

TABLE 8.3 Influence of Easily Polarizable Groups in Nitrogen of Hexamethonium Derivatives (*14*)

Compound	Curarizing Activity Arbitrary Units
I Hexamethonium $(CH_3)_3\overset{\oplus}{N}(CH_2)_6\overset{\oplus}{N}(CH_3)_3$	1

	Curarizing Activity Arbitrary Units
II 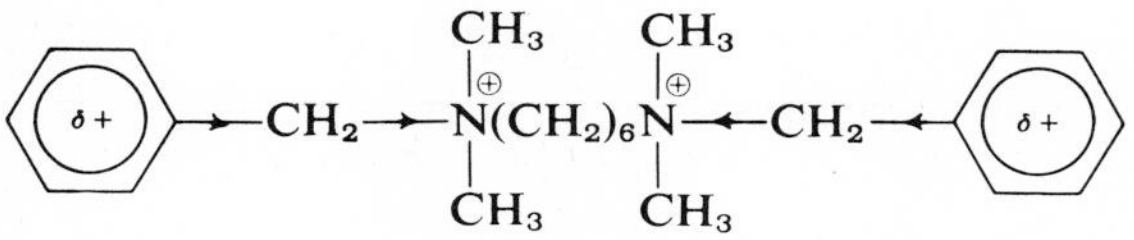	40
III 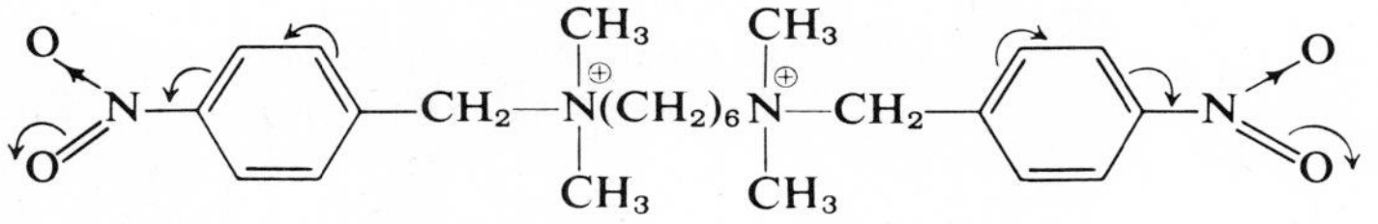	100

Reprinted by permission of the Williams and Wilkins Company.

relaxant it is 40 times more active. This last charge $\delta+$ becomes even stronger when the aromatic ring contains a highly electrophilic group such as the nitro group, in the *para* position; this new derivative, compound III, is almost inactive as a ganglionic blocker; as a muscle relaxant, however, it is 100 times more active than hexamethonium.

TABLE 8.4 Curarimimetic Drugs, Hexacarbacholine Analogs and Others with the C-16 Structure (*14*)

Reprinted by permission of the Williams and Wilkins Company.

Likewise, there are curarimimetics where the distance between the two quaternary nitrogens is about 20 Å and the chain that separates them has 16 atoms (C-16 structure) (Table 8.4).

On the other hand, due to the electronic effects of the substituents in quaternary nitrogens, compounds having a chain of 12 atoms between these nitrogens can present distances of 20 Å between the induced $\delta+$ charges (Table 8.5). These also manifest curarimimetic activity.

TABLE 8.5   Curare-like Activity in the Series of Benzoquinonium Derivatives (14)

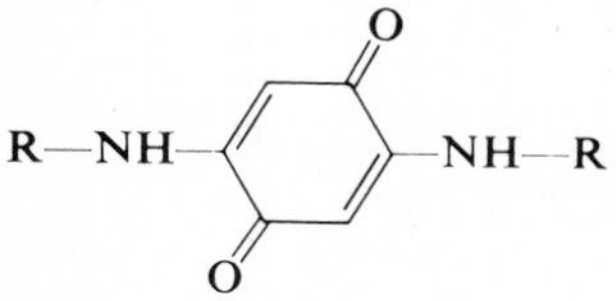 R	Number of Atoms between Quaternary Nitrogens $\overset{\oplus}{N} \cdots \overset{\oplus}{N}$	Number of Atoms between Induced $\delta+$ Charges 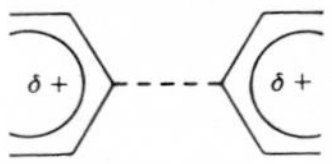	Curare-like Activity (Tubocurarine = 1)
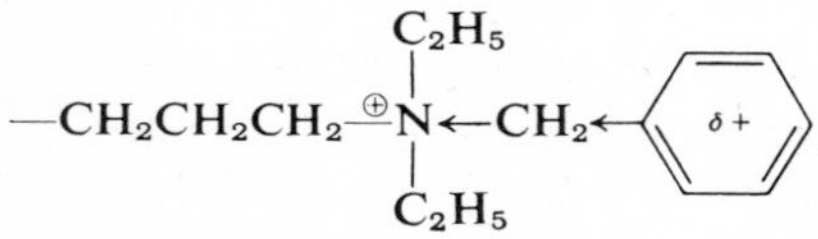 $-CH_2CH_2CH_2-\overset{\oplus}{N}\leftarrow CH_2\leftarrow$ (Benzoquinonium)	12	16	1
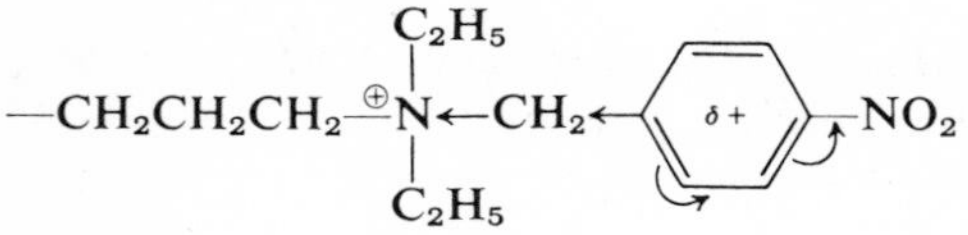 $-CH_2CH_2CH_2-\overset{\oplus}{N}\leftarrow CH_2\leftarrow \cdots NO_2$	12	16	4
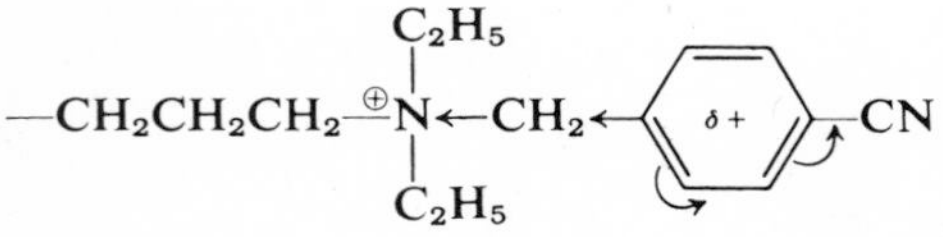 $-CH_2CH_2CH_2-\overset{\oplus}{N}\leftarrow CH_2\leftarrow \cdots CN$	12	16	4
Tubocurarine			1

Reprinted by permission of the Williams and Wilkins Company.

These results led researchers to reformulate their hypotheses about cholinergic receptors. Taking into account the role of the esterophilic points of the receptor, Rybolovlev suggested a receptor scheme that can accommodate compounds of both the C-10 and the C-16 structures (Figure 8.31).

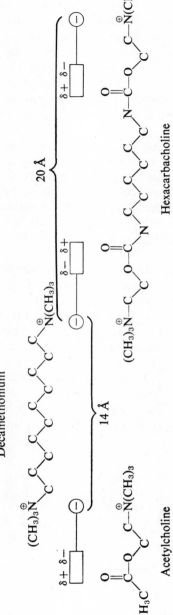

Fig. 8.31. Interaction of drugs with cholinergic receptors (*14*). (Reprinted by permission of the Williams and Wilkins Company.)

227

On the postsynaptic membrane the disposition of the receptors is "head to head" and "tail to tail"; the head is the anionic site, and the tail is the esterophilic site of the receptor. Acetylcholine interacts with two points: one, anionic (through the cationic head); the other, esterophilic (by means of the ester group). Decamethonium interacts with two anionic points, through the two cationic heads. Hexacarbacholine interacts with four points: two anionic (by means of cationic heads) and two esterophilic (through the ester groups).

Compound KB-72, which possesses a C-16 structure, prolonged curare-like action, and considerable anticholinesterase activity, interacts in the manner shown in Figure 8.32.

Koelle (68) proposed that the protein of a cholinergic receptor has a tetrameric structure; that is, the receptor is constituted of four subunits, disposed as shown in Figure 8.33. It was therefore suggested that the neighboring receptors are arranged on the postsynaptic membrane in such a way that the distance between the anionic points corresponds to the internitrogen distances in decamethonium. The pore of the postsynaptic membrane, in the Waser hypothesis (112,113), has a diameter of 14 Å. This is the distance between nitrogens in the C-10 structure. On the axis of the 10-atom chain (represented by the side of the square), between the anionic groups there are no dipolar groups, so that muscle relaxants with a corresponding structure can interact only with the anionic points.

Still in accordance with Rybolovlev, compounds of the decamethonium type—which do not contain esterophilic groups—interact with the receptor only through the anionic points of the C-10 structure. In this structure the ester group is not essential; there are several muscle relaxants of this type that do not possess it (115). The important factor is the presence of two anionic points; compounds with only one have a very reduced potency (Table 8.6). Note that some of these compounds, although having a C-10 structure, possess only one quaternary nitrogen and not two, and lack the ester group.

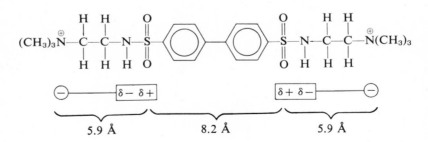

Fig. 8.32.   Interaction of the compound KB-72 with its receptor site (14). (Reprinted by permission of the Williams and Wilkins Company.)

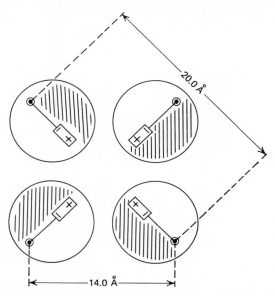

Fig. 8.33. Tetrameric arrangement of cholinoreceptor subunits (*14*). (Reprinted by permission of the Williams and Wilkins Company.)

On the other hand, still with reference to Figure 8.33, on the axis of the 16-atom chain (represented by the diagonal of the square), the two esterophilic dipolar groups are located between two anionic points, so that curarimimetics of a complementary structure can interact with two anionic points, and two positive ends and two negative ends of dipoles—that is, with six different points, as is the case with hexacarbacholine and its derivatives.

The lack of symmetry in Figure 8.33, as marked by the shaded area, serves to indicate the asymmetry of primary and secondary structures of the protein molecules. The C-10 structure (represented by the side of the square) is also asymmetric. The molecule of the muscle relaxant will therefore bind to different parts of the two component subunits of the C-10 structure (light area and shaded area). This explains why a muscle relaxant with an asymmetric structure can have greater activity than one with a symmetric structure (Table 8.7).

The C-16 structure is, however, symmetric. For this reason asymmetric muscle relaxants of this type are less potent than the symmetric ones (Table 8.8).

Note that in most of the maps of drug-receptor interactions discussed in this Section V the ester oxygen atom of acetylcholine, cholinergics and cholinergic blocking agents is represented as being *partially positive*, in keeping with the usual manner of considering the π-electron system only. Based

TABLE 8.6 Succinylcholine Derivatives with the C-10 Structure (123)

Structure	Curarizing Dose, Rabbit (Head-Drop Dose, mg/kg Intravenously)
$(CH_3)_3\overset{\oplus}{N}$—C—C—O—$\overset{\overset{\displaystyle O}{\|}}{C}$—C—C—$\overset{\overset{\displaystyle O}{\|}}{C}$—O—C—C—$\overset{\oplus}{N}(CH_3)_3$	0.15
$(CH_3)_3\overset{\oplus}{N}$—C—C—C—C—C—C—$\overset{\overset{\displaystyle O}{\|}}{C}$—O—C—C—$\overset{\oplus}{N}(CH_3)_3$	0.15
$(CH_3)_3\overset{\oplus}{N}$—C—C—C—C—C—C—C—C—C—C—$\overset{\oplus}{N}(CH_3)_3$	0.1
$(CH_3)_3\overset{\oplus}{N}$—C—C—$\overset{\overset{\displaystyle O}{\|}}{C}$—O—C—C—O—$\overset{\overset{\displaystyle O}{\|}}{C}$—C—C—$\overset{\oplus}{N}(CH_3)_3$	0.1
$(CH_3)_3\overset{\oplus}{N}$—C—C—O—$\overset{\overset{\displaystyle O}{\|}}{C}$—C—C—$\overset{\overset{\displaystyle O}{\|}}{C}$—O—C—C—H	10.0
$(CH_3)_3\overset{\oplus}{N}$—C—C—C—C—C—C—C—C—C—C—H	5.0

TABLE 8.7 Role of Asymmetry of Muscle-Relaxant Molecule of the C-10 Structure in Its Pharmacological Action (14)

Structure	Activity in Arbitrary Units
$(CH_3)_3\overset{\oplus}{N}$—C—C—O—$\overset{\overset{\displaystyle O}{\|}}{C}$—C—C—$\overset{\overset{\displaystyle O}{\|}}{C}$—O—C—C—$\overset{\oplus}{N}(CH_3)_3$	1
$(CH_3)_3\overset{\oplus}{N}$—C—C—$\overset{\overset{\displaystyle H}{\|}}{N}$—$\overset{\overset{\displaystyle O}{\|}}{C}$—C—C—$\overset{\overset{\displaystyle O}{\|}}{C}$—O—C—C—$\overset{\oplus}{N}(CH_3)_3$	1.8
$(CH_3)_3\overset{\oplus}{N}$—C—C—$\overset{\overset{\displaystyle H}{\|}}{N}$—$\overset{\overset{\displaystyle O}{\|}}{C}$—C—C—$\overset{\overset{\displaystyle O}{\|}}{C}$—$\overset{\overset{\displaystyle H}{\|}}{N}$—C—C—$\overset{\oplus}{N}(CH_3)_3$	Inactive

TABLE 8.8 Potency of Muscle-Relaxant Isomers of the C-10 Structure (*14*)

Compound	Potency

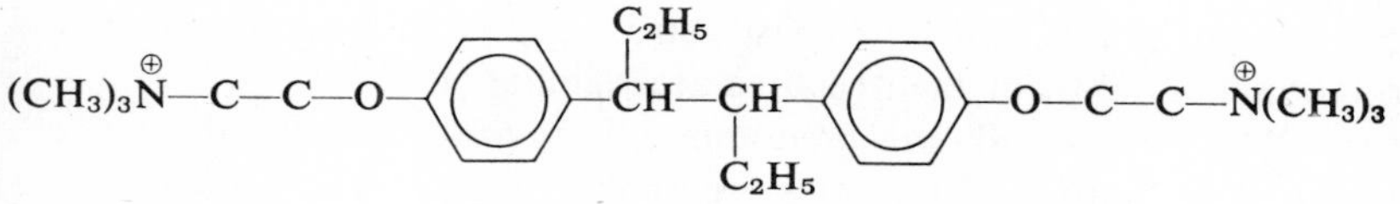

$(CH_3)_3\overset{\oplus}{N}$—C—C—O—[benzene ring]—$\underset{C_2H_5}{\overset{C_2H_5}{CH}}$—CH—[benzene ring]—O—C—C—$\overset{\oplus}{N}(CH_3)_3$ 1

$(CH_3)_3\overset{\oplus}{N}$—C—C—O—[benzene ring]—C—$\underset{C_3H_7}{CH}$—[benzene ring]—O—C—C—$\overset{\oplus}{N}(CH_3)_3$ 0.07

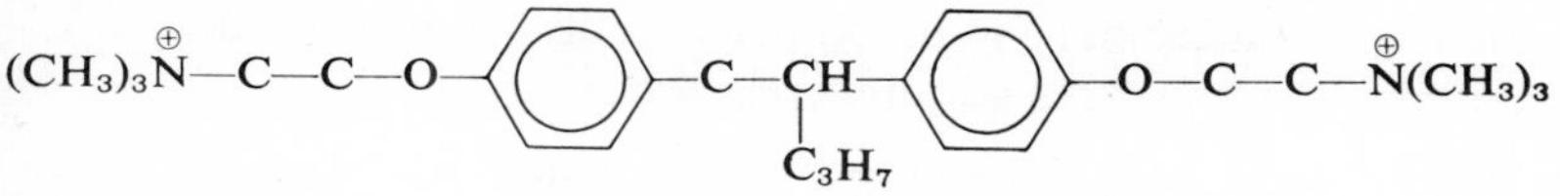

Reprinted by permission of the Williams and Wilkins Company.

on molecular-orbital calculations in which the total valence electron composition of the atom was considered in a point-charge model, Kier (*117*) concluded that the net total charge on that atom in acetylcholine is *slightly negative*:

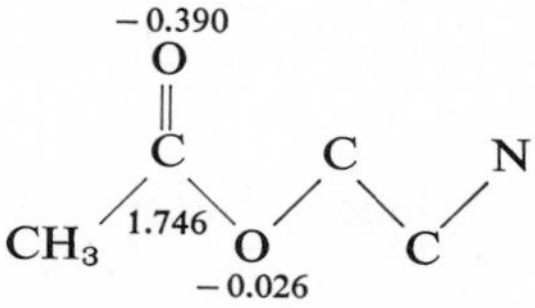

Therefore, according to Kier it is incorrect to consider the referred ester oxygen atom as a partially positively charged atom. It remains to be seen how this finding will affect the future attempts to propose the topography for cholinergic receptors.

VI. ADRENERGIC RECEPTORS

On the basis of pharmacological action, the adrenergics can be classified into three categories: those that act directly, those that act indirectly, and those that may act either way. The activity of the first group results from their complexation with specific receptors. Those of the second group act by liberating catecholamines, especially norepinephrine, from their storage areas; the last group shows mixed activity.

It is admitted that there are at least two receptors for adrenergics: α-adrenergic receptors and β-adrenergic receptors (124–127). Lands and co-workers (128) postulated, however, the existence of two β-receptors. There are authors who defend the existence of other adrenergic receptors, named γ and δ (129). There is no conclusive evidence whether the differences between α- and β-receptors are related to basic structural characteristics, flexible conformational variants, or their relative accessibility (106).

The α-adrenergic receptors are predominantly involved in smooth-muscle excitation and relaxation of the intestine and glandular cells, whereas the β-receptors are associated with the inhibition of smooth-muscle tonus (including that of the intestine) and the stimulation of the myocardium (130).

There are therefore two types of adrenergic drugs:

1. The α-adrenergic ones, the prototype of which is norepinephrine, although phenylephrine is the specific one.

2. The β-adrenergic ones, the prototype and specific one being isoproterenol (isoprenaline).

Epinephrine, by acting on both α- and β-receptors, has both α- and β-adrenergic properties (131). This can be schematically shown as follows (65):

norepinephrine ⟶ α-receptor ⟶ excitation of smooth muscle

epinephrine ⟶ β-receptor, heart, metabolism ⟶ cardiac and metabolic activation

isoproterenol ⟶ β-receptor, smooth muscle ⟶ inhibition of smooth-muscle blocking

Similarly there are two adrenergic blocking agents: α-adrenergic blocking agents and β-adrenergic blocking agents. Those of the first type inhibit the action of α-adrenergics; those of the second, the action of β-adrenergics.

The fundamental structure of the majority of adrenergics and of various adrenergic blocking agents is

$$HO-\underset{HO}{\bigcirc}-\overset{\beta}{C}H-\overset{\alpha}{C}H-NH-$$

Experiments have shown that the amino group in the adrenergic drugs is of special significance for the intrinsic activity on α-receptors, whereas the catechol nucleus—mainly the phenolic hydroxy groups—seems to be of particular relevance to the intrinsic activity on β-receptors (132).

Epinephrine possesses both characteristics, and for this reason it has α- and

α blocking agents: phenoxybenzamine, phentolamine

β blocking agents: dichloroisoproterenol, alprenolol, practolol (β-specific) propanolol,

β-adrenergic properties. In fact it contains the following structural components:

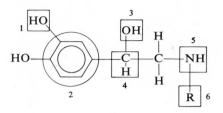

Each of these components contributes to the affinity for the receptor and to the α- and β-adrenergic activity. The phenolic hydroxy groups assist in the fixation to the β-adrenergic-receptor site, through electrostatic forces; removal of these groups results in a considerable decrease in β-adrenergic activity, but not in α-adrenergic activity. The aromatic ring, attaching itself to the receptor by van der Waals forces, is also essential for β-adrenergic activity, although not for α-adrenergic activity. The alcoholic hydroxy group in the (−)-isomer allows another electrostatic bond with the receptor. This might explain why (−)-epinephrine is 45 times more active as a bronchodilator than (+)-epinephrine (in isoproterenol the ratio of this activity between the (−)- and (+)-isomers is 800). The β-carbon, which in the series of β-phenethylamines can form a carbonium ion, helps in the interaction of the drug with the receptor. Finally, the presence of an amino group is essential, especially for α-adrenergic activity, owing to its interaction in a cationic form with the receptor's anionic phosphate group; the substitution of the amino group by OCH_3 results in a product devoid of adrenergic activity; likewise, the bulkier the alkyl substituent on the nitrogen, the greater will be the affinity of the resulting compounds with β-receptors, and the less the affinity with α-receptors (*133*).

On the basis of kinetic studies, Triggle (*134*) suggested that β-haloethylamines alkylate the α-adrenergic receptor at two sites (Figure 8.34).

Although the most potent β-adrenergics are actually catecholamines, there are aminic compounds in which the aromatic groups are not at all similar to a catecholic system; nevertheless they exert β-adrenergic activity. This throws doubt on any mechanism that ascribes a vital role to the catechol group (*135*).

One of the first representations of a receptor site for adrenergics (Figure 8.35) was given by Easson and Stedman (*136*), who suggested that only (−)-epinephrine could enter into complete contact with the receptor, attaching to it by three parts, whereas the optical isomer (+)-epinephrine would attach only by two parts. Hence (−)-epinephrine is much more active than (+)-epinephrine (*3,28*).

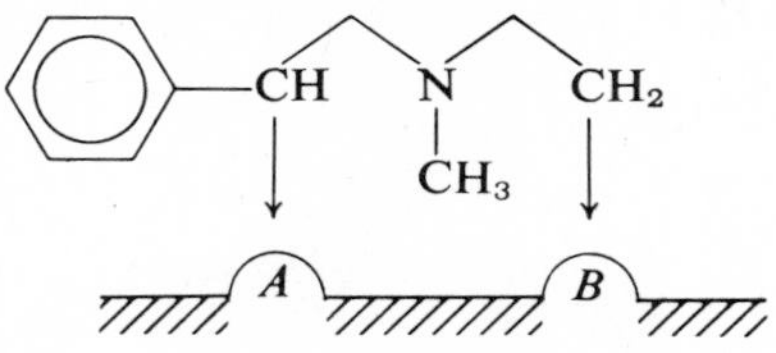

Fig. 8.34.   Interaction of β-haloethylamines with α-adrenergic receptor (*134*).

An analogous hypothesis, but including more details, was advanced by Barlow (*1*). The structure of α- and β-adrenergic receptors that he proposed is shown in Figure 8.36.

Belleau (*137*), on his part, proposed a still more detailed model. Like Barlow's, it incorporates both sites, α and β, into a sole receptor. The anionic site is a phosphate group. The α, or excitatory, effect results from the formation of an ionic pair at the anionic site, as occurs with epinephrine; the β, or inhibitory effect, is a consequence of the chelating action of the phenolic hydroxy group (Figure 8.37).

Bloom and Goldman (*135*), in a later hypothesis, suggested that the basic types of adrenergic regulation result fundamentally from two different phosphorolytic enzyme systems: ATPase activated by magnesium and adenylcyclase. Both use ATP as the normal substrate. According to these authors, the adrenergic receptors consist of enzyme–substrate complexes, their agonism being the process that facilitates the utilization of the substrate. In interacting with a catecholamine the receptor is destroyed and subsequently regenerated through complexation with the enzyme of another

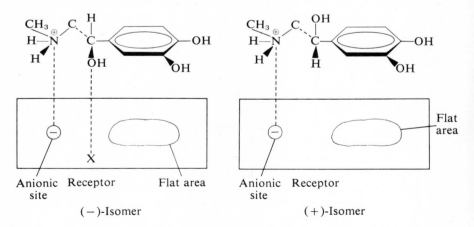

Fig. 8.35.   Interaction of epinephrine isomers with receptor (*28*).

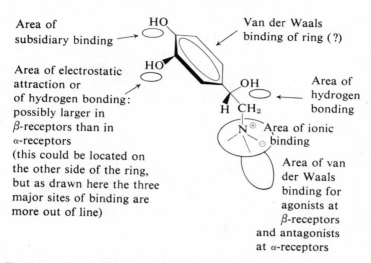

Area of subsidiary binding →

HO

Van der Waals binding of ring (?)

Area of electrostatic attraction or of hydrogen bonding: possibly larger in β-receptors than in α-receptors (this could be located on the other side of the ring, but as drawn here the three major sites of binding are more out of line)

HO

OH
H CH₂
N⊕
⊖

Area of hydrogen bonding

Area of ionic binding

Area of van der Waals binding for agonists at β-receptors and antagonists at α-receptors

Fig. 8.36. Hypothetical structure of α- and β-adrenergic receptors (*1*).

molecule of ATP substrate. The catecholamines are thus catalysts of an ATP cleavage; the nature of the catalytic process is determined by the protein metallic ion system to which the nucleotide is attached. This concept of a

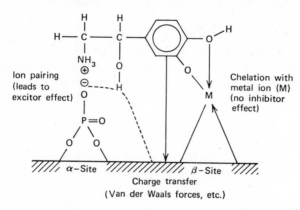

Ion pairing (leads to excitor effect)

Chelation with metal ion (M) (no inhibitor effect)

α–Site   β–Site

Charge transfer
(Van der Waals forces, etc.)

Fig. 8.37. Interaction of norepinephrine with the α- and β-sites of the adrenergic receptor. Ion-pair formation results in a predominantly excitatory effect regardless of the chelation that takes place at the β-site. With epinephrine, the methyl substituent in the amino group causes some steric hindrance, but it does not prevent entirely ionic bond formation at the α-site; this explains why epinephrine exerts excitatory and inhibitory effects. In the case of isoproterenol, however, it can complex only with the β-site because the much bulkier isopropyl group prevents the formation of an ionic bond at the α-site; for this reason isoproterenol manifests no excitatory effects (*137*). (Reprinted with permission.)

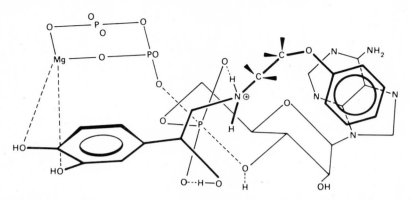

Fig. 8.38. Spatial representation of β-agonism. Catalytic surface of adenylcyclase enzyme binding ATP is not shown (*135*).

dynamic receptor leads to the conclusion that the α- and β-adrenergic receptors, although showing considerable structural similarity, in view of the involvement with ATP at the active site in both cases, are distinct entities. Thus the interaction of a β-agonistic molecule, an indispensable part of which is the amino group, could be represented by Figures 8.38 and 8.39. These models, however, have several weak features, some of which were pointed out by Belleau (*138*).

In a more recent paper Belleau (*138*) summarized the structural characteristics of α- and β-interactions in the following manner: for an active complexation at the α-receptor it is essential that catecholamine possess a small cationic head, such as an ammonium or methylammonium; a substituent bulkier than the methyl group, such as the isopropyl group in isoproterenol,

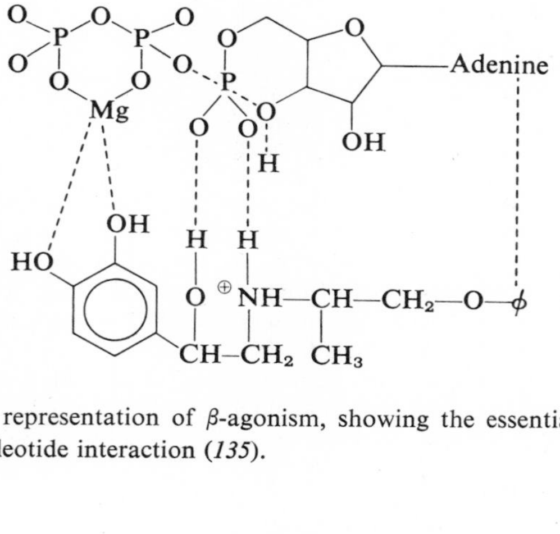

Fig. 8.39. Planar representation of β-agonism, showing the essential features of the catecholamine–nucleotide interaction (*135*).

Nonpolar region

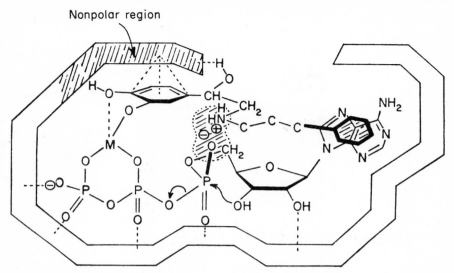

Fig. 8.40. Adenylcyclase or β-receptor activation by N-aralkyl-catecholamine *(138)*. (Reprinted by permission of the Williams and Wilkins Company.)

prevents the formation of the ionic pair at the α-ionic site, but favors the activation of the β-receptor. The catechol system contributes significantly to the activation of the β-receptor.

In the same paper Belleau *(138)* emphasized that his representation of adrenergic receptors (Figure 8.40) could be applicable only when the regulatory site of adenylcyclase for catecholamines constitutes an integral part of the ATP binding surface. There is no direct evidence that this actually occurs.

In a series of graphs accompanied by an explanatory text, Belleau presented a hypothetical model of the α-adrenergic receptor surface and proposed mechanisms through which interaction with drugs would occur. He also presented a model of the β-adrenergic receptor, showing how it would complex with agonists and antagonists. Figures 8.41, 8.42, and 8.43 are some of the several schemes presented by Belleau *(139)*.

Robison and co-workers *(140)* postulated that both α- and β-receptors are related to adenylcyclase. On the basis of this assumption, these researchers presented two simplified models of adrenergic receptors, one of which is shown in Figure 8.44.

Following a mathematical approach to the problem of adrenergic receptors, on the basis of molecular-orbital calculations, Kier deduced the preferred conformations of ephedrine isomers *(141)* and of norepinephrine *(142)*, and proposed a pattern of complementary features to represent the α-adrenergic receptor (Figure 8.45).

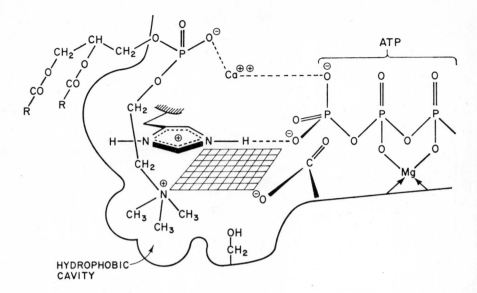

Fig. 8.41. Hypothetical α-adrenergic-receptor surface (resting state) as part of a lipoprotein complex (*139*). (Reprinted by permission of the New York Academy of Sciences.)

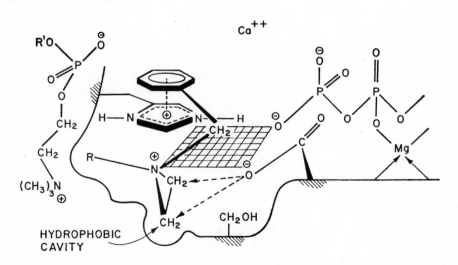

Fig. 8.42. Addition complex between α-adrenergic receptor and dibenamine analogs (*139*). (Reprinted by permission of the New York Academy of Sciences.)

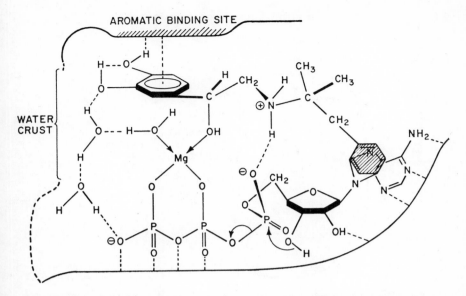

Fig. 8.43. Schematic interaction of β-sympathomimetic drug with adenylcyclase (π-bonding with adenine?) (*139*). (Reprinted by permission of the New York Academy of Sciences.)

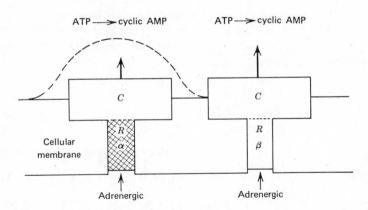

Fig. 8.44. Possible model of adenylcyclase as related to adrenergic receptors. Both adenylcyclase molecules are essentially similar with respect to catalytic activity, but are localized in such a way that cyclic AMP (adenosine- 3′,5′-phosphate) levels may increase in different parts of the cell. The adenylcyclase molecule is represented as consisting of at least two distinct subunits: *R*, the regulatory subunit, facing the extracellular fluid; *C*, the catalytic subunit, the active center of which is in contact with the interior of the cell (*140*). (Reprinted by permission of the New York Academy of Sciences.)

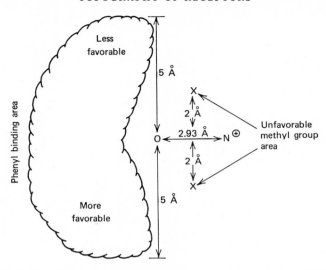

Fig. 8.45. Postulated β-adrenergic-receptor features based on preferred conformations of norepinephrine and ephedrine isomers (*141*). (Reprinted by permission of the Williams and Wilkins Company and of the author.)

Very recently Belleau and co-workers (*143*) found specific and profound irreversible inhibition of the catecholamine adrenergic α-receptor by carbamates of the 1,2- and 1,4-dihydroquinoline series. In order to explain the mechanism of action of these agents, Belleau proposed a cross-link formation between the carboxy function of the hypothetical receptor and a sterically accessible nucleophile on the active surface (*143*):

By considering that the common functionality in some adrenergic agents is a 4-hydroxybenzyl alcohol or amine, system which can undergo quinone methide formation, Larsen (*144*) proposed the following mechanism for the interaction between these drugs and their receptors: stereoselective activation of the benzylic hydroxyl I*a*, elimination of the benzylic hydroxyl or its activated derivative, *in situ* generation of the quinone methide I*b*, and finally reaction of the latter with an external receptor nucleophile. This mechanism is as shown below.

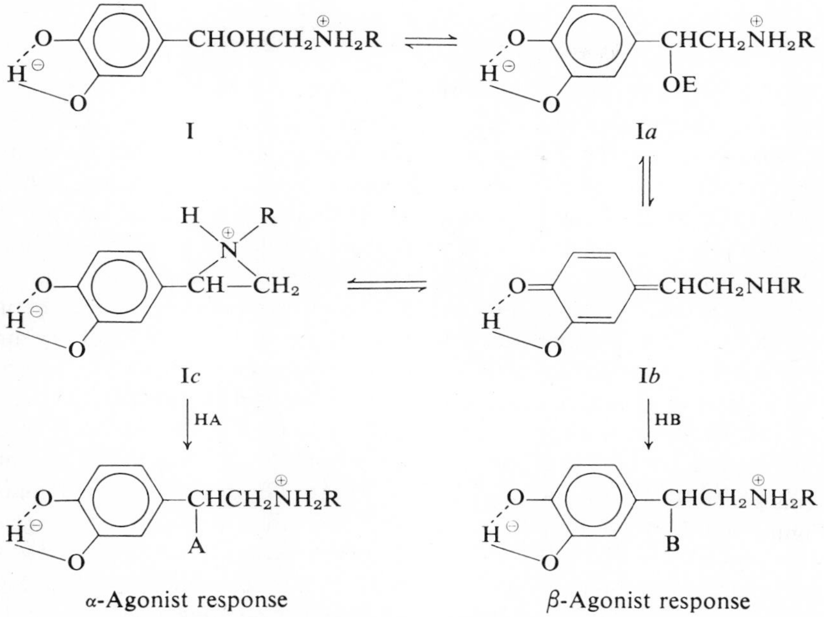

α-Agonist response   β-Agonist response

According to Larsen's hypothesis, catecholamines having a small substituent on the amino nitrogen atom and therefore able to form an aziridine ring are α-adrenergic agonists. The presence of a bulky group on that atom either makes more difficult or prevents the formation of an aziridine ring by internal cyclization; hence eventually these drugs mediate only β-adrenergic response. The amino substituent thus determines the relative availability of the two reactive species I*b* and I*c*, accountable for β- and α-adrenergic responses, respectively.

However, besides other criticisms that can be made to Larsen's hypothesis it must be recalled that the chemical structure of several adrenergic agents (125), some of which do not even have the catecholic system (135), does not allow the formation of the proposed common activated complex.

Details on adrenergics and adrenergic blocking agents as well as on the hypothetical interactions of these two groups of drugs with their respective receptors can also be found in recent monographs (133,134,145–152).

VII. HISTAMINE RECEPTORS

The pharmacology of histamine has been the object of systematic and complete studies (153), and its most important aspects were reviewed recently (154).

$$
\begin{array}{c}
CH_2 \\
\;CH_2 \\
H-N \bigcirc N \cdots H - NH_2 \\
\oplus
\end{array}
$$

Taking into consideration preliminary studies (*155*) especially those related to the fact that at physiological pH histamine ionizes, behaves as a cation and forms an intramolecular hydrogen bond, and also that histamine action is inhibited by derivatives of arginine, histidine, and guanidine, Rocha e Silva (*153*) assumed that histamine fits the receptor and attaches to it by means of two poles: the imino group of the imidazole ring and the free amino group of the side chain. The first one forms a transitory bond with the polarized carbonyl group of a peptide linkage of the receptor; the second one forms a hydrogen bonding with a protein residue of histidine or of arginine (Figure 8.46). Other forces, mainly hydrophobic, can assist in the interaction.

Later studies gave support to this theory. According to Bloom and Goldman (*135*), the histamine-receptor interaction involves a phosphoryl group transfer process; histamine-like substances function as catalysts of enzymic reactions by direct interaction with the substrate. On the basis of the remarkable physiological parallelism of histamine-like substances, adrenergic agents and cholinergic agents, Bloom and Goldman proposed for histamine the hypothetical receptor shown in Figure 8.47. In this conception the monoester phosphate substrate is very similar to the corresponding in acetylcholine, whereas the role of agonist seems to be analogous to the process involved in the α-receptor system.

Noting that the structural requirements for a histamine receptor in the ileum of the guinea pig were different from those for a histamine receptor in the uterus or in the stomach, Ash and Schild (*156*) concluded that there should be at least two types of histamine receptors.

Recently, through molecular-orbital calculations, Kier (*157*) predicted that

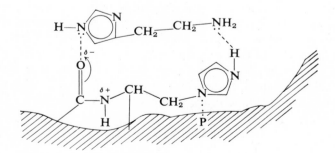

Fig. 8.46.   Schematic representation of histamine receptor (*153*).

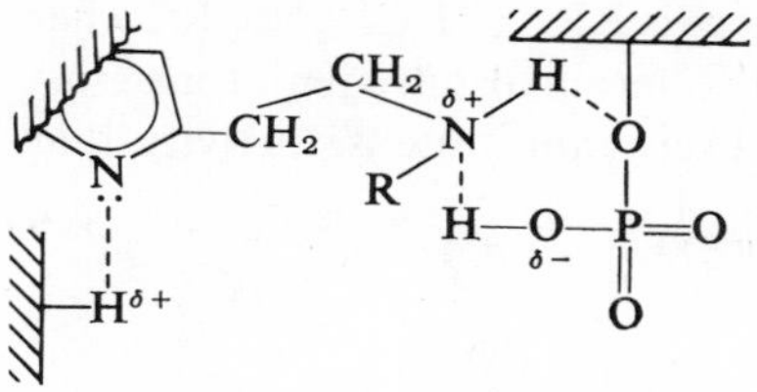

Fig. 8.47. Hypothetical receptor of histamine (*135*).

histamine has the ability to exist in two preferred conformations (shown in Chapter 5, Section II.A). He therefore postulated that histamine can elicit two distinct biological responses, depending on the presence of one or the other complementary receptor. The H^1 receptor would be complementary to the internitrogen relationship

$$\sum N \xleftrightarrow{4.55\text{Å}} N^{\oplus}$$

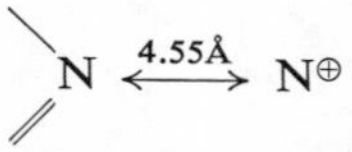

whereas the H^2 receptor would be complementary to the internitrogen relationship

$$\sum N \xleftrightarrow{3.60\text{Å}} N^{\oplus}$$

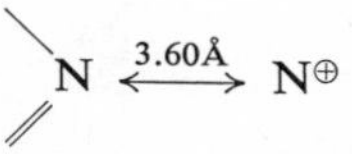

This dual action also occurs, as it was already seen, in the case of acetylcholine. As analogous calculations show, acetylcholine also exists in two conformations: muscarinic and nicotinic (Section V of this chapter).

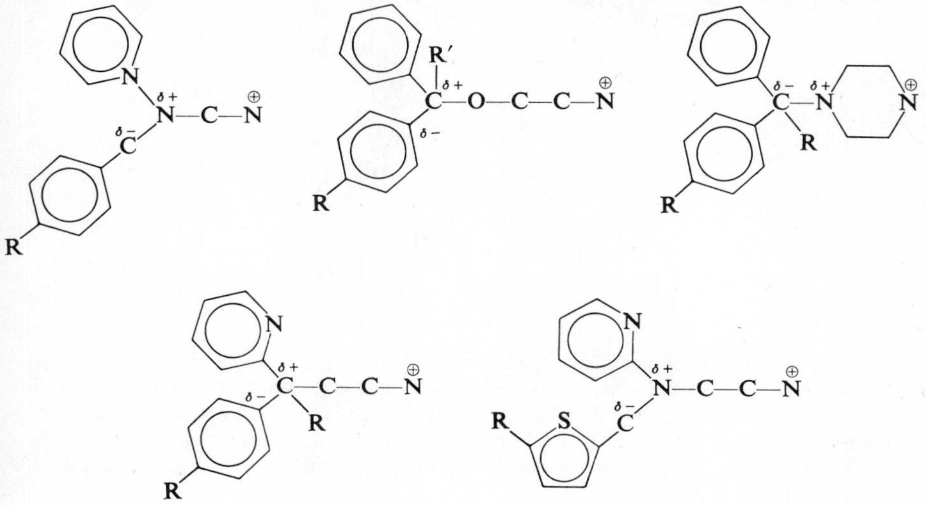

It is believed that antihistaminic agents act by a competitive mechanism for the histamine-receptor site. The formula of the antihistaminic agents that act as competitive inhibitors is $RRXCH_2CH_2NR'R''$, where X stands for nitrogen, oxygen, or carbon. The terminal nitrogen atom must be a tertiary one; the dimethyl derivatives exert more intense activity than other homologs; the

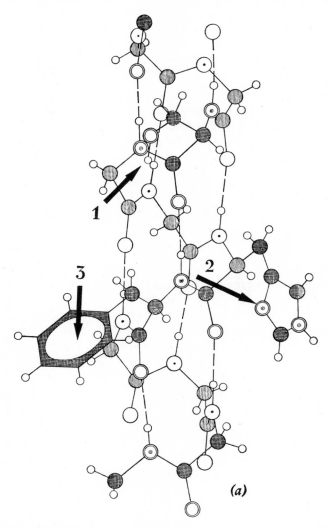

Fig. 8.48. α-Helix polypeptide receptor model showing three anchorage sites: (1) serine—OH; (2) histidine—N_3; (3) phenylalanine–phenyl group. Small circles: hydrogen atoms; large shaded circles: carbon atoms; large open circles: oxygen atoms; centered circles: nitrogen atoms; broken lines: hydrogen bonds. (b) Receptor model accommodating histamine. (c) Receptor model accommodating 4-methyldiphenhydramine (*159*). (Reprinted with permission.)

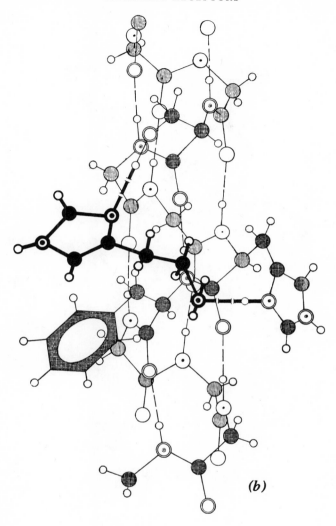

(b)

alkyl chain between X and N, for optimal activity, must have two carbon atoms; optimal activity is obtained when R and R′ are aromatic; the introduction of groups with a −*I* inductive effect into the *para* position of the R phenyl enhances the potency. Summing up, an antihistaminic agent of this type will have an ionizable amino group and a central dipole (*63*).

Steric factors influence antihistaminic activity. For instance, in triprolidine the pyridyl and pyrrolidyl groups are in a *trans* position in the more active

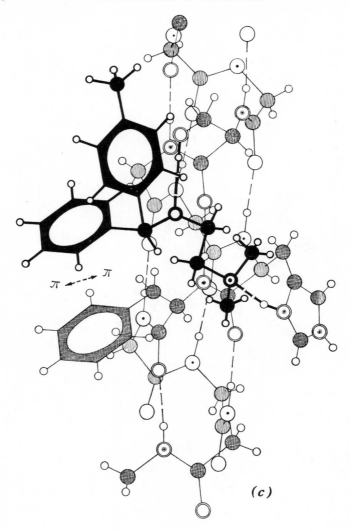

(c)

isomer; of all the optical isomers of *p*-methylbenzhydryl-2-dimethylamino-ethyl ether, the dextrorotatory form is three to four times more active than the levorotatory isomer.

In order to explain the interaction of an antihistaminic agent with its receptor, Harms and Nauta (*158*) proposed that it consists of (a) an anionic site that attaches to a protonated aliphatic group and (b) a flat region—at a more or less fixed distance—that accommodates one of the aromatic rings, which is approximately coplanar with the lateral chain.

In a later paper Nauta and co-workers (*159*) suggested a detailed model of the histamine receptor (Figure 8.48). It is depicted as composed of a polypeptide chain in the α-helix configuration. The complexation of receptor and antihistaminic agent is claimed to occur at three points:

1. A phenyl group of a phenylalanylhistidyl residue of the α-helix interacts with an aromatic ring of the drug.

2. An imidazole ring of the same residue attaches to the —NH(CH$_3$)$_2$ group of the drug.

3. A hydroxy group, for instance, of the neighboring serine of the receptor, forms a hydrogen bond with the ether oxygen of the drug.

According to Barlow (*1*), the antihistaminic agent triprolidine and others of the same type (e.g., isothipendyl) attach to a receptor surface such as the one shown in Figure 8.49. Note that in triprolidine the distance between the nitrogen atoms is 4.80 ± 0.2 Å (very close to 4.55 Å, found for one of the preferred conformations of histamine), and the pyridyl ring is coplanar with the olefin bond (*157*). However, in the light of new facts, especially those related to the configuration of (+)-pheniramine, the topography of the receptor could also be a mirror image of the one represented in Figure 8.49 (*160*). Antihistaminic agents would have, therefore, two receptor sites (Figure 8.50).

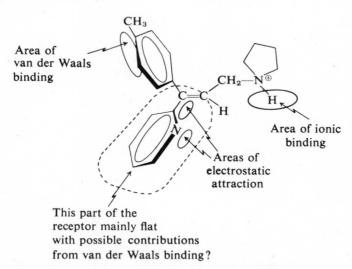

Fig. 8.49. Receptor for antihistaminic agents. The interaction is through electrostatic attraction, ionic binding, and van der Waals forces (*1*).

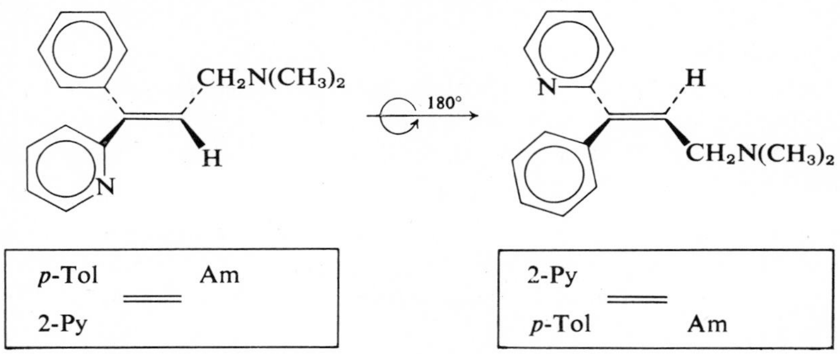

Fig. 8.50. The two receptor areas of antihistaminic agents (*160*). (Reproduced with permission of the copyright owner.)

In order to obtain evidence for this hypothesis the synthesis of anti-histaminic agents with rigid structure is in progress.

VIII. SEROTONIN RECEPTOR

Serotonin has been thoroughly studied (*161–165*). However, even extensive and systematic research, such as carried out by Offermeier and Ariëns (*166*), failed to give insight into the chemical structure of its hypothetical receptors.

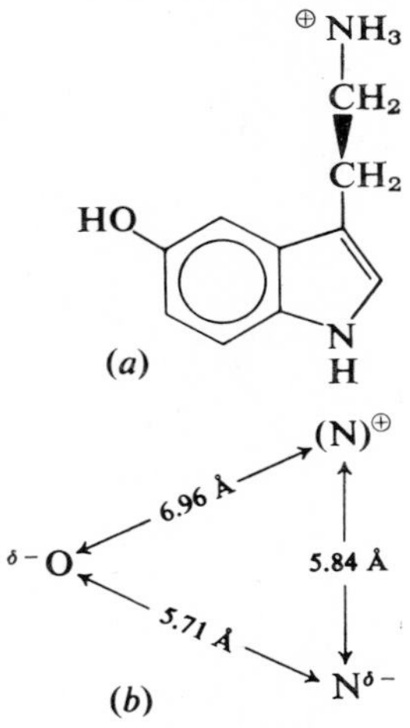

Fig. 8.51. Serotonin receptor: (*a*) preferred conformation of serotonin; (*b*) structural features proposed as being complementary to the serotonin receptor (*167*). (Reproduced with permission of the copyright owner.)

Gaddum described these as being of two types: M, blocked by morphine, and D, blocked by dibenzyline (*162*).

Recently, however, from molecular-orbital calculations, Kier (*167*) concluded that serotonin exists in only one preferred conformation and deduced a complementary pattern of forces on the proposed receptor (Figure 8.51).

IX. RECEPTORS OF MONOAMINE OXIDASE INHIBITORS

The monoamine oxidase (MAO) inhibitors possess, as characteristic structures, a planar π-system (aromatic ring) and a cationic head with analogous arrangement to the natural substrates of this enzyme, such as epinephrine, norepinephrine, tyramine, and DOPA, or to that of the imino intermediary that would be formed through oxidation of the amine (*168,169*).

Kinetic studies (*170,171*) led to the conclusion that the rate-determining step of oxidation of amines catalyzed by MAO is the abstraction of an α-hydrogen and that the two hydrogen atoms attached to the α-carbon are not equivalent for the enzyme, this being the reason for the interaction between MAO and its inhibitors being generally depicted as a "three-point accommodation": through the two α-hydrogens and the only amine function (*169*). Sometimes, however, only a "two-point accommodation" is possible. For instance, owing to the relative lack of specificity of MAO toward the enantiomers of such inhibitors as amphetamine, pheniprazine, tranylcypromine, and α-alkyltryptamines, it seems that in the interaction of these with the enzyme only a sole substituent is involved besides the amino group attached to the α-carbon. Likewise the very fact that 1-methyl-2-phenylcyclopropylamine, a potent MAO inhibitor, has no α-hydrogen atom is evidence that it is not essential for this attachment (*168*).

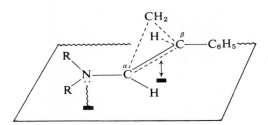

Fig. 8.52. Postulated mode of interaction between 2-phenylcyclopropylamine and MAO. The drug complexes with the enzyme either through the unshared electron pair of the amino group or more likely through the electrostatic interaction between the positively charged ammonium ion form of the amine and a negative group of the enzyme (*168*). (Reprinted by permission of the American Chemical Society.)

Reasoning thusly, and not disregarding the role of the aromatic ring, Belleau and Moran (*169*) suggested that the interaction between 2-phenylcyclopropylamine and MAO occurs mainly as a result of the high electron density

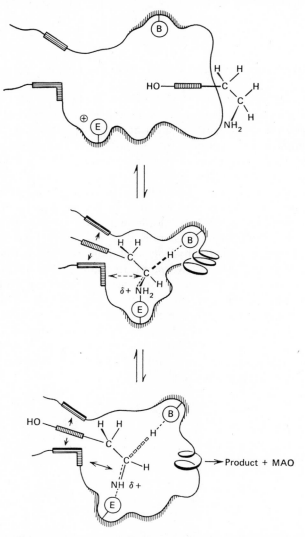

Fig. 8.53. Interaction between tyramine and monoamine oxidase. The weakening of an α-C—H bond allows the substrate to induce a conformational change in the enzyme; this opens the possibility of interaction between acceptor B and α-H; furthermore the polarizable C⋯N bond interacts with the enzyme surface (*169*). (Reprinted by permission of the New York Academy of Sciences and of the authors.)

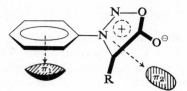

Fig. 8.54. Hypothetical interaction between *N*-arylsydnones and MAO by means of π-electrons in two regions (*172*). (Reprinted by permission of the American Chemical Society.)

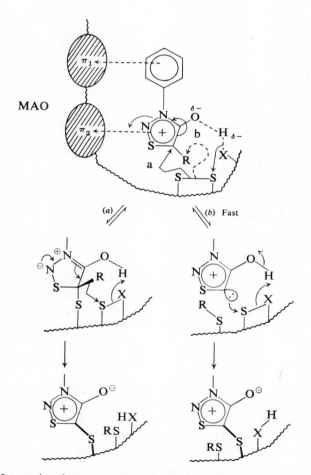

Fig. 8.55. Interaction between anhydrothiadiazolium hydroxides and hypothetical MAO (*173*). (Reprinted by permission of the American Chemical Society.)

present in the bond that binds the α- and β-carbons of the cyclopropane, and not as a consequence of the direct interactions of the α-substituents (excepting the amino group) with the enzyme. The high affinity of this drug for the receptor therefore results from electronic and steric properties, since MAO is rigorously stereospecific toward the α-hydrogen of substrates but only slightly stereoselective toward β-substituents and inhibitors in general (Figure 8.52).

On the basis of the deuterium isotope effects in their experiments designed to study the chemical mechanism of MAO, Belleau and Moran proposed that tyramine–MAO complexation occurs as represented in Figure 8.53.

Recently a novel MAO-inhibitor class has been described—namely, heterocyclic mesoionic compounds. The first group of this class is represented by N-arylsydnones (*172*), which contain an aromatic ring and a basic function; the latter one is the carbonyl oxygen of sydnone. It is claimed that the moderate action of these new chemical compounds both *in vitro* and *in vivo* results from noncompetitive interaction between either the carbon 4 or the carbonyl carbon and a nucleophilic function of the enzyme (Figure 8.54).

Another group of that class of mesoionic compounds is constituted by anhydro-1,2,3-thiadiazolium hydroxides (*173*). Some of these inhibited MAO both *in vitro* and *in vivo*. In an attempt to explain their biological action by accommodating them within the framework of the hypothetical requirements for MAO inhibition (*169*), it was postulated that the aromatic ring interacts with the π-electron binding surfaces of the enzyme, and the anionic charge (which acts primarily through the *exo*-oxygen) is so situated as to permit binding with an electrophilic enzyme group (Figure 8.55).

X. RECEPTOR OF PHENOTHIAZINE TRANQUILIZERS

After studying a series of tranquilizers with a phenothiazine nucleus, Gordon and co-workers (*174*) postulated that these tranquilizers interact with cellular receptor sites in the central nervous system. The receptor that was proposed for compounds of the prochlorperazine type is shown in Figure 8.56.

In that model portion *A* has a low order of specificity in the longitudinal direction but a high order along the transverse axis; this seems to indicate that the molecule fits into a rather narrow slot. It is believed that the highest degree of structural specificity is in the position *B* of the molecule; when R is CH$_3$, the molecule has greater activity, perhaps because the methyl group, being relatively bulky, restricts the possibility of rotation and thus facilitates the attachment of the drug to the receptor by three points. Portion *C* shows the same structural requirements as those of the three-carbon side chain but

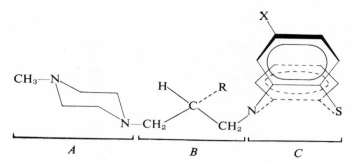

Fig. 8.56. Possible conformation of prochlorperazine-type molecule interacting with receptor surface (*174*).

allows considerable variation in the nature of X; the function of the X-group is to influence the resonance forms of the ring system and/or the electron density of the sulfur, since it is removed from the receptor surface (*171, 174–176*), as the phenothiazine ring system has a fold along the nitrogen–sulfur axis (*177*). Further, considering the results obtained through structural variations in chlorpromazine, it is presumed that the diethylamino and piperidino groups must have definite widths (*171*).

For information on the pharmacology and chemical structure of substituted phenothiazines, see a recent review (*178*).

see also Schenker, E. & Harbst, H." Phenothiazine und Azaphenothiazine als Heilmittel" in Fortschritte der Arzneimittelforschung, vol V. Ed., E. Jucker. Basel · Stuttgart: Birkhäuser Verlag, 1963.

XI. DIURETIC RECEPTORS

Diuretics belong to different chemical classes. They are not, however, structurally nonspecific drugs. The biological response they produce is directly related to their chemical structure. However, they act through different mechanisms (*179*). Each class of diuretics interacts with different receptors (*180*). It was thought that the receptor of organomercurial diuretics would be like the one shown in Figure 8.57.

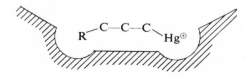

Fig. 8.57. Proposed interaction of organomercurial diuretics with receptor.

However, since many organomercurial diuretics cannot be accommodated by this receptor model, it is now assumed that the active species is the mercuric ion, which attaches specifically to two receptor sites, one being a sulfhydryl and the second another sulfhydryl or a phenolic hydroxy group, amino group, carboxyl group, or imidazole ring, through the mechanism represented in Chapter 7, Section II (181).

Sulfamido as well as benzothiadiazino diuretics attach to the active center of a carbonic anhydrase molecule by a competitive mechanism as represented in Figure 7.14 (Chapter 7, Section V), due to the structural analogy between the carbonic acid and the sulfamido group. This group must not contain substituents, otherwise it may lose or have diminished diuretic action as a result of a weakened attachment to the receptor. Details on the interaction of sulfamido diuretics with carbonic anhydrase have been obtained by Fridborg and co-workers by the X-ray diffraction method (Chapter 6, Section III).

XII. STEROID RECEPTORS

The molecules of steroids are relatively inflexible, because their structure is flat and rigid. The manner in which they interact with their receptors was suggested by Bush (182).

In the case of glucocorticoids, gestagens, and possibly other types of steroid hormones, Bush claims that the intrinsic action results not from a chemical reaction but from relatively firm "physical" association with their receptors that involves *little or no movement of the parts of the molecules that are in close apposition.* In consequence the portion of the receptor that interacts with other molecules or groups (or with other parts of the same molecule, if large enough) is prevented from doing so *by the mere presence of the steroid.*

To explain the mode of action of androgens, Wolff and collaborators (183) suggested that in the steroid–receptor complex the steroid is in contact with the receptor surface in two discrete areas: the β-face of rings A, B, and C, and the α-face of ring D, as shown in Figure 8.58. The two principal binding sites are the A-ring, where a π-bond is formed, and the 17 β-function, which can be attached by hydrogen bonding mainly (184), hydrophobic bonding, and other nonbonded interactions. The remaining surfaces of the molecule complex with the receptor through hydrophobic interactions or van der Waals forces. Wolff et al. claimed that the effect of the steroid is to induce a conformational change in the receptor, since no chemical reaction as such takes place. Crystallographic measurements of estriol seem to give support to this model (185).

In a recent book, in which are reviewed critically the several theories

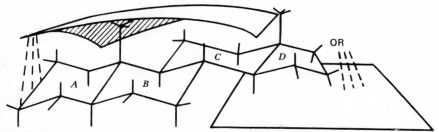

Fig. 8.58. Simultaneous interaction of the androgen molecule with two spatially separate surfaces at the receptor site (*183*). (Reprinted by permission of the American Chemical Society.)

presented thus far on structure-activity relationships in hormone steroids, Vida postulates that the *steroid-receptor interaction is a three-dimensional attachment.* Androgens-receptor interaction, for instance, involves all rings of these steroids, not only their α and β faces (α of *A* and *D*; β of *B*, *C* and *D*) but their peripheral sides as well (*186*).

In the case of the 2-nitroestrone-3-methyl ether it was suggested that its complexation with the receptor occurs between the *A*- or *B*-rings and an aromatic group of the enzyme, probably a tyrosyl residue. The interaction of these rings with the aromatic ring of the enzyme is either hydrophobic or through π-electrons or through both types. Furthermore the nitro group attaches to the hydroxy group of the tyrosyl residue by means of hydrogen bonding reinforcing the complexation. This effect is increased if the methyl group engages in hydrophobic interactions with alkyl residues on the receptor surface (*187*).

On the basis of the preferred conformations of progesterone, corticosterone, and cortisol as deduced from molecular-orbital calculations, some of which were experimentally confirmed through infrared and nuclear-magnetic-resonance techniques (*188*), Kier (*189*) proposed a complementary receptor of cortisol (Figure 8.59). He claims that his model can explain how cortisol might interfere with both serotonin and histamine, functioning as an antagonist if these amine receptors were involved in directing the inflammatory response. In a later paper Kier and Whitehouse (*190*) postulated that 17-β-hydroxycorticoids and some nonsteroid anti-inflammatory drugs, such as

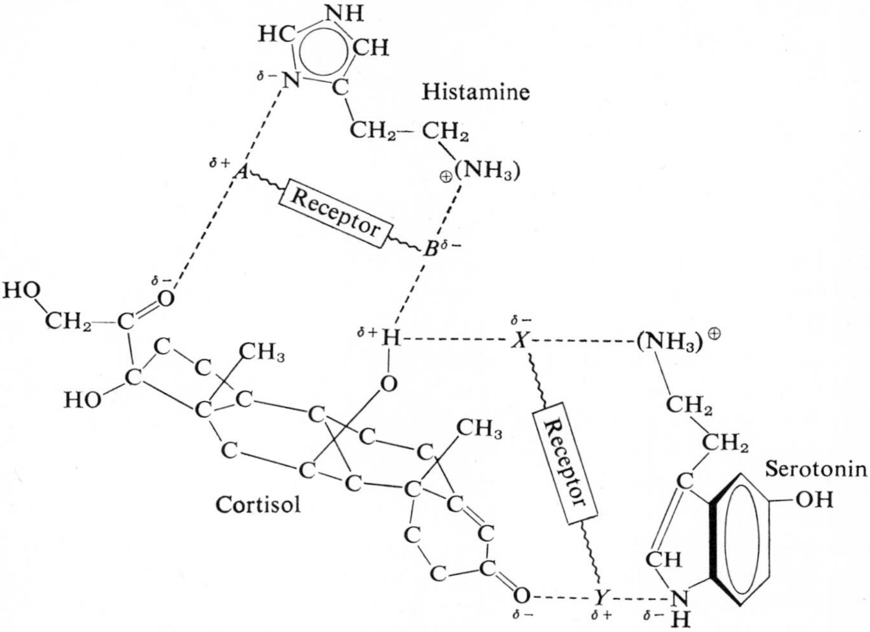

Fig. 8.59. Relationship of key atoms of cortisol in calculated preferred conformation to histamine and serotonin in their preferred conformations. A simultaneous engagement of the cortisol with the receptors is not intended to be implied (*189*). (Reprinted by permission of the American Chemical Society and of the author.)

indomethacin, phenylbutazone, the fenamic acids, and salicylates, have common receptor(s), since the latter mimic cortisol in suppressing acute inflammation in experimental animals and have some similar structural features that allow them to bind to certain receptors for histamine and serotonin, although they might act by an allosteric inhibition mechanism and not necessarily as competitive antagonists of the inflammagenic amines.

A recent monograph has analyzed several other aspects of gestagens (*191*).

XIII. RECEPTORS OF POLYCYCLIC CARCINOGENIC AGENTS

In Chapter 5, Section IV, we examined some structural aspects of carcinogens, mainly the electronic charge distribution in the polycyclic hydrocarbons. It was seen that these attach to the cellular constituent through the *K*- or *L*-regions. The molecules are flat and elongated in shape, and the hypothetical surface that corresponds to them is shown in Figure 8.60.

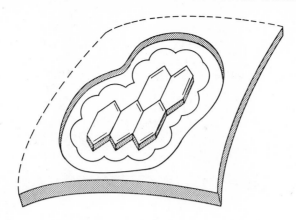

Fig. 8.60. A schematic representation of the receptor-surface site of carcinogens (*192*).

According to Arcos and Arcos (*192*), such hydrocarbons penetrate between the layers of polypeptide chains linked by hydrogen bonds and form compounds of inclusion, as shown in Figure 8.61. It is quite possible that in these inclusion compounds interaction occurs through charge transfer (*192*).

Carcinogenic azo compounds, on the other hand, interact with functional groups of the endoplasmic membrane (Figure 8.62).

Details on cancer research may be found elsewhere (*193,194*).

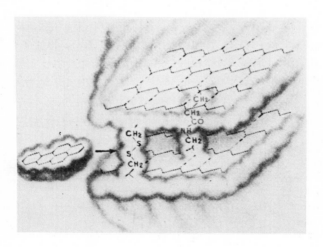

Fig. 8.61. Carcinogen–protein interaction involving the formation of molecular inclusion (*192*).

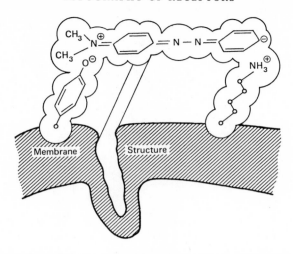

Fig. 8.62. Interaction of 4-dimethylaminoazobenzene with functional groups on an endoplasmic membrane surface through electrostatic attraction with the phenolic hydroxyl of tyrosine and the ε-amino nitrogen of lysine. Another possibility is the intervention of the electron-rich β-azo nitrogen, through either charge transfer or secondary interactions. Protonation of the β-azo nitrogen may result in covalent-bond formation. Interaction is therefore with more than one functional group (*192*).

REFERENCES

1. R. B. Barlow, *Introduction to Chemical Pharmacology*, 2nd ed., Methuen, London, 1964.
2. W. C. Holland, R. L. Klein, and A. H. Briggs, *Introduction to Molecular Pharmacology*, Macmillan, New York, 1964.
3. J. R. diPalma, Ed., *Drill's Pharmacology in Medicine*, 3rd ed., McGraw-Hill, New York, 1965.
4. B. M. Bloom, *Ann. Rep. Med. Chem.*, **2**, 227 (1967).
5. A. Goldstein, L. Aronow, and S. M. Kalman, *Principles of Drug Action*, Harper and Row, New York, 1968.
6. B. L. Vallee and J. F. Riordan, *Ann. Rev. Biochem.*, **38**, 733 (1969).
7. S. Ehrenpreis, J. H. Fleisch, and T. W. Mittag, *Pharmacol. Rev.*, **21**, 131 (1969).
8. H. G. Mautner, *Ann. Rep. Med. Chem.*, **4**, 230 (1969).
9. S. J. Singer, *Advan. Prot. Chem.*, **22**, 1 (1967).
10. J. F. Moran, M. May, H. Kimelberg, and D. J. Triggle, *Mol. Pharmacol.*, **3**, 15, 28 (1967).
11. J.-P. Changeux, T. R. Podleski, and L. Wofsy, *Proc. Natl. Acad. Sci. U.S.*, **58**, 2063 (1967).
12. I. Silman and A. Karlin, *Science*, **164**, 1420 (1969).
13. H. G. Mautner, *Pharmacol. Rev.*, **19**, 107 (1967).

14. N. V. Khromov-Borisov and M. J. Michelson, *Pharmacol. Rev.*, **18**, 1051 (1966).
15. E. E. Smissman, W. L. Nelson, J. B. LaPidus, and J. L. Day, *J. Med. Chem.*, **9**, 458 (1966).
16. P. D. Armstrong, J. G. Cannon, and J. P. Long, *Nature*, **220**, 65 (1968).
17. M. R. Boots and S. G. Boots, *J. Pharm. Sci.*, **58**, 553 (1969).
18. J. P. Glusker, *J. Mol. Biol.*, **38**, 149 (1968).
19. M. F. Perutz, *European J. Biochem.*, **8**, 455 (1969).
20. D. M. Chipman and N. Sharon, *Science*, **165**, 454 (1969).
21. O. Jardetzky, *Advan. Chem. Phys.*, **7**, 499 (1964).
22. J. J. Fischer and O. Jardetzky, *J. Am. Chem. Soc.*, **87**, 3237 (1965).
23. M. Mandel, *J. Biol. Chem.*, **240**, 1586 (1965).
24. D. H. Meadows, J. L. Markley, J. S. Cohen, and O. Jardetzky, *Proc. Natl. Acad. Sci. U.S.*, **58**, 1307 (1967).
25. O. Jardetzky, "The Study of Drug Binding Sites by Nuclear Magnetic Relaxation," in E. J. Ariëns, Ed., *Physico-Chemical Aspects of Drug Action*, Pergamon, Oxford, 1968, pp. 189–191.
26. D. R. H. Gourley, *Progr. Drug Res.*, **7**, 11 (1964).
27. A. H. Beckett and A. F. Casy, *J. Pharm. Pharmacol.*, **6**, 986 (1954).
28. A. H. Beckett, *Progr. Drug Res.*, **1**, 455 (1959).
29. A. H. Beckett and A. F. Casy, *Progr. Med. Chem.*, **2**, 43 (1962).
30. A. H. Beckett and A. F. Casy, *Progr. Med. Chem.*, **4**, 171 (1965).
31. J. Fridrichsons, M. F. Mackay, and A. McL. Mathieson, *Tetrahedron Letters*, 2887 (1968).
32. P. A. J. Janssen and C. A. M. van der Eycken, "The Chemical Anatomy of Potent Morphine-like Analgesics," in A. Burger, Ed., *Drugs Affecting the Central Nervous System*, Dekker, New York, 1968, pp. 25–60.
33. P. S. Portoghese and D. L. Larson, *J. Pharm. Sci.*, **57**, 711 (1968).
34. P. S. Portoghese, A. A. Mikhail, and H. J. Kupferberg, *J. Med. Chem.*, **11**, 219 (1968).
35. A. F. Casy, *J. Med. Chem.*, **11**, 188 (1968).
36. A. F. Casy and M. M. A. Hassan, *J. Med. Chem.*, **11**, 601 (1968).
37. A. F. Casy and A. P. Parulkar, *J. Med. Chem.*, **12**, 178 (1969).
38. R. A. Hardy, Jr., and M. G. Howell, "Synthetic Analgetics with Morphine-like Actions," in G. deStevens, Ed., *Analgetics*, Academic, New York, 1965, pp. 179–279.
39. W. R. Martin, *Pharmacol. Rev.*, **19**, 463 (1967).
40. L. L. Smith, *J. Pharm. Sci.*, **55**, 101 (1966).
41. P. S. Portoghese and D. A. Williams, *J. Pharm. Sci.*, **55**, 990 (1966).
42. P. S. Portoghese and D. A. Williams, *J. Med. Chem.*, **12**, 839 (1969).
43. A. F. Casy and M. M. A. Hassan, *Can. J. Chem.*, **47**, 1587 (1969).
44. N. B. Eddy, *Chem. Ind.*, 1462 (1959).
45. E. L. May and E. M. Fry, *J. Org. Chem.*, **22**, 1366 (1957).
46. E. E. Smissman and M. Steinman, *J. Med. Chem.*, **9**, 455 (1966); *ibid.*, **10**, 1054 (1967).
47. D. E. Koshland, Jr., "Mechanisms of Transfer Enzymes," in P. D. Boyer, H. Lardy, and K. Myrbäck, Eds., *The Enzymes*, 2nd ed., Vol. I, Academic, New York, 1959, pp. 305–346.

48. B. Labouesse, B. H. Havsteen, and G. P. Hess, *Proc. Natl. Acad. Sci. U.S.*, **48**, 2137 (1962).

49. H. Parker and R. Lumry, *J. Am. Chem. Soc.*, **85**, 483 (1963).

50. B. Belleau, *J. Med. Chem.*, **7**, 776 (1964).

51. L. Stryer, *Ann. Rev. Biochem.*, **37**, 25 (1968).

52. D. E. Koshland, Jr., "Regulatory Control Through Conformation Changes in Proteins," in G. Weber, Ed., *Advances in Enzyme Regulation*, Vol. VI, Pergamon, Oxford, 1968, pp. 291–301.

53. S. N. Timasheff and G. D. Fasman, Eds., *Structure and Stability of Biological Macromolecules*, Dekker, New York, 1969.

54. P. S. Portoghese, *J. Med. Chem.*, **8**, 609 (1965).

55. P. S. Portoghese, *J. Pharm. Sci.*, **55**, 865 (1966).

56. D. E. Koshland, Jr., *Federation Proc.*, **23**, 719 (1964).

57. K. W. Bentley, D. G. Hardy, B. Meek et al., *J. Am. Chem. Soc.*, **89**, 3267, 3273, 3281, 3293, 3303, 3312 (1967).

58. L. S. Harris and W. L. Dewey, *Ann. Rep. Med. Chem.*, **2**, 33 (1967).

59. M. W. Whitehouse, *Biochem. Pharmacol.*, Sp. Suppl., 293 (1968).

60. T. Y. Shen, *Topics Med. Chem.*, **1**, 29 (1967).

61. P. T. Thyrum, R. J. Luchi, and E. M. Thyrum, *Nature*, **223**, 747 (1969).

62. J. Büchi, *Grundlagen der Arzneimittelforschung und der synthetischen Arzneimittel*, Birkhauser, Basel, 1963.

63. E. J. Ariëns, Ed., *Molecular Pharmacology*, Vol. I, Academic, New York, 1964.

64. G. B. Koelle, W. W. Douglas, and A. Carlsson, Eds., *Pharmacology of Cholinergic and Adrenergic Transmission*, Pergamon, Oxford, 1965.

65. G. Kuschinsky and H. Lüllmann, *Kurzes Lehrbuch der Pharmakologie*, Thieme, Stuttgart, 1967.

66. K. S. Cole, *Membranes, Ions and Impulses*, University of California Press, Berkeley, 1968.

67. J. J. Lewis, *An Introduction to Pharmacology*, 3rd ed., Williams and Wilkins, Baltimore, 1964.

68. G. B. Koelle, Ed., *Cholinesterase and Anticholinesterase Agents. Handbuch der experimentellen Pharmakologie*, Vol. XV, Springer, Berlin, 1963.

69. W. S. Root and F. G. Hofmann, Eds., *Physiological Pharmacology*, Vol. III, Academic, New York, 1967.

70. A. Burger, Ed., *Drugs Affecting the Peripheral Nervous System*, Dekker, New York, 1967.

71. J. Durell, J. T. Garland, and R. O. Friedel, *Science*, **165**, 862 (1969).

72. B. Belleau and G. Lacasse, *J. Med. Chem.*, **7**, 768 (1964).

73. J. C. Kellett, Jr., and C. W. Hite, *J. Pharm. Sci.*, **54**, 883 (1965).

74. A. W. Solter, *J. Pharm. Sci.*, **54**, 1755 (1965).

75. E. E. Smissman and G. S. Chappell, *J. Med. Chem.*, **12**, 429, 432 (1969).

76. A. H. Beckett, *Ann. N.Y. Acad. Sci.*, **144**, 675 (1967).

77. T. R. Podleski, *Biochem. Pharmacol.*, **18**, 211 (1969).

78. M. Martin-Smith, G. A. Smail, and J. B. Stenlake, *J. Pharm. Pharmacol.*, **19**, 561 (1967).

79. F. G. Canepa, P. Pauling and H. Sörum, *Nature*, **210**, 907 (1966).

80. B. Belleau, *Advan. Drug Res.*, **2**, 89 (1965).
81. S. Ehrenpreis, "Drug-Macromolecular Interactions: Implications for Pharmacological Activity," submitted for publication in *Progress in Drug Research*.
82. S. Ehrenpreis, *Ann. N.Y. Acad. Sci.*, **144**, 720 (1967).
83. J. C. Watkins, *J. Theoret. Biol.*, **9**, 37 (1965).
84. R. F. Steiner, *The Chemical Foundations of Molecular Biology*, Van Nostrand, Princeton, N.J., 1965.
85. W. Leuzinger and A. L. Baker, *Proc. Natl. Acad. Sci. U.S.*, **57**, 446 (1967).
86. W. Leuzinger, A. L. Baker, and E. Cauvin, *Proc. Natl. Acad. Sci. U.S.*, **59**, 620 (1968).
87. W. Leuzinger, M. Goldberg, and E. Cauvin, *J. Mol. Biol.*, **40**, 217 (1969).
88. W. B. Neely, *Mol. Pharmacol.*, **1**, 137 (1965).
89. T. R. Podleski and D. Nachmansohn, *Proc. Natl. Acad. Sci. U.S.*, **56**, 1034 (1966).
90. I. B. Wilson, *Ann. N.Y. Acad. Sci.*, **144**, 664 (1967).
91. P. Pauling, "The Structure of Molecules Active in Cholinergic Systems," in A. Rich and N. Davidson, Eds., *Structural Chemistry and Molecular Biology*, Freeman, San Francisco, 1968, pp. 555–565.
92. C. J. Cavallito, *Ann. N.Y. Acad. Sci.*, **144**, 900 (1967).
93. L. W. Cunningham, *Science*, **125**, 1145 (1957).
94. R. M. Krupka and K. J. Laidler, *Nature*, **190**, 916 (1961).
95. F. G. Canepa, *Ann. N.Y. Acad. Sci.*, **144**, 918 (1967).
96. N. Engelhard, K. Prchal, and M. Nenner, *Angew Chem. Int. Ed. Engl.* **6**, 615 (1967).
97. J.-P. Changeux, *Mol. Pharmacol.*, **2**, 369 (1966).
98. R. J. Kitz and L. T. Kremzner, *Mol. Pharmacol.*, **4**, 104 (1968).
99. A. Karlin, *Proc. Natl. Acad. Sci. U.S.*, **58**, 1162 (1967).
100. A. Karlin and E. Bartels, *Biochim. Biophys. Acta*, **126**, 525 (1966).
101. A. Karlin and M. Winnik, *Proc. Natl. Acad. Sci. U.S.*, **60**, 668 (1968).
102. J. B. Kay and J. B. Robinson, *J. Pharm. Pharmacol.*, **21**, 145 (1969).
103. A. Cammarata and R. L. Stein, *J. Med. Chem.*, **11**, 829 (1968).
104. B. Belleau, *Ann. N.Y. Acad. Sci.*, **144**, 705 (1967).
105. B. Belleau, H. Tani, and F. Lie, *J. Am. Chem. Soc.*, **87**, 2283 (1965).
106. C. J. Cavallito, *Ann. Rev. Pharmacol.*, **8**, 39 (1968).
107. A. Bebbington and R. W. Brimblecombe, *Advan. Drug Res.*, **2**, 143 (1965).
108. L. B. Kier, *Mol. Pharmacol.*, **3**, 487 (1967).
109. W. C. Bowman, M. J. Rand, and G. B. West, *Textbook of Pharmacology*, Blackwell, Oxford, 1968.
110. S. G. Kuznetsov and S. N. Golikov, *Synthetic Atropine-like Substances*, U.S. Joint Publications Research Service, Washington, D.C., 1963.
111. E. J. Ariëns, *Farmaco, (Pavia), Ed. Sci.*, **23**, 52 (1968).
112. P. G. Waser, *Actualités Pharmacol.*, **16**, 169 (1963).
113. P. G. Waser, *Farmaco, (Pavia), Ed. Sci.*, **23**, 513 (1968).
114. P. G. Waser, *Advan. Drug Res.*, **3**, 81 (1966).
115. J. B. Stenlake, *Progr. Med. Chem.*, **3**, 1 (1963).
116. J. Crow, O. Wassermann, and W. C. Holland, *J. Med. Chem.*, **12**, 764 (1969).
117. L. B. Kier, *Mol. Pharmacol.*, **4**, 70 (1968).
118. T. O. Soine, "Autonomic Blocking Agents and Related Drugs," in C. O. Wilson,

O. Gisvold, and R. F. Doerge, Eds., *Textbook of Organic Medicinal and Pharmaceutical Chemistry*, 5th ed., Lippincott, Philadelphia, 1966, pp. 468–546.

119. D. A. Kharkevich, *Ganglion-Blocking and Ganglion-Stimulating Agents*, Pergamon, Oxford, 1967.

120. J. P. Long, F. P. Luduena, B. F. Tullar, and A. M. Lands, *J. Pharmacol. Exptl. Therap.*, **117**, 29 (1956).

121. J. M. van Rossum, *Int. J. Neuropharmacol.*, **1**, 97, 403 (1962).

122. J. P. Long, "Structure-Activity Relationships of the Reversible Anticholinesterase Agents," in G. B. Koelle, Ed., *Cholinesterases and Anticholinesterase Agents. Handbuch der experimentellen Pharmakologie*, Vol. XV, Springer, Berlin, 1963, pp. 374–427.

123. D. Bovet, "Rapports entre constitution chimique et activité pharmacodynamique dans quelques séries de curares de synthèse," in D. Bovet, F. Bovet-Nitti, and G. B. Marini-Bettòlo, Eds., *Curare and Curare-like Agents*, Elsevier, Amsterdam, 1959, pp. 252–287.

124. P. Pratesi and E. Grana, *Advan. Drug Res.*, **2**, 127 (1965).

125. R. P. Ahlquist, *J. Pharm. Sci.*, **55**, 359 (1966).

126. R. P. Ahlquist, *Ann. N.Y. Acad. Sci.*, **139**, 549 (1967).

127. E. J. Ariëns, *Ann. N.Y. Acad. Sci.*, **139**, 606 (1967).

128. A. M. Lands, A. Arnold, J. P. McAuliff, F. P. Luduena, and T. G. Brown, Jr., *Nature*, **214**, 597 (1967).

129. R. F. Furchgott, *Pharmacol. Rev.*, **11**, 429 (1959).

130. R. P. Ahlquist, *Ann. Rev. Pharmacol.*, **8**, 259 (1968).

131. S. E. Epstein and E. Braunwald, *N. Engl. J. Med.*, **275**, 1106, 1175 (1966).

132. E. J. Ariëns, *Advan. Drug Res.*, **3**, 235 (1966).

133. J. H. Biel and B. K. B. Lum, *Progr. Drug Res.*, **10**, 46 (1966).

134. D. J. Triggle, *Advan. Drug Res.*, **2**, 173 (1965).

135. B. M. Bloom and I. M. Goldman, *Advan. Drug Res.*, **3**, 121 (1966).

136. L. H. Easson and E. Stedman, *Biochem. J.*, **27**, 1257 (1933).

137. B. Belleau, "An Analysis of Drug-Receptor Interactions," in K. J. Brunings, Ed., *Modern Concepts in the Relationship Between Structure and Pharmacological Activity*, Pergamon, Oxford, 1963, pp. 75–99.

138. B. Belleau, *Pharmacol. Rev.*, **18**, 131 (1966).

139. B. Belleau, *Ann. N.Y. Acad. Sci.*, **139**, 580 (1967).

140. G. A. Robison, R. W. Butcher, and E. W. Sutherland, *Ann. N.Y. Acad. Sci.*, **139**, 703 (1967).

141. L. B. Kier, *J. Pharmacol. Exptl. Therap.*, **164**, 75 (1968).

142. L. B. Kier, *J. Pharm. Pharmacol.*, **21**, 93 (1969).

143. B. Belleau, V. DiTullio, and D. Godin, *Biochem. Pharmacol.*, **18**, 1039 (1969).

144. A. A. Larsen, *Nature*, **224**, 25 (1969).

145. J. R. Vane, G. E. W. Wolstenholme, and M. O'Connor, *Adrenergic Mechanisms*, Little, Brown, Boston, 1960.

146. E. Marley, *Advan. Pharmacol.*, **3**, 167 (1964).

147. A. L. A. Boura and A. F. Green, *Ann. Rev. Pharmacol.*, **5**, 183 (1965).

148. E. Muscholl, *Ann. Rev. Pharmacol.*, **6**, 107 (1966).

149. Second Catecholamine Symposium, *Pharmacol. Rev.*, **18**, 1–803 (1966).

150. W. S. Root and F. G. Hofmann, Eds., *Physiological Pharmacology*, Vol. IV, Academic, New York, 1967.

151. N. E. Andén, A. Carlsson, and J. Häggendal, *Ann. Rev. Pharmacol.*, **9**, 119 (1969).

152. M. S. K. Ghouri and T. J. Haley, *J. Pharm. Sci.*, **58**, 511 (1969).

153. M. Rocha e Silva, Ed., *Histamine and Antihistaminics. Handbuch der experimentellen Pharmakologie*, Vol. XVIII/I, Springer, Berlin, 1966.

154. G. Kahlson and E. Rosengren, *Ann. Rev. Pharmacol.*, **5**, 305 (1965).

155. M. Rocha e Silva, *Arch. Intern. Pharmacodyn.*, **128**, 355 (1960).

156. A. S. F. Ash and H. O. Schild, *Brit. J. Pharmacol.*, **27**, 427 (1966).

157. L. B. Kier, *J. Med. Chem.*, **11**, 441 (1968).

158. A. F. Harms and W. Th. Nauta, *J. Med. Pharm. Chem.*, **2**, 57 (1960).

159. W. Th. Nauta, R. F. Rekker, and A. F. Harms, "Diarylcarbinol Ethers: Structure Activity Relationships. A Physico-Chemical Approach," in E. J. Ariëns, Ed., *Physico-Chemical Aspects of Drug Action*, Pergamon, Oxford, 1968, pp. 305–325.

160. G. Hite and A. Shafi'ee, *J. Pharm. Sci.*, **56**, 1041 (1967).

161. V. Erspamer, *Progr. Drug Res.*, **3**, 151 (1961).

162. L. Gyermek, *Pharmacol. Rev.*, **13**, 399 (1961).

163. P. A. Shore, *Pharmacol. Rev.*, **14**, 531 (1962).

164. S. Garattini and L. Valzelli, *Serotonin*, Elsevier, Amsterdam, 1965.

165. V. Erspamer, Ed., *5-Hydroxytryptamine and Related Indolealkylamines. Handbuch der experimentellen Pharmakologie*, Vol. XIX, Springer, Berlin, 1966.

166. J. Offermeier and E. J. Ariëns, *Arch. Intern. Pharmacodyn.*, **164**, 192, 216 (1966).

167. L. B. Kier, *J. Pharm. Sci.*, **57**, 1188 (1968).

168. B. Belleau and J. Moran, *J. Med. Pharm. Chem.*, **5**, 215 (1962).

169. B. Belleau and J. Moran, *Ann. N.Y. Acad. Sci.*, **107**, 822 (1963).

170. E. A. Zeller, Ed., "New Reflections on Monoamine Oxidase Inhibition," *Ann. N.Y. Acad. Sci.*, **107**, 809–1158 (1963).

171. M. Gordon, Ed., *Psychopharmacological Agents*, 2 vols., Academic, New York, 1964, 1967.

172. D. P. Cameron and E. H. Wiseman, *J. Med. Chem.*, **11**, 820 (1968).

173. E. H. Wiseman and D. P. Cameron, *J. Med. Chem.*, **12**, 586 (1969).

174. M. Gordon, L. Cook, D. H. Tedeschi, and R. E. Tedeschi, *Arzneimittel-Forsch.*, **13**, 318 (1963).

175. M. Gordon, P. N. Craig, and C. L. Zirkle, "Molecular Modification in the Development of Phenothiazine Drugs," in F. W. Schueler, Ed., *Molecular Modification in Drug Design*, Advances in Chemistry Series, Vol. 45, American Chemical Society, Washington, D.C., 1964, pp. 140–147.

176. M. Gordon, *Topics Med. Chem.*, **2**, 97 (1968).

177. K. Stach and W. Pöldinger, *Progr. Drug Res.*, **9**, 129 (1966).

178. E. F. Domino, R. D. Hudson, and G. Zografi, "Substituted Phenothiazines: Pharmacology and Chemical Structure," in A. Burger, Ed., *Drugs Affecting the Central Nervous System*, Dekker, New York, 1968, pp. 327–397.

179. M. Goldberg, "The Physiology and Pathophysiology of Diuretic Agents," in W. F. M. Fulton, Ed., *Modern Trends in Pharmacology and Therapeutics*, Vol. I, Appleton-Century-Crofts, New York, 1967, pp. 41–75.

180. J. M. Sprague, *Topics Med. Chem.*, **2**, 1 (1968).

181. E. J. Cafruny, *Pharmacol. Rev.*, **20**, 89 (1968).

182. I. E. Bush, *Pharmacol. Rev.*, **14**, 317 (1962).

183. M. E. Wolff, W. Ho, and R. Kwok, *J. Med. Chem.*, **7**, 577 (1964).

184. I. E. Bush, *Brit. Med. Bull.*, **18**, 141 (1962).

185. A. Cooper, D. A. Norton, and H. Hauptman, *Acta Cryst.*, **B25**, 814 (1969).

186. J. A. Vida, *Androgens and Anabolic Agents: Chemistry and Pharmacology*, Academic New York, 1969.

187. L. L. Engel, A. M. Stoffyn, and J. F. Scott, "The Role of Molecular Configuration in the Interaction of Steroid Hormones with Coenzymes and Enzymes," in L. Martini and A. Pecile, Eds., *Hormonal Steroids*, Vol. I, Academic, New York, 1964, pp. 291–299.

188. W. G. Cole and D. H. Williams, *J. Chem. Soc. (C)*, 1849 (1968).

189. L. B. Kier, *J. Med. Chem.*, **11**, 915 (1968).

190. L. B. Kier and M. W. Whitehouse, *J. Pharm. Pharmacol.*, **20**, 793 (1968).

191. K. Junkmann, Ed., *Die Gestagene. Handbuch der experimentellen Pharmakologie*, Vol. XXII/I and II, Springer, Berlin, 1968, 1969.

192. J. C. Arcos and M. Arcos, *Progr. Drug Res.*, **4**, 407 (1962).

193. H. Busch, Ed., *Methods in Cancer Research*, 4 vols., Academic, New York, 1967, 1968.

194. J. C. Arcos, M. F. Argus, and G. Wolf, *Chemical Induction of Cancer*, 3 vols., Academic, New York, 1968–

THEORIES OF DRUG ACTION

The realization that significant conformational changes can and probably do occur in receptor systems as the result of their binding drugs as substrates, inhibitors, allosteric effectors, or otherwise, suggests one very good reason why it is so difficult to conceive their nature merely by assuming molecular complementarity with interacting drugs. More direct means of gaining insight are clearly needed. Perhaps the best such means presently available involves the extrapolation of newer knowledge and concepts regarding the structure of proteins, the regulation of enzyme activity, and the nature of feedback control mechanism at the molecular level.

Barry M. Bloom

I. NATURE OF PHARMACOLOGICAL ACTION

According to what has been reported in Chapter 2, the action of drugs results either from their physicochemical properties (as in the case of structurally nonspecific drugs) or from their chemical structure (as in structurally specific drugs). The former, exemplified by general anesthetics and certain narcotics (*1*) (e.g., aliphatic alcohols), act in relatively large doses, presumably by forming a monomolecular layer over the whole area of some cells of the organism. The structurally specific drugs, however, act in very small doses, and it is deduced that their activity results from complexation with specific receptors localized in certain molecules of the organism (2–4).

The last statement is based on various considerations, mainly the following mathematical calculations (5). One mole of a drug contains 6.02×10^{23} molecules. If the molecular weight of this drug is 200, 1 mg (often the effective dose) will contain

$$\frac{6 \times 10^{23}}{200 \times 10^3} = 3 \times 10^{18} \text{ molecules}$$

The human organism is made up of about 3×10^{13} cells. Therefore each cell will be acted on by

$$\frac{3 \times 10^{18}}{3 \times 10^{13}} = 1 \times 10^5 \text{ molecules of drug}$$

One erythrocyte has been found to contain approximately 1×10^{10} molecules. On the assumption that the same number of molecules is found in each cell, it is deduced that for each molecule of drug there are

$$\frac{1 \times 10^{10}}{1 \times 10^5} = 1 \times 10^5 = 100,000 \text{ molecules of the human body}$$

Clark (6) has calculated that ouabain fixed to the cells of the heart ventricle isolated from the toad would cover only 2.5% of the cellular surface and that the area covered by a dose of acetylcholine sufficient to reduce by 50% the heart beat of the same animal corresponds to only 0.016% of the surface of the ventricular cells (4).

Simple calculations such as the foregoing indicate that structurally specific drugs do not act on all molecules of the body but only on certain ones— precisely those that, as is generally assumed, constitute the receptor of the drug. In regard to the way this interaction might take place and for the mode of drug action various theories have been proposed: occupancy, rate, induced fit, and macromolecular perturbation. These theories are briefly considered here. Recent progress in studies of the biology of nucleic acids, the tertiary and quaternary structure of proteins, the nature of enzymes, and the mechanism by which they act permit us to describe—in more precise terms than could be done heretofore—possible modes of drug action at the molecular level (7).

II. OCCUPANCY THEORY

Formulated by Clark (8) and Gaddum (9), the occupancy theory states, in essence, that the intensity of pharmacological effect is directly proportional to the number of receptors occupied by the drug. According to this theory, drug–receptor interactions follow closely Langmuir's adsorption isotherm (10). This has been confirmed by various authors (11–17). These interactions, which comply with the law of mass action, may be represented by the equation

$$R + D \underset{k_2}{\overset{k_1}{\rightleftharpoons}} RD \longrightarrow E$$

where R is a receptor, D a molecule of the drug, RD the drug–receptor complex, E the pharmacological effect, and k_1 and k_2 the rate constants of adsorption and desorption, respectively.

The number of occupied receptors depends on the concentration of the drug in the compartment of the receptor and on the total number of receptors (R_t) in the unity of area or of volume. The drug effect will become much more intense as the number of occupied receptors increases; hence maximal action will correspond to the occupation of all receptors (4,18).

The effect of pharmacological action will be proportional to the concentration of RD, so that

$$E = k_3[RD] \tag{I}$$

where k_3 is the factor of proportionality. In the state of equilibrium

$$\frac{[R][D]}{[RD]} = \frac{k_2}{k_1} = K_D$$

where K_D is the dissociation constant of the complex. The total concentration of the receptors will be

$$[R_t] = [R] + [RD]$$

and

$$K_D = \frac{[R_t - RD][D]}{[RD]} \quad \text{or} \quad \frac{[RD]}{[R_t]} = \frac{[D]}{[D] + K_D} = \frac{1}{1 + (K_D/[D])}$$

When all receptors are occupied, the biological effect will be maximal:

$$E_m = k_3[R_t] \tag{II}$$

By dividing Equation I by Equation II, we obtain

$$\frac{E}{E_m} = \frac{[RD]}{[R_t]}$$

Hence

$$E = \frac{E_m[D]}{[D] + K_D} \tag{III}$$

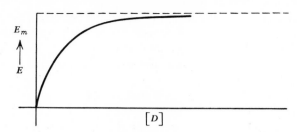

Fig. 9.1. Effect produced by drug–receptor interaction versus concentration of drug.

Equation III can be represented by Figure 9.1. This equation is identical to the classical equation of Michaelis–Menten,

$$V = \frac{V_m[S]}{K_m[S] + K_m} \tag{IV}$$

which gives the rate V of an enzymic reaction as a function of the concentration of the substrate $[S]$, of the maximal rate V_m, and of the dissociation constant K_m of the enzyme–substrate complex. By representing Equation IV graphically, we obtain Figure 9.2.

The theory of occupancy is applicable when the drug–receptor interaction is identical for all drugs considered; that is, when all of them can produce the same maximal response, independent of dose. Nevertheless certain drugs— such as some congeners of acetylcholine—never elicit maximal response, even though the dose is increased indefinitely. In this case it is proven that the biological effect is neither subject to the law of mass action nor dependent on the affinity of drugs for their receptors (*19*).

With the purpose of offering an explanation for this and other incongruences, Ariëns (*11*) and Stephenson (*20*) proposed some modifications to the theory of occupancy. According to these authors, drug–receptor interactions comprise two stages: (a) complexation of the drug with its receptor and (b) production of effect. For a chemical compound to manifest biological

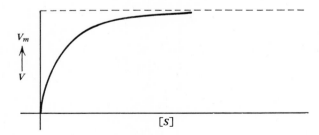

Fig. 9.2. Rate of an enzymic reaction versus concentration of substrate.

activity it is necessary not only that it have *affinity* for the receptor, owing to complementary structural characteristics, but also another property called *intrinsic activity* by Ariëns and *efficacy* by Stephenson. This latter property, intrinsic activity or efficacy, would be a measure of the ability of the drug–receptor complex to produce the biological effect.

The mathematical expression of Ariëns' theory is stated by the following equation:

$$E_D = \alpha[RD] = \frac{\alpha[R_t]}{1 + (K_D/[D])} \tag{V}$$

where E_D is the effect produced by a drug, and α can vary from 1 (in the case of a full agonist) to 0 (in the case of a competitive antagonist).

Stephenson (20) presented the following equation:

$$E = f(S) = f\left(\frac{e[RD]}{[R_t]}\right) = f\left[\frac{e}{1 + (K_D/[D])}\right] \tag{VI}$$

where the effect E is a positive function f of the stimulus S, which in turn is equal to the efficacy e multiplied by the fraction of the total receptors occupied by the drug. When e is zero, a pure competitive antagonist is involved; when e is sufficiently high, it may happen that a fraction of receptors is not occupied —this fraction constitutes the "spare receptors" (21). According to Waud (22), probably it is a case of "spare cells" and not of "spare receptors," since the antagonist, being applied for a short time, would block only the superficial cells, and not the deep ones. On the basis of experimental results, Moran and co-workers (23) concluded that there is no existing evidence for "spare receptors" in rat vas deferens adrenergic α-receptor systems.

In more recent papers Ariëns and co-workers (13,16) have used an equation similar to that of Stephenson; that is,

$$\frac{E_D}{E_m} = f\frac{S_D}{S_m} = f\left(\frac{\alpha[RD]}{[R_t]}\right) \tag{VII}$$

where E_D/E_m is the effect in relationship to the maximal effect obtainable by the biological system, and S_D/S_m is the relative intensity of the stimulus; in certain circumstances α can be greater than unity.

According to the Ariëns–Stephenson theory, the agonists as well as the antagonists have strong affinity for the receptor, and this enables them to form the drug–receptor complex. However, only the agonists have the ability of giving origin to the stimulus—that is, have intrinsic activity, or efficacy. Therefore, by plotting the intensity of biological effect versus the concentration of the drugs (Figure 9.3), those that present curves of similar shapes are considered as having equal intrinsic activity. Otherwise, the greater the affinity of the drugs for the receptor, the lesser will be the concentration that

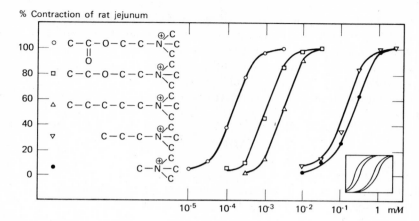

Fig. 9.3. Biological effect produced by a series of quaternary ammonium compounds on the rat jejunum (*14*). (Reprinted with permission of the Editor.)

causes analogous effects. If, on the other hand, the curves are of different shapes, it will mean that their intrinsic activities are different, even though the affinities remain identical (Figure 9.4); such drugs are *dualists*, according to Ariëns, or *partial agonists*, according to Stephenson. Drugs of low intrinsic activity are antagonists, and they can be used to antagonize drugs with greater intrinsic activity (*4*).

Antagonists are drugs that bind strongly to the receptor—that is, they have great affinity for it, but are devoid of activity. It is possible to transform an agonist into an antagonist through appropriate structural modifications, such as the addition or removal of certain chemical groups (Figure 9.5).

In spite of its appeal, the occupancy theory, even with the changes introduced by Ariëns and Stephenson, cannot explain satisfactorily why drugs

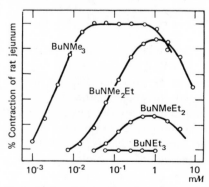

Fig. 9.4. Biological effect produced by salts of pentyltrialkylammonium on the rat jejunum (*14*). (Reprinted with permission of the Editor.)

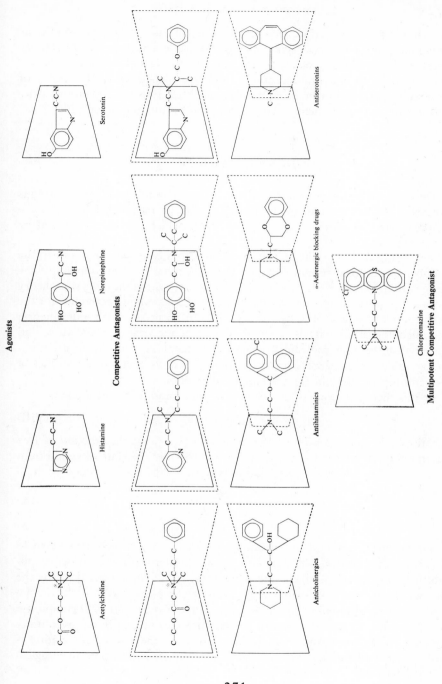

Fig. 9.5. Relationship between structure and action of agonists and their competitive antagonists (*17*). (Reprinted by permission of the New York Academy of Sciences.)

271

vary in their type of action; that is, why one acts as agonist and another as antagonist, although both can occupy the same receptor, as the theory assumes. Its failure to elucidate the mechanism of drug action at the molecular level in terms of chemical structure is the chief deficiency of the theory of occupancy (24,25). Furthermore, mathematical analysis has shown that drug action cannot be explained by simple receptor-occupation models (26).

III. RATE THEORY

On the basis of the postulate of Croxatto and Huidobro (27) that a drug is efficient only at the moment of encounter with its receptor, Paton and co-workers have advanced a rate theory (28-30), which has been espoused by other authors (21).

According to Paton, the activation of receptors is proportional not to the number of occupied receptors but to the total number of encounters of the drug with its receptor per unit time. Unlike previous theories, the rate theory does not require the formation of a stable Michaelis–Menten complex for the activation of the receptor by a drug (25). In accordance with the theory, pharmacological activity is a function only of the *rate* of association and dissociation between molecules of drug and receptors, and not of formation of a stable drug–receptor complex (29). Each association constitutes a "quantum" of stimulus for the biological reaction.

In this theory the rate of association (A) is expressed by the equation

$$A = k_1[D](1 - p) \qquad \text{(VIII)}$$

where $[D]$ is concentration of the drug, and $(1 - p)$ is the fraction of free receptors (p is the fraction of occupied receptors). In the state of equilibrium —that is, when the rate of association is equal to the rate of dissociation,

$$A = \frac{k_2}{1 + \dfrac{(k_1/k_2)}{[D]}} \qquad \text{(IX)}$$

Equation IX is analogous to Equations VI and VII, which are related to the occupancy theory. The difference is that the term for stimulus S is substituted by association rate A and the efficacy (or intrinsic activity) e, by the dissociation constant k_2 of the drug–receptor complex.

In the case of agonists the rates both of association and dissociation are fast (the latter faster than the former) and produce several impulses in unity of time. When we consider antagonists, however, the rate of association is fast but that of dissociation is slow, which explains their pharmacological action. This has some experimental basis, because it has been shown that, before causing blockade, antagonists produce a short stimulating effect (*30*). In short, agonists are characterized by high (and variable) dissociation rates, partial agonists by intermediate dissociation rates, and antagonists by low dissociation rates as a consequence of stronger adherence to the receptor and of greater difficulty in being withdrawn from it because they are larger in size when compared with agonists and partial agonists (*30*).

In this aspect Paton's theory diverges from that of Croxatto and Huidobro (*27*). Although the latter authors might have suggested that drug–receptor interaction depends on the "superficial complementarity" between both, they assumed that an antagonist acts on a site that is different from the site of action of an agonist, since the chemical structures of many potent antagonists are different from those of agonists.

As in the case of the occupancy theory, the rate theory has been widely criticized because it presents several inconsistencies, and it does not allow interpretations of various experimentally observed facts. For instance, contrary to what Paton assumes, the agonist has characteristics that favor the formation of a complex that does not rapidly dissociate (*31*). Further, the rate theory, as well as the occupancy theory, cannot explain, through interpretation of phenomena that take place at the molecular level, why one drug acts as an agonist while another structurally similar one acts as an antagonist. Both theories, as well as many others that have been proposed, lack a plausible physicochemical basis for the interpretation of phenomena involving receptors at the molecular level (*24,25*).

In an effort to refute criticisms of the rate theory Paton and Rang (*29*) proposed as an alternative the *dissociation theory*. In this new theory the dissociation-rate constant is a function not of the intensity of the binding forces but of the extent to which the drug molecule disturbs the secondary protein structure. Relating stimulus to rate of dissociation, and this rate being proportional to the occupation of receptors, the dissociation theory is not formally different from the occupancy theory (*29*).

In 1966, Mackay (*32*) gave mathematical expression to the occupation and rate theories, analyzing, on this basis, the interactions of receptors with antagonists, partial agonists, and full agonists. Thron and Waud (*33*) have proposed, on the basis of kinetic observations, that the action of atropine is limited by the *rate of access* to the receptor region, and not by the rate of the atropine–receptor interaction.

IV. INDUCED-FIT THEORY

Although it is not yet known how an enzyme works, everything leads us to believe that stability, activation, and particularly the effects of inactivation may often be induced by environmental factors, especially by substrates and

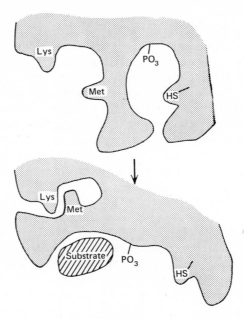

Fig. 9.6. Schematic illustration of the effect that a conformational change of phospho-glucomutase causes on the reactivity of amino acid residues of this enzyme. The binding of substrate is seen to cause an unfolding leading to the exposure of an SH residue and the burying of methionine and lysine residues (*52–54*).

cofactors, these effects being probably related to conformational changes (*34,35*). In the study of the conformational changes that enzymes and other macromolecules undergo several techniques are used. They are mainly optical rotatory dispersion (*36–41*), circular dichroism (*37,39,41,42*), and X-ray diffraction (*43*). These techniques were utilized, for instance, to determine the conformational change of α-chymotrypsin as it interacts with its natural substrate and with inhibitors (*44–49*).

The hypothesis of induced conformational changes in enzymes has been advanced by several authors. For example, Koshland (*50*) suggested that the active site of an isolated crystalline enzyme does not necessarily need to have a morphology that is complementary to that of the substrate, being a kind of negative thereof, but that it acquires such morphology only after interacting with the substrate, which induces such a conformational change. Likewise, he listed the characteristics that distinguish substrate–enzyme, haptene–antibody, and drug–receptor interactions (*51*):

1. The main attractive forces are hydrophobic bonds, electrostatic bonds, hydrogen bonds and chelation.

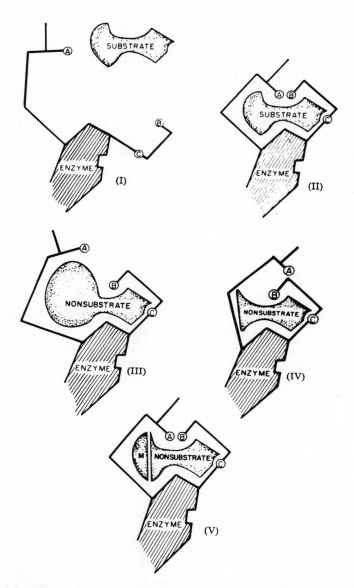

Fig. 9.7. Schematic model of plastic active-site mechanism. Black lines indicate protein chains containing catalytic groups A and B and binding group C. The diagram I shows substrate and enzyme dissociated. Diagram II represents substrate with induced change of protein chains to bring A and B into proper alignment for reaction. Diagram III shows that a bulky group added to the substrate prevents proper alignment of A and B. The decrease in volume of substrate, as it is observed in IV, produces an analogous result. The introduction of a small molecule M in the nonsubstrate can transform it into a substrate, as in V, and activate an enzymic reaction (*53–55*). (Reprinted by permission of the publishers.)

275

2. The main repulsive forces are electrostatic repulsions and steric hindrance.

3. The three-dimensional protein geometry determines different combinations of these forces in individual cases.

4. The sequence of amino acids in a protein plays a fundamental role in determining this three-dimensional geometry.

5. Only a small fraction of amino acid residues are directly involved in the specificity of the interaction, but some that are far from the active site play a role in determining the necessary geometry of the essential amino acids.

On the basis of these suppositions, Koshland (52,53) advanced the hypothesis that, in combining with an enzyme, the substrate induces a change in its conformation; this results in an enzymically active orientation of the

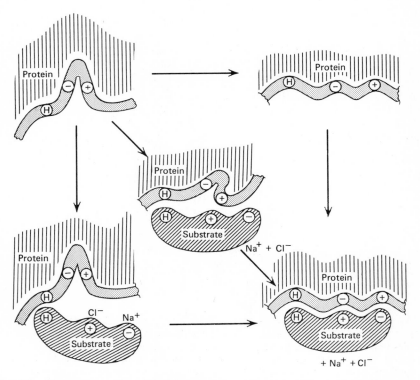

Fig. 9.8.   Illustrative example of changes in conformation of an enzyme induced by a substrate. In this diagram H, $\oplus$, and $\ominus$ represent hydrophobic and electrostatic attractions between protein chain, substrate molecule, and solution ions. The complex formed can be dissociated and the protein refolded to its initial conformation by an unfolding process similar to the folding (56). (Reprinted with permission of Annual Reviews, Inc.)

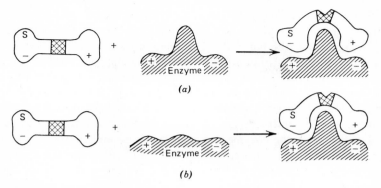

Fig. 9.9. Schematic representation of the strain induced on the substrate by (*a*) a rigid enzyme; (*b*) an enzyme in which conformation changes on binding of substrate (*56*). (Reprinted with permission of Annual Reviews, Inc.)

catalytic groups (Figure 9.6). The biological effect of such combination is thus a consequence not only of the strong binding between the substrate and the enzyme but mainly of the induction of an appropriate conformational change. It is assumed that the active site of the enzyme is flexible—or, better, plastic or elastic—and not rigid (*34*). With increase or decrease in substrate volume therefore it can be avoided that the catalytic groups of the active site may be aligned (necessary condition for enzymic action), and this leads to inactivation of the enzyme (Figure 9.7).

Another representation of conformational changes in enzymes is presented in Figure 9.8.

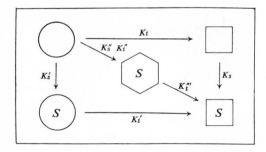

Fig. 9.10. Conformational changes of a protein monomer induced by substrate. In the pathway $K_t K_s$ initial protein conformation change is followed by the binding of substrate to the new conformation; in the pathway $K_s' K_t'$ substrate binds first and protein conformation change occurs afterward; pathway $K_s'' K_t''$ involves simultaneous conformation change and binding followed (K_t''') by further isomerization to final conformation (*56*). (Published with permission of Annual Reviews, Inc.)

Koshland and Neet (56) postulated that conformational changes can occur not only in the enzyme but also in the substrate, so that proper alignment of catalytic groups may be more easily attained, even though this may cause a strain in the substrate (Figure 9.9). These conformational changes can take place by several pathways, as schematically illustrated in Figure 9.10.

The induced-fit theory has been proposed only to explain enzymic action on substrates. However, a similar enzyme activating or deactivating effect can be produced by a drug. This effect may be produced through complexation of a drug with the enzyme's normal substrate and subsequent increase or decrease in its volume. It may also be caused by interaction of a drug with an enzyme, not necessarily with its catalytic groups at the active site, but

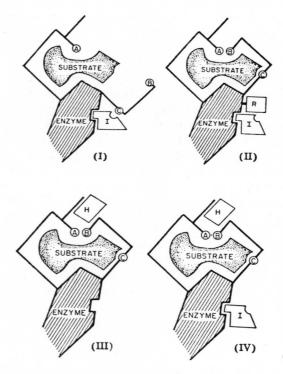

Fig. 9.11. The effect of inhibitors and activating agents on the elastic active site of the enzyme. In diagram I the inhibitor I attracts group C and prevents proper alignment of a catalytic group B, causing inhibition, which may be competitive, if the B chain is involved in complexation, or noncompetitive, if it is not involved. In diagram II reagent R prevents juxtaposition of group C with inhibitor I, nullifying its effect without changing its affinity for the active site. In diagram III the hormone H stabilizes the active conformation by attracting chains containing A and B. In diagram IV the hormone H overcomes the effect of the inhibitor I by attracting chains containing A and B (53).

with any binding group at a modifier site (57,58) or at an allosteric site (59), as discussed in Chapter 6. The binding group is situated in the receptor, which, instead of having fixed and rigid morphology, is *elastic*; that is, not only can it be deformed or altered but also it has the ability to return to the original form after being deformed (34). The receptor, therefore, is dynamic (60). Inhibition caused by an inactivator can be prevented through the effect either of a reactant that hinders juxtaposition of inhibitor with the binding group of the enzyme or of an activating hormone, which stabilizes the active conformation of the enzyme by attracting catalytic groups so that they can be properly aligned to carry out their function (Figure 9.11).

This hypothesis, based on the deep conformational perturbation that attends the complexation of substrate with an enzyme or of a reagent with a protein (61–65), gave origin to the *induced-fit* theory, which has been also invoked to explain the mode of action of drugs. In accordance with it, when a drug comes in touch with a receptor, which usually is part of a protein molecule, it causes a reversible perturbation or change in the protein's tertiary structure. This change, which in certain instances is allosteric transition (59), causes the observed biological effect.

In conformity with the induced-fit theory, interaction of the drug should not necessarily be with an enzyme—it may be with a noncatalytic protein. If the interaction is with an enzyme, it may be not only at its active site but also at its allosteric site (Figure 9.12).

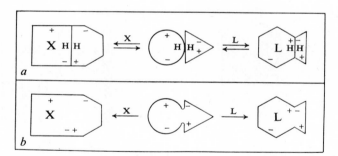

Fig. 9.12. Conformational changes of an enzyme induced by the binding of different ligands to its allosteric site. X and L represent ligands and can be inhibitors or activators, respectively; by binding at an allosteric site they influence the conformation and stability of the adjacent catalytic unit. (*a*) In the center the unliganded form of the enzyme, consisting of two subunits of the polypeptide chain held together by hydrophobic interactions; positive and negative charges are too far apart to interact. Binding of X to a subunit produces in it a conformational change, which in turn induces a conformational change in the adjacent subunit. Binding of L to this same subunit causes a different conformational change, which in turn stabilizes a different conformational change of the adjacent subunit. (*b*) A similar situation, but hydrophobic interactions are replaced by covalent bonds (56). (Published with permission of Annual Reviews, Inc.)

Both in the case of enzymes and of noncatalytic proteins, interaction of substrate or drug with them causes perturbations in their conformations. Koshland (*53*) described this effect in the following words:

The substrate is like a spider at the center of the web. It can change the conformation near the center and start a perturbation which will cause a change in a far distant corner of the web. It follows, of course, that a change in a far distant corner of the web may be felt by the spider at the center.

He assumed, in short, that the active site of an enzyme is not necessarily the "complement" of the substrate, but it becomes so when an enzyme–substrate complex is formed, which induces a structure suitable to it (Figure 9.13).

By adapting the induced-fit theory to the rate theory, it could be stated that, if drug–receptor complexation results in such a conformation that a

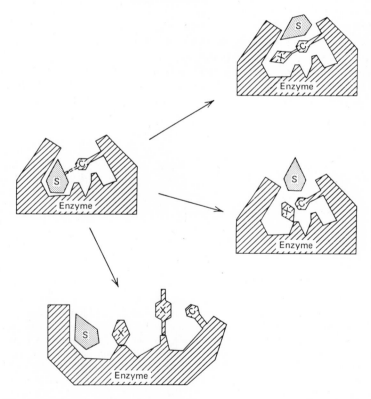

Fig. 9.13. Several modes of inactivation of an enzyme through specific chemical modification. The modifying reagent (X), a catalytically active constituent of the enzyme (C), and the substrate (S), are indicated in this illustration. [Adapted from (*66*).]

drug binds less strongly and dissociates more easily, it is an agonist; if, however, the complexation does not result in a change in conformation, the binding will be stable and an antagonist rather than an agonist is involved.

Recently Koshland and co-workers (55,56) have formulated a variant of the induced-fit theory in order to explain cooperative effects—the phenomenon that binding of one ligand molecule somehow accelerates binding of subsequent ones. Thus binding of the first ligand to a polymeric protein (which may be an enzyme containing the receptor) induces a conformational change in one of its subunits. A change in the shape of this subunit affects the stability of the remaining subunits. The resulting energy of stabilization makes possible stronger binding of the next molecules (Figure 9.14).

Analogous theories, also based on conformational changes in macromolecules, have been advanced in recent years. One of them, that of Changeux and co-workers (67), instead of assuming that conformational alterations of the protomers that constitute the macromolecules are induced, that is, consecutive to the binding of ligands, postulates that they not only precede the ligand binding but are not fundamentally different whether the ligand is bound or not.

Another theory has been proposed by Wyman, who introduced the concept of allosteric linkage to allosteric binding potential, which, although it applies to any system, is especially relevant to a macromolecule containing a number

Number of S bound		2		3	4
Formula	A_3BS	$A_2B_2S_2$		AB_3S_3	B_4S_4
Number of ways of arranging S	4	4	2	4	1
Number of AB pair interactions	2	2	4	2	0
Number of BB pair interactions	0	1	0	2	4

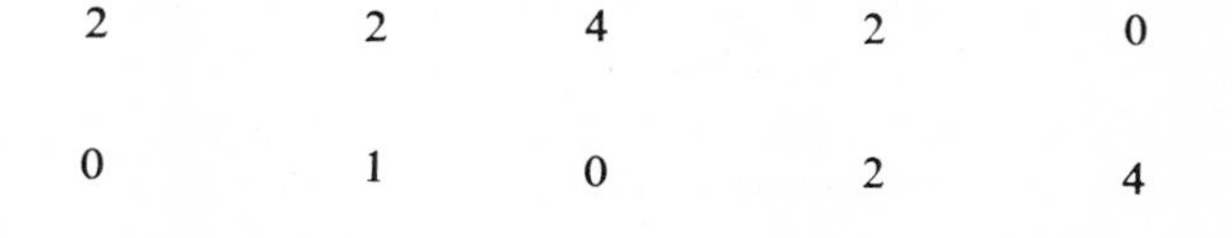

Fig. 9.14. Schematic illustration of a model to explain cooperative effects. In the case of a bound ligand, subunit exists in conformation A, denoted by circle. By binding to ligand S, conformation A is changed to conformation B, denoted by square. In the case of additional favorable interaction when two squares are adjacent, the ligands subsequent to the first bound ligand will be stabilized by the favorable interaction of adjacent squares. Thus binding of the second, third, and fourth ligands will be substantially easier (54–56). (Reprinted by permission of the publishers.)

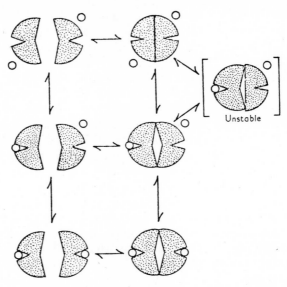

Fig. 9.15. Schematic representation of a two-dimensional, two-subunit protein, with the strong cooperative interactions between its two ligand binding sites. The subunits have a high ligand affinity but offer a relatively poor steric fit for inter-subunit binding. When the unliganded subunits combine, they are distorted to increase the strength of inter-subunit bonding. This reduces the ligand affinity by constricting the ligand-binding crevice. Attachment of one ligand to the dimer forces the liganded subunit into its open conformation. There is then nothing to hold the partner subunit in its strained conformation, so it opens and becomes highly reactive toward the ligand (*70*).

of interacting sites for several different ligands (*68*). Wyman suggested an allosteric model that is physically equivalent to that proposed by Changeux and co-workers (*67*), but differs in that his model involves "mixed" conformations, since each protomer can exist in either one of two forms or states (*69*).

Seeking to give support to the theories of Monod et al. (*35*) and of Wyman (*68*), and to shed some light on the general mechanism for cooperative allosteric interactions, Noble (*70*) postulated that inter-subunit binding energy accounts for these interactions (Figure 9.15).

V. MACROMOLECULAR PERTURBATION THEORY

In 1964 another theory of mode of action of drugs, the macromolecular perturbation theory, was proposed by Belleau (*24*). Very similar to the induced-fit theory, it may be considered an application of that theory to some classes of drugs. It is based on the following two facts and one assumption:

1. Drug–receptor interactions very often follow the law of mass action, mainly in relation to competitive antagonism.

2. Formation of the drug–receptor complex is attended by change in free energy, whence it is deduced that this complexation takes place with chemical modification in the receptor due to vibrational and electronic energies.

3. Conformational changes in proteins that act as receptors convert them from inactive species to ones capable of catalyzing reactions with substrates (*34*).

Taking into account the conformational adaptability of enzymes (and the receptors would be enzymes of a particular sort), Belleau reasoned that in the interaction of a drug with the protein component two general types of perturbation can occur in the complex:

1. Specific conformational perturbation, or specific ordering, which makes possible the adsorption of certain molecules related to the substrate; this is the case of an agonist.

2. Nonspecific conformational perturbation, or nonspecific disordering, which may serve to accommodate other classes of extraneous molecules; this is the case of an antagonist.

If the drug has both characteristics—that is, if it contributes to specific as well as to nonspecific macromolecular perturbation—a mixture of two complexes will result. This explains the partial stimulating action of the drug or the case of the partial agonist or antagonist.

The macromolecular perturbation theory, developed by Belleau in a more recent review (*25*), assumes that, when a small molecule M_s that is structurally closely related to the natural regulator (or neurotransmitter) forms an addition complex with the regulatory site, the protein undergoes a change from its resting state P to a conformationally rearranged active state P^*:

$$P + M_s \rightleftharpoons P^*M_s \qquad\qquad (X)$$

In this specifically rearranged form the receptor efficiently catalyzes the transformation of a substrate molecule A into a product B:

$$P^*M_s + A \rightleftharpoons P^*M_sA \longrightarrow P^*M_s + B \qquad\qquad (XI)$$

the latter being essential for the initiation of a stimulus. The contrary will occur if another molecule, M_i, due to its chemical structure, leads to an unfavorable conformation $P^\ddagger$. The receptor will not act as an efficient catalyst for the conversion of A to B and this will result in competitive antagonism:

$$P + M_i \rightleftharpoons P^{\ddagger}M_i$$

$$P^{\ddagger}M_i + A \rightleftharpoons P^{\ddagger}M_iA \nrightarrow P^{\ddagger}M_i + B \tag{XII}$$

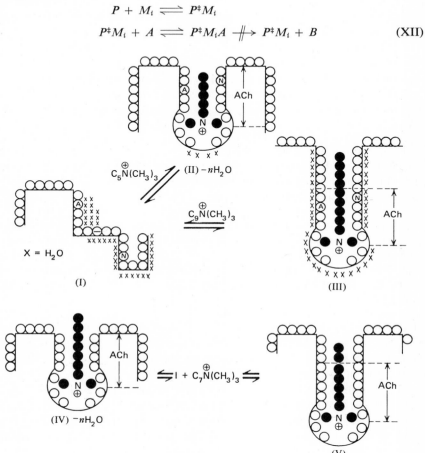

Fig. 9.16. Schematic representation of the interaction of trimethylammonium alkyl derivatives with muscarinic receptor. The light circles denote hydrophobic residues; the black circles, alkyl groups; the symbol X, the molecules of water of hydration; A and N, the reactive species representing the specific binding site for acetylcholine and other muscarinic agents. In diagram I protein chains are in the resting state. Diagram II shows the specific conformational perturbation caused by pentyltrimethylammonium as it interacts with the protein through hydrophobic forces. Diagram III shows the non-specific conformational perturbation that results from hydrophobic interactions with the four more methylene groups of nonyltrimethylammonium in relation to pentyltrimethyl-ammonium. Diagrams IV and V denote the equilibrium mixture of P^*M_{si} and P^*M_i complexes formed with heptyltrimethylammonium, molecule of the M_{si} type *(24)*. (Reprinted by permission of the American Chemical Society.)

The conformational transition from an ordered to a disordered arrangement may be abrupt (if the compounds have very different structures) or gradual (as in a homologous series). In the latter case it is possible that some molecules (M_{si}) transform P into an equilibrium mixture of $P*$ and $P^{\ddagger}$ complexes:

$$P^{\ddagger}M_{si} \rightleftharpoons P + M_{si} \rightleftharpoons P*M_{si} \qquad \text{(XIII)}$$

This possibility is presented when the changes of free energy in the process of formation of the two kinds of complexes are of comparable magnitudes. Such compounds will act as partial agonists.

The macromolecular perturbation theory was proposed by Belleau (24) to explain the interaction of alkyltrimethylammonium ions with the muscarinic receptor, which he assumed to be the acetylated acetylcholinesterase (Figure 9.16). The drugs used can be represented by the general formula $R\overset{+}{N}(CH_3)_3$.

In the above experiment group R varied from 1 to 12, and the thermodynamic parameters shown in Table 9.1 were obtained. Belleau considered that in this homologous series hydrophobic interactions and formation of ionic pairs are the more important forces in establishing binding with the receptor. In this experiment he observed that ions in which the R-group

TABLE 9.1 Thermodynamic Parameters for the Binding of $H[CH_2]_n\overset{\oplus}{N}(CH_3)_3$ on Acetylcholinesterase (25,71)

n	$\Delta G°$ (kcal/mole)	$\Delta H°$ (kcal/mole)	$\Delta S°$ (e.u.)	Perturbation	Contracture (%) (Muscarinic)[a]
1	-3.59	-6.60	-10.1	Ordering	100
2	-3.81	-6.45	-8.9	Ordering[b]	100
3	-3.92	-6.32	-8.1	Ordering	100
4	-4.20	-5.22	-3.4	Ordering	100
5	-3.76	-5.40	-5.5	Ordering	100
6	-3.92	-4.55	-2.1	Ordering[b]	100
7	-4.08	-4.49	-1.4	$\pm$ Ordering	60–80[c]
8	-4.34	-4.40	-0.2	$\pm$ Ordering	20–40[c]
9	-4.53	-4.40	$+0.44$	$\pm$ Disordering	5–10[c]
10	-4.97	-4.26	$+2.4$	Disordering	0[d]
11	-5.37	-2.76	$+9.1$	Disordering[b]	0[d]
12	-5.85	-2.75	$+10.4$	Disordering	0[d]

[a] Data from literature (12,20,28).
[b] Interpolated.
[c] Partial stimulants, partial antagonists.
[d] Antagonists.

contains from one to six carbon atoms stimulate muscarinic receptor, owing to the possibility of binding to the receptor's apolar regions through hydrophobic forces, which causes a specific perturbation in its structure. Ions that have from 9 to 12 carbon atoms in the R-group, however, induce a nonspecific conformational perturbation as a result of association with an additional segment of the protein, at the periphery of its catalytic surface, and therefore manifest antagonistic action. Ions that have seven or eight carbon atoms in the R-group act as partial agonists because, being able to induce a specific as well as a nonspecific perturbation, they form an equilibrium mixture of the two kinds of complexation.

Belleau's hypothesis does not need to assume the existence of affinity and intrinsic activity, and it is in complete agreement with several subsequent experimental data and results, because it offers a plausible physicochemical basis for the explanation of phenomena that involve a receptor at the molecular level (7). For example, Portoghese (72) has verified that at least two groups of analgetics derived from morphine, although having configuration opposite to that of several other congeners, exhibit similar pharmacological action. He therefore concluded that these analgetics interact with a receptor identical to that for other morphine congeners but that the exact nature of the interaction should differ; this can be explained by assuming that the receptor complexes with one group of drugs in its normal conformation and with another in its perturbed conformation. To explain the similar inhibitory potency of both *cis* and *trans* isomers of esters of choline and β-triethylammoniopropionic acid as anticholinesteratic agents, Kay and Robinson (73) assumed that either these compounds bind to the receptor area in different conformations or that different modes of binding are operative or the two series of compounds do not bind to the enzyme receptor area in the same manner.

On the basis of experimental data obtained in more recent work, Belleau advanced further support to his macromolecular perturbation theory (74).

REFERENCES

1. P. Rossignol, *Actualités Pharmacol.*, **17**, 85 (1964).
2. A. Albert, *Selective Toxicity*, 3rd ed., Wiley, New York, 1965.
3. Z. M. Bacq, et al., *Pharmacodynamie Biochimique*, 2nd ed., Masson, Paris, 1961.
4. R. B. Barlow, *Introduction to Chemical Pharmacology*, 2nd ed., Methuen, London, 1964.
5. M. Litter, *Farmacologia*, 2nd ed., El Ateneo, Buenos Aires, 1961.
6. A. J. Clark, *The Mode of Action of Drugs on Cells*, Williams and Wilkins, Baltimore, 1933.
7. B. M. Bloom, *Ann. Rep. Med. Chem.*, **1**, 236 (1966).

8. A. J. Clark, *J. Physiol.*, **61**, 530, 547 (1926).

9. J. H. Gaddum, *J. Physiol.*, **61**, 141 (1926); *ibid.*, **89**, 7P (1937).

10. I. Langmuir, *J. Am. Chem. Soc.*, **40**, 1361 (1918).

11. E. J. Ariëns, *Arch. Intern. Pharmacodyn.*, **99**, 32 (1954).

12. E. J. Ariëns, J. M. van Rossum, and A. M. Simonis, *Pharmacol. Rev.*, **9**, 218 (1957).

13. E. J. Ariëns, J. M. van Rossum, and P. C. Koopman, *Arch. Intern. Pharmacodyn.*, **127**, 459 (1960); *ibid.*, **136**, 385 (1962).

14. E. J. Ariëns and A. M. Simonis, *J. Pharm. Pharmacol.*, **16**, 137, 289 (1964).

15. E. J. Ariëns, Ed., *Molecular Pharmacology*, Vol. I, Academic, New York, 1964.

16. A. M. Simonis, *Farmaco*, *(Pavia)*, *Ed. Sci.*, **20**, 53 (1965).

17. E. J. Ariëns and A. M. Simonis, *Ann. N.Y. Acad. Sci.*, **144**, 842 (1967).

18. J. M. van Rossum, *Advan. Drug Res.*, **3**, 189 (1966).

19. B. Belleau and G. Lacasse, *J. Med. Chem.*, **7**, 768 (1964).

20. R. P. Stephenson, *Brit. J. Pharmacol.*, **11**, 379 (1956).

21. R. F. Furchgott, *Ann. Rev. Pharmacol.*, **4**, 21 (1964).

22. D. R. Waud, *Pharmacol. Rev.*, **20**, 49 (1968).

23. J. F. Moran, C. R. Triggle, and D. J. Triggle, *J. Pharm. Pharmacol.*, **21**, 38 (1969).

24. B. Belleau, *J. Med. Chem.*, **7**, 776 (1964).

25. B. Belleau, *Advan. Drug Res.*, **2**, 89 (1965).

26. L. D. Homer, *J. Theoret. Biol.*, **17**, 399 (1967).

27. R. Croxatto and F. Huidobro, *Arch. Intern. Pharmacodyn.*, **106**, 207 (1956).

28. W. D. M. Paton, *Proc. Roy. Soc.* (*London*), Ser. B, **154**, 21 (1961).

29. W. D. M. Paton and H. P. Rang, *Advan. Drug Res.*, **3**, 57 (1966).

30. W. D. M. Paton and J. P. Payne, *Pharmacological Principles and Practice*, Churchill, London, 1968.

31. A. Burger and A. P. Parulkar, *Ann. Rev. Pharmacol.*, **6**, 19 (1966).

32. D. Mackay, *J. Pharm. Pharmacol.*, **18**, 201 (1966).

33. C. D. Thron and D. R. Waud, *J. Pharmacol. Exptl. Therap.*, **160**, 91 (1968).

34. S. Grisolia, *Physiol. Rev.*, **44**, 657 (1964).

35. J. Monod, J. Wyman, and J.-P. Changeux, *J. Mol. Biol.*, **12**, 88 (1965).

36. C. Djerassi, *Optical Rotatory Dispersion: Applications to Organic Chemistry*, McGraw-Hill, New York, 1960.

37. P. Crabbé, *Optical Rotatory Dispersion and Circular Dichroism in Organic Chemistry*, Holden-Day, San Francisco, 1965.

38. N. Greenfield, B. Davidson, and G. D. Fasman, *Biochemistry*, **6**, 1630 (1967).

39. G. Snatzke, Ed., *Optical Rotatory Dispersion and Circular Dichroism in Organic Chemistry*, Sadtler Research Laboratories, Philadelphia, 1967.

40. C. F. Chignell, *Mol. Pharmacol.*, **5**, 244 (1969).

41. W. B. Gratzer and D. A. Cowburn, *Nature*, **222**, 426 (1969).

42. L. Velluz, M. Legrand, and M. Grosjean, *Optical Circular Dichroism: Principles, Measurements, and Applications*, Verlag Chemie, Weinheim, 1965.

43. J. P. Glusker, *J. Mol. Biol.*, **38**, 149 (1968).

44. H. Neurath, J. A. Rupley, and W. J. Dreyer, *Arch. Biochem. Biophys.*, **65**, 243 (1956).

45. K. Imahori, A. Yoshida, and H. Hashizume, *Biochim. Biophys. Acta*, **45**, 380 (1960).

46. B. W. Matthews, P. B. Sigler, R. Henderson, and D. M. Blow, *Nature*, **214**, 652 (1967).

47. S. G. Cohen and A. Milovanovič, *J. Am. Chem. Soc.*, **90**, 3495 (1968).
48. B. Belleau and R. Chevalier, *J. Am. Chem. Soc.*, **90**, 6864 (1968).
49. J. McConn, G. D. Fasman, and G. P. Hess, *J. Mol. Biol.*, **39**, 551 (1969).
50. D. E. Koshland, Jr., *Proc. Natl. Acad. Sci. U.S.*, **44**, 98 (1958).
51. D. E. Koshland, Jr., *Biochem. Pharmacol.*, **8**, 57 (1961).
52. D. E. Koshland, Jr., J. A. Yankeelov, Jr., and J. A. Thoma, *Federation Proc.*, **21**, 1031 (1962).
53. D. E. Koshland, Jr., *Federation Proc.*, **23**, 719 (1964).
54. D. E. Koshland, Jr., *Federation Proc.*, **27**, 907 (1968).
55. D. E. Koshland, Jr., G. Némethy, and D. Filmer, *Biochemistry*, **5**, 365 (1966).
56. D. E. Koshland, Jr., and K. E. Neet, *Ann. Rev. Biochem.*, **37**, 359 (1968).
57. J. Botts and M. Morales, *Trans. Faraday Soc.*, **49**, 696 (1953).
58. C. Cennamo, *J. Theoret. Biol.*, **21**, 260 (1968).
59. J. Monod, *Endocrinology*, **78**, 412 (1966).
60. B. M. Bloom and I. M. Goldman, *Advan. Drug Res.*, **3**, 121 (1966).
61. K. U. Linderstrøm-Lang and J. A. Schellman, "Protein Structure and Enzyme Activity," in P. D. Boyer, H. Lardy, and K. Myrbäck, Eds., *The Enzymes*, Vol. I, 2nd ed., Academic, New York, 1959, pp. 443–510.
62. R. Lovrien, *J. Am. Chem. Soc.*, **85**, 3677 (1963).
63. I. A. Rose, *Ann. Rev. Biochem.*, **35**, 23 (1966).
64. C. H. W. Hirs, Ed., "Enzyme Structure," in S. P. Colowick and N. O. Kaplan, Eds., *Methods in Enzymology*, Vol. XI, Academic, New York, 1967.
65. C. M. Venkatachalam and G. N. Ramachandran, *Ann. Rev. Biochem.*, **38**, 45 (1969).
66. S. Bernhard, *The Structure and Function of Enzymes*, Benjamin, New York, 1968.
67. J.-P. Changeux, J. Thiéry, Y. Tung, and C. Kittel, *Proc. Natl. Acad. Sci. U.S.*, **57**, 335 (1967).
68. J. Wyman, *J. Am. Chem. Soc.*, **89**, 2202 (1967).
69. J. Wyman, *J. Mol. Biol.*, **39**, 523 (1969).
70. R. W. Noble, *J. Mol. Biol.*, **39**, 479 (1969).
71. B. Belleau, *Ann. N.Y. Acad. Sci.*, **144**, 705 (1967).
72. P. S. Portoghese, *J. Med. Chem.*, **8**, 609 (1965).
73. J. B. Kay and J. B. Robinson, *J. Pharm. Pharmacol.*, **21**, 145 (1969).
74. B. Belleau and J. L. Lavoie, *Can. J. Biochem.*, **46**, 1397 (1968).

10

MECHANISMS OF DRUG ACTION

A fundamental understanding of the mechanism of action of a drug can come only from a biochemical or biophysical approach.

Jack R. Cooper

I. PRINCIPAL MECHANISMS OF ACTION

Many attempts have been made to propose a general theory on the mechanism of action of drugs. This desideratum, however, becomes more and more remote, as new knowledge accumulates (*1*). It is assumed, nevertheless, that the majority of the drugs act at the molecular level by one of the three following mechanisms (*2*):

1. Inhibition of enzymic systems or alteration of the specificity of the enzymes.
2. Alteration of molecules that serve as templates.
3. Alteration of the permeability of biological membranes.

II. ACTION OF DRUGS ON ENZYMES

Until recently it was thought that drugs exerted their effects through action on an enzyme, a coenzyme, a prosthetic group, or on factors that affect them (*1*). Danielli (*3*) postulated that drugs could influence enzymic reactions by acting as carrier molecules to accelerate a controlled reaction, activators, inhibitors, prosthetic groups, coenzymes, cosubstrates, removers of substrates through change in the structure of a specific substrate. Although several examples of drugs that act by such mechanisms are already known, cases in which this has been unequivocally proven are not numerous.

All enzyme inhibitions result from the interaction of the drug with some component of the enzyme system. Taking into account the component primarily involved in inhibition, Webb (*4*) has presented the following classification for the sites of inhibition:

I. Reaction of inhibitor with apoenzyme
  A. Chemical reaction with specific protein groups: these groups, such as sulfhydryl, amino, or phenolic groups, may react irrespective of their position relative to the active center.
  B. Specific reaction with sites on the apoenzyme: the specificity of interaction here resides in the spatial pattern of matter and charge over the site rather than in a simple chemical group.
    1. Substrate site
    2. Coenzyme site
    3. Activator site
  C. Generalized adsorption onto the protein surface: a relatively nonspecific and weak interaction by substances, frequently nonpolar or amphotropic compounds, that associate with the protein side chains and may interfere with binding of any component.
  D. Denaturation of the protein: an alteration of the basic protein structure, usually by substances reacting with those protein groups responsible for the bonds holding the polypeptide fabric in a specific orientation.
  E. Hydrolysis of apoenzyme: the breaking of peptide bonds in the protein, generally by proteolytic enzymes, giving rise to fragments of the apoenzyme that may be partially or completely inactive.
II. Reaction of inhibitor with substrate: the binding or the subsequent transformations of the substrate are hindered.
III. Reaction of inhibitor with coenzyme: generally the ability of the coenzyme to participate in the reaction is reduced, although the affinity for the apoenzyme may also be decreased.
IV. Reaction of inhibitor with activator.
V. Reaction of inhibitor with enzyme-complex: combination with the enzyme–substrate, enzyme–coenzyme, or enzyme–activator complex,

although there is not necessarily a reaction with any of the individual components.

VI. Entry of inhibitor into the reaction sequence: the inhibitor may be acted upon by the enzyme so that it undergoes reactions similar to substrate, thus reducing the amount of substrate reacted or causing a subsequent block if a normal transfer reaction is slowed.

VII. Reaction of inhibitor with linking components in an enzyme aggregate: dissociation of enzyme units in a complex system by interaction with substances, perhaps nonprotein in nature, functioning structurally in the spatial orientation of these units.

Several reviews (5–11) as well as large volumes (4,12–16) give some examples of drugs that act on enzymes, whether activating or inhibiting them. But, in order to assume that a drug acts on a particular enzyme it must be proved that (5) (a) the enzyme involved is inhibited in the intact living cell; (b) the blockade of the enzyme will explain quantitatively the drug effect; (c) the enzymic inhibition occurs with an amount of drug not greater than that necessary to produce the action. It is accepted, for instance, that physostigmine acts through the inhibition of cholinesterases because (a) the natural substrate of cholinesterases accumulates in intoxicated tissues; (b) the intoxication symptoms can be produced by acetylcholine if properly applied; (c) considering that dissociation of the drug-enzyme complex is slow, the intoxicated tissues can be removed and triturated, and the enzymatic inhibition shown *in vitro*.

A. Activation of Enzymes

In order to exert maximal activity enzymes need various components, such as apoenzymes (protein constituents), coenzymes, cofactors, and substrates. Coenzymes are vitamin derivatives and cofactors are inorganic ions.

It was shown that electrolytes such as Na^+, K^+, Rb^+, Cs^+, Mg^{2+}, Ca^{2+}, Zn^{2+}, Cd^{2+}, Cr^{2+}, Cu^{2+}, Mn^{2+}, Fe^{2+}, Co^{2+}, Ni^{2+}, and Al^{3+}, whose atomic numbers vary from 11 to 55, activate one or more enzymes in the body. But there is not an absolute specificity in the activation of enzymes by metallic ions. In this activation, however, an important role is played by complex stability, stereochemical factors, size, charge, and electronic properties of the metallic ions. Therefore drugs that can provide such inorganic ions act by activating enzymes. Such a process can be visualized in two ways. The ion can interact with an enzyme inhibitor preventing enzyme deactivation or it can interact with an enzyme directly altering its conformation and charge.

Activation in turn can result from three different mechanisms (17):

1. Formation of a complex between the enzyme and the metallic ion, as

occurs in peptidases. It is assumed that in this case the complex is the sole catalytically active species:

$$E + M \xrightleftharpoons{K_{[E][M]}} EM$$

$$EM + S \underset{k_2}{\overset{k_1}{\rightleftharpoons}} EMS \xrightarrow{k_3} EM + P$$

where S is the substrate and P the product.

The reaction rate can be represented by

$$V = k_3 \frac{[E]}{1 + K_m/[S] + K_m/K_{[E][M]}[M][S]} \tag{I}$$

where K_m is the Michaelis–Menten constant.

2. Formation of the substrate–metal complex, which is assumed to be the real substrate that reacts with the enzyme:

$$S + M \xrightleftharpoons{K_{[S][M]}} SM$$

$$E + SM \underset{k_2}{\overset{k_1}{\rightleftharpoons}} ESM \xrightarrow{k_3} E + PM$$

The rate is expressed by the equation

$$V = k_3 \frac{[E]}{1 + K_m/[S] + K_m/K_{[S][M]}[M][S]} \tag{II}$$

This, kinetically, is identical to the representative equation of mechanism 1, differing from it only in the dissociation constant.

3. Combination of a metal with the enzyme–substrate complex. The rate equation is similar to the preceding one (Equation II), and for this reason it is difficult to make a distinction between the two.

Other types of drugs increase enzymic activity through an induced adaptation mechanism. This phenomenon acquires special relevance in microbial systems. A classical example is the activation of penicillinase induced by penicillin itself. Another example is provided by barbiturates, which stimulate their own oxidation by activating some enzymes.

On the other hand, heavy metals, such as Hg^{2+}, Cu^{2+}, Ni^{2+}, Pb^{2+}, Zn^{2+}, Co^{2+}, Cd^{2+}, Mn^{2+}, Mg^{2+}, Ca^{2+}, and Ba^{2+}, can cause inhibition of enzymes, often with highly toxic effects to the human or animal body. In chemotherapy the aim is to poison the parasite selectively, without causing damage to the host. The association constants of these metals with amino and carboxy groups of amino acids have this order: $Hg^{2+} > Cu^{2+} > Ni^{2+} > Pb^{2+} > Zn^{2+} > Co^{2+} > Cd^{2+} > Mn^{2+} > Mg^{2+} > Ca^{2+} > Ba^{2+}$. With cysteine Co^{2+} and Co^{3+} form chelates through sulfhydryl and amino groups; the same seems to happen between Zn^{2+} and cysteine (*17*). The poisoning subsequent to inter-action of metallic ions with enzymes results from their complexation with one or more of the following groups existing in any living cell and in many or most enzymes: —OH, —COOH, —PO_3H_2, —SH, —NH, imidazole ring (*18*).

B. Inhibition of Enzymes

In biochemistry the effect produced by an inhibitor is called a *biochemical lesion*, an expression used originally (*19*) to designate perturbation in brain metabolism and function by a deficiency of vitamin B_1, and nowadays employed to mean any disturbance of metabolism by agents acting directly on metabolic systems (*4,20*). An obvious example of a biochemical lesion is the toxic effect of cyanide on cytochrome oxidase (*15*).

The action of inhibitors on living systems results in modification of energy flow (*4*). The main routes of this flow are indicated in Figure 10.1. An inhibitor can interfere with one or more of these routes, in the following ways:

1. By preventing the entrance of substrates into the cell through alteration of permeability or depression of transport systems.
2. By exerting action on the degradative reactions in which the substrates are oxidatively broken down to products.
3. By hindering the formation of high-energy phosphates.
4. By hampering the biosynthesis of protoplasmic components.

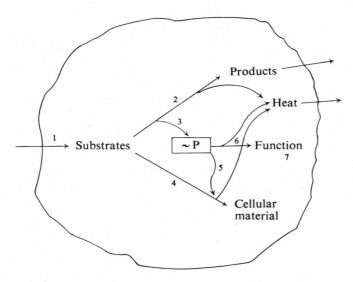

Fig. 10.1. Schematic representation of the basic energy flow through a cell. [Adapted from (*4*).]

5. By preventing the utilization of the high-energy substances by these synthetic processes.

6. By operating on the reactions involved in the utilization of energy.

7. By acting directly on the functional systems themselves.

Interference with any of these routes alters the biochemical morphology and functional phenomena necessary for the life of the cell and for the playing of the cell's role in the life of the whole organism (4).

Among drugs that act as inhibitors of enzymes may be mentioned some cholinergic blocking agents [acetylcholinesterase inhibitors (21)], some psychoanaleptics [monoamine oxidase inhibitors (22)], certain diuretics [carbonic anhydrase inhibitors (23)], several antibiotics (24–29), besides other groups of drugs (1,4,12). Table 10.1 lists some examples of enzyme inhibitors.

The inhibition caused by drugs can be (15) reversible or irreversible. It is reversible when it is characterized by an equilibrium between the enzyme and the inhibitory drug; in this case the efficiency of the drug is usually expressed by the constant K_i, which is the reciprocal of the affinity of the inhibitor for the enzyme; an example is the action of malonate on succinate dehydrogenase. The inhibition is irreversible when it increases with time, provided that the inhibitory drug is present in excess; the efficiency of the drug is then expressed not by an equilibrium constant but by a rate constant, which determines the fraction of the inhibited enzyme in a given lapse of time by a certain concentration of the inhibitor; an example of such inhibition is the action of cyanide on xanthine oxidase.

An inhibitory drug can affect the enzymic process in two ways: (a) by altering the affinity of the enzyme E for substrate S; (b) by interfering with the rate at which the enzyme–substrate complex dissociates into products (4):

$$
\begin{array}{ccc}
 & \text{ES} \xrightarrow{k} \text{E} + \text{P} & \\
K_s \nearrow & & \searrow \alpha K_i \\
\text{E} & & \text{EIS} \xrightarrow{\beta k} \text{EI} + \text{P} \\
K_i \searrow & & \nearrow \alpha K_s \\
 & \text{EI} &
\end{array}
$$

$$ \text{E} + \text{S} \rightleftharpoons \text{ES} \xrightarrow{k} \text{E} + \text{P} \qquad K_s = \frac{(E)(S)}{(ES)} $$

$$ \text{E} + \text{I} \rightleftharpoons \text{EI} \qquad K_i = \frac{(E)(I)}{(EI)} $$

$$ \text{EI} + \text{S} \rightleftharpoons \text{EIS} \xrightarrow{\beta k} \text{EI} + \text{P} \qquad \alpha K_s = \frac{(EI)(S)}{(EIS)} $$

$$ \text{ES} + \text{I} \rightleftharpoons \text{EIS} \xrightarrow{\beta k} \text{EI} + \text{P} \qquad \alpha K_i = \frac{(ES)(I)}{(EIS)} $$

In the equations above K_i is the constant of the inhibitory drug and K_s the dissociation constant for the enzyme–substrate complex; α represents the alteration in affinity and β, the alteration in the decomposition rate of the complex induced by the inhibitory drug; the values of α and β determine whether the drug acts as an activator or an inhibitor. The following relations can be written:

$$(E_t) = (E) + (ES) + (EI) + (EIS)$$

$$v_i = k(ES) + \beta k(EIS)$$

By combining these relations with the preceding ones, Equation III is obtained (4):

$$v_i = V_m \frac{(S)[\alpha K_i + \beta(I)]}{(S)(I) + \alpha[K_i(S) + K_s(I) + K_s K_i]} \tag{III}$$

in which v_i is the enzymic-reaction rate in the presence of the inhibitory drug and $V_m = k(E_t)$ is the maximal rate. The *fractional inhibition i*, which may be defined as $i = 1 - a$, a being the fractional activity, is expressed by the equation

$$i = \frac{(I)[(S)(1 - \beta) + K_s(\alpha - \beta)]}{(I)[(S) + \alpha K_s] + K_i[\alpha(S) + \alpha K_s]} \tag{IV}$$

By considering the different values of α and β, five characteristic types of inhibition can be distinguished (4):

1. Completely competitive inhibition ($\alpha = \infty$ and $\beta = 0$): the inhibitor completely prevents the combination of the substrate with the enzyme.

$$v_i = V_m \frac{(S)}{(S) + K_s[1 + (I)/K_i]}$$

$$i = \frac{(I)}{(I) + K_i[1 + (S)/K_s]}$$

2. Partially competitive inhibition ($\infty > \alpha > 1$ and $\beta = 1$): the inhibitor hinders only partially the binding of the substrate to the enzyme and does not affect the complex-dissociation rate.

$$v_i = V_m \frac{(S)}{(S) + K_s\{[\alpha(I) + \alpha K_i]/[(I) + \alpha K_i]\}}$$

$$i = \frac{(I)(\alpha - 1)}{(I)[\alpha + (S)/K_s] + \alpha K_i[1 + (S)/K_s]}$$

TABLE 10.1 Some Representative Inhibitors of Enzymes [a,b] (30)

Inhibitor	Sensitive Group	Mechanism of Action	Type of Reaction	Representative Sensitive Enzyme
p-Chloromercuribenzoate	Sulfhydryl	$RS\overline{|H\ Cl|}HgC_6H_4COOH$ or $RS\overline{|H\ HO|}HgC_6H_4COOH$	Mercaptide formation	Urease
Iodoacetamide (also iodoacetate)	Sulfhydryl (amino group also)	$RS\overline{|H\ I|}CH_2CONH_2$	Alkylation	Papain
N-Ethylmaleimide	Sulfhydryl	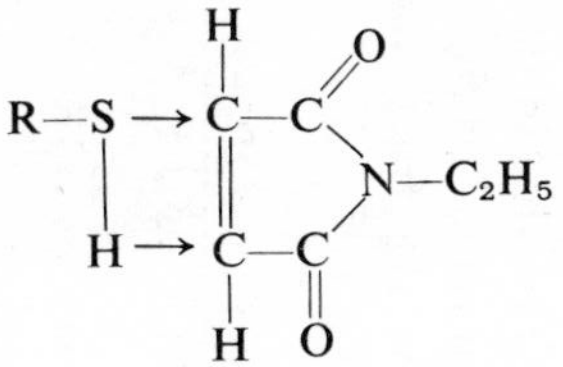 (ring structure, maleimide N–C_2H_5 addition)	Addition	Myosin
Iodosobenzoate	Sulfhydryl	$R-S\overline{|H}$ $O\ IC_6H_4COOH$ / $R-S\overline{|H}$	Oxidation	Triose phosphate dehydrogenase
Trivalent arsenicals	Sulfhydryl	$R-S\overline{|H\ Cl|}$ As·R / $R-S\overline{|H\ Cl|}$	Mercaptide formation	Succinoxidase
Ferricyanide	Sulfhydryl	$2RSH \rightarrow R-S-S-R$	Oxidation	β-Amylase

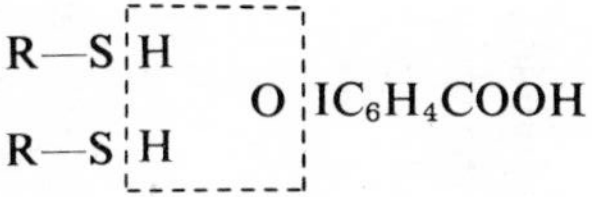

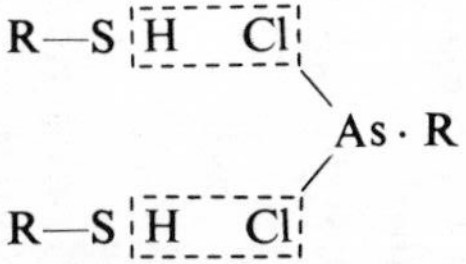

296

Inhibitor	Point of attack	Reaction	Effect	Enzyme
Iodine	(Sulfhydryl, aromatic residues)	2RSH + I$_2$ → R—S—S—R + 2HI	Oxidation Iodination	Lactic dehydrogenase
Heavy-metal cations (Hg, Ag, etc.)	(Sulfhydryl, anions)	Mercaptylation RCOO$^{\ominus}$ + M$^{\oplus}$ → RCOO$^{\ominus}$M$^{\oplus}$	Mercaptide formation Salt formation	Glutamic dehydrogenase
Cyanide, azide	Metalloporphyrins; metals	Attachment to metals	Metal inactivation	Tyrosinase, catalase
Carbon monoxide	Metalloporphyrins	Attachment to metals (iron–porphyrin complex is photodissociable)	Metal inactivation	Cytochrome oxidase
Chelating agents (citrate, oxalate, pyrophosphate, ethylenediamine tetraacetate, etc.)	Metals	Removal of metal	Metal inactivation	Aspartase
Fluoride	Metals; magnesium–protein complex	Mg-fluorophosphate or Mg-fluoride; Mg-protein	Metal inactivation	Enolase
Alkoxyhalogeno-phosphates (diisopropylfluorophosphate, DFP, etc.)	Serine or imidazole?	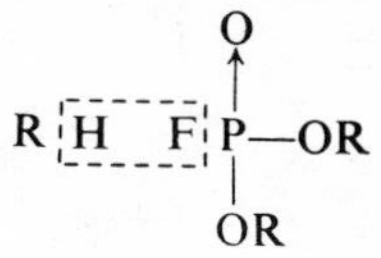 R—[H F]—P—OR with O and OR	Phosphorylation	Cholinesterase
Arsenate	Organic phosphate bond with $\Delta F_{\text{hydrolysis}} > 4000$ cal	Competitive acceptor against phosphate	Arsenolysis	Phospho-transacetylase

[a] Further data are available in references 4, 13, 15, 31.

[b] The table does not include nonspecific inhibitors, such as the macroanionic and macrocationic substances.

297

3. Completely noncompetitive inhibition ($\alpha = 1$ and $\beta = 0$): the inhibitor does not alter the binding of the substrate to the enzyme but prevents decomposition of the ES complex into products.

$$v_i = V_m \frac{K_i}{(I) + K_i} \frac{(S)}{(S) + K_s}$$

$$i = \frac{(I)}{(I) + K_i}$$

4. Partially noncompetitive inhibition ($\alpha = 1$ and $0 < \beta < 1$): the binding of the substrate to the enzyme is not altered, but the rate of breakdown of the EIS complex is slower than that of the ES complex.

$$v_i = V_m \frac{\beta(I) + K_i}{(I) + K_i} \frac{(S)}{(S) + K_s}$$

$$i = (1 - \beta) \frac{(I)}{(I) + K_i}$$

5. Mixed inhibition ($\infty > \alpha > 1$ and $\beta = 0$): the inhibitor reduces the affinity of the enzyme for the substrate, preventing dissociation of the EIS complex.

$$v_i = V_m \frac{\alpha K_i}{(I) + \alpha K_i} \frac{(S)}{(S) + K_s\{[\alpha(I) + \alpha K_i]/[(I) + \alpha K_i]\}}$$

$$i = \frac{(I)}{(I) + K_i\{[\alpha(S) + \alpha K_s]/[(S) + \alpha K_s]\}}$$

A particular case of this last type of inhibition occurs when α is less than 1: this is *uncompetitive inhibition*.

Although there are five types of inhibition, for the sake of simplicity only three main types of inhibition are usually mentioned: competitive, noncompetitive, and uncompetitive (*1,8,15,30–33*).

1. Competitive Inhibition. In competitive inhibition the drug competes with the substrate for the same site of the enzyme and combines with it reversibly (Figure 10.2). In this process, therefore, the relative concentrations of the substrate and of the drug are of fundamental importance, because they determine the degree of inhibition. Actually in the presence of excess substrate the drug is displaced from the receptor, which is then occupied by the substrate, as indicated below:

$$E + S \rightleftharpoons ES$$

$$E + I \rightleftharpoons EI$$

$$EI + S \longrightarrow ES + I$$

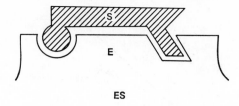

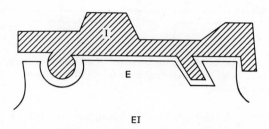

Fig. 10.2. Schematic representation of competitive inhibition.

An example of this type of inhibition is the effect of eserine on acetylcholinesterase. This type of inhibition is expressed by the following equation (*34*):

$$K_i = (I_t) \frac{(E_t - EI - ES)}{EI}$$

where K_i is the constant of inhibitory drug, I_t is the total drug, and E_t the total enzyme. Because of the difficulty of determining the maximal rate V_m, it is preferred to use the reciprocal of the preceding equation, as follows (*35*):

$$\frac{1}{V} = \left[1 + \frac{I}{K_i}\right]\left[\frac{K_m}{V_m}\frac{1}{S_t}\right] + \frac{1}{V_m}$$

where K_m is the Michaelis–Menten constant (equivalent to K_s in the simplified equation) and V_m is the maximal rate.

By plotting the inverse of the rate as a function of the inverse of the substrate concentration, the graph of Figure 10.3 is obtained. It is observed that in the absence of an inhibitor the slope of the straight line is smaller than in the presence of an inhibitor, although both lines intercept the $1/V$ axis at the same point. This means that K_m varies, whereas V_m remains constant. Therefore, in the presence of an inhibitory drug but low concentration of a substrate, the enzymic-reaction rate decreases. On the other hand, the reaction can again proceed at the original maximal rate when the inhibitor concentration is kept constant and the substrate concentration is increased.

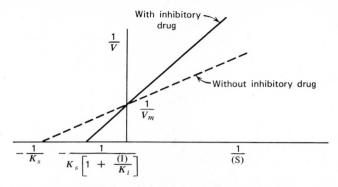

Fig. 10.3. Competitive inhibition. In the presence of an inhibitor the angular coefficient of the straight line is reduced by a factor equal to $[1 + (I)/K_i]$, although the maximal rate V_m may remain unchanged.

2. Noncompetitive Inhibition. In noncompetitive inhibition the drug combines with the enzyme or with an enzyme–substrate complex with equal ease, but at a site different from that to which the substrate is attracted. This indicates that the inhibitor binds itself to different sites on the enzyme, and not to the catalytic center—that is, the active site. This fact has been experimentally confirmed: it was shown that many allosteric enzymes can become insensitive to allosteric inhibitors without losing catalytic activity (*36*). Such inhibition, which is usually reversible and not affected by substrate concentration, depends solely on drug concentration and on the dissociation constant K_i of this inhibitor; a substrate never displaces the inhibitor even at high concentrations. Though purely noncompetitive inhibition is very unusual, the effect of isoflurophate on cholinesterase action is an example (*4*). Presently noncompetitive inhibition is considered as being related to allosteric phenomena.

$$E + I \rightleftharpoons EI$$

$$EI + S \rightleftharpoons EIS \longrightarrow EI + P$$

Graphically, this type of inhibition can be represented by Figure 10.4. The mathematical equation that expresses noncompetitive inhibition is

$$K_i = I_t \frac{(E_t - EI)}{EI}$$

This equation differs from the one corresponding to competitive inhibition by not including ES. This is so because there is no competition between the inhibitory drug and the substrate, and consequently the interaction of the enzyme with the inhibitor is not affected by the amount of enzyme that is combined with the substrate.

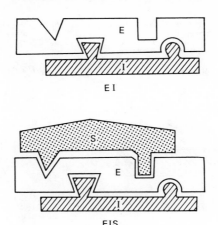

Fig. 10.4. Schematic representation of noncompetitive inhibition.

The rate is expressed by the relation

$$\frac{1}{V} = \left(1 + \frac{I}{K_i}\right)\left(\frac{K_m}{V_m}\frac{1}{S_t} + \frac{1}{V_m}\right)$$

The plot of $1/V$ as a function of $1/(S)$ is shown in Figure 10.5. It can be seen that, contrary to what happens in competitive inhibition, K_m remains constant, whereas the maximal rate V_m and the reaction rate V decrease.

3. Uncompetitive Inhibition. *Anticompetitive*, or *uncompetitive*, *inhibition*, more properly named *coupling inhibition*, is a particular form of mixed inhibition. In this relatively rare type of inhibition the drug combines only

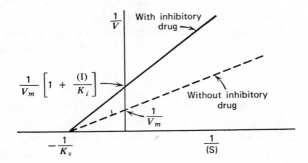

Fig. 10.5. Noncompetitive inhibition. In the presence of only the substrate as well as in the presence of different concentrations of the inhibitory drug K_m remains constant, while the angular coefficient of the straight line is reduced by a factor equal to $[1 + (I)/K_i]$.

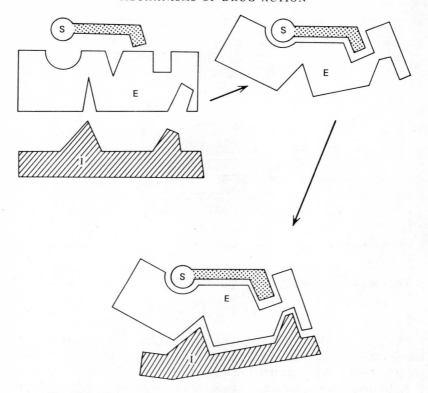

Fig. 10.6. Schematic representation of uncompetitive inhibition.

with the enzyme–substrate complex (not with the free enzyme, as occurs in noncompetitive inhibition) at a site different from the one with which the substrate is combined. Enzymes that have several sites of bonding are called *allosteric* (*37–39*). Examples of this type of inhibition are the actions of azide on the oxidized form of cytochrome oxidase (*40*) and of hydrazine on pepsin (*1,4*).

$$E + S \rightleftharpoons ES \xrightarrow{I} ESI$$

It was indicated in Chapter 6 that the active site of enzymes is not necessarily rigid, but flexible or elastic. This flexibility can occur either during the tension caused by denaturing agents or during enzymic action itself (*41,42*). In the case of uncompetitive inhibition it is assumed that such flexibility or elasticity manifests itself as shown in Figure 10.6.

The plot of $1/V$ as a function of $1/(S)$ (Figure 10.7) shows that the straight lines are parallel. This means that both maximal rate V_m and K_m vary.

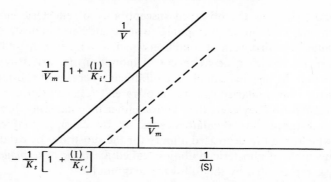

Fig. 10.7. Uncompetitive inhibition. In this type of inhibition both the maximal rate and the Michaelis–Menten constant undergo variation, being both these values reduced by a factor equal to $[1 + (I)/K_i']$.

C. Allosteric Inhibition

The classical concept of enzymic inhibition by an antimetabolite can be represented by the following scheme (*43*):

antimetabolite A
inhibition
↓

$$\text{metabolite A} \xrightarrow{\quad \text{enzyme A} \quad} \text{metabolite B}$$

The antimetabolite is similar in structure to a given metabolite, and this characteristic of complementarity allows it to combine with the active site of the enzyme, altering the enzyme–substrate complex dissociation. This mechanism is valid for enzymes in general, with the exception of allosteric enzymes.

Due to the unusual kinetic and structural characteristics of the allosteric enzymes, Monod and co-workers (*44*) have proposed the following model for them:

1. All are polymers, made up of one or more identical subunits and, therefore, can exist in at least two different conformational states.
2. Each one of the identical subunits has a single catalytic site, specific for the substrate, and a separate allosteric site for each allosteric effector (inhibitor or activator).
3. For each conformational state the catalytic and allosteric sites have equal affinities for their respective ligands.
4. The various conformational states of the enzyme are in mutual dynamic equilibrium.
5. The transition from one state to another occurs with simultaneous alterations in all the identical subunits within a particular molecule.

This model explains the observed susceptibility of allosteric enzymes to association and dissociation in response to substrate and to allosteric agents, and to change in environmental conditions, such as temperature and pH (*36*).

Based on this model, a new concept of inhibition has arisen recently. It was shown that the enzyme can also be inhibited by chemical substances that have no structural similarity with the substrate. These substances are called *allosteric inhibitors*. They exert their action either by competing directly with activator substances for regulatory sites or by causing conformational changes, which result in decreased affinity for the substrates by catalytic sites (*36*). An example of allosteric inhibition, called *feedback* or *terminal product inhibition*, is represented by the following diagram (*43*):

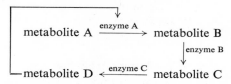

In a series of reactions catalyzed by enzymes only the first enzyme A is inhibited, due to the accumulation of the terminal metabolite D. The interaction of the inhibitor, the metabolite D, with the enzyme A is not necessarily at the same site that interacts with the substrate—that is, with its active site; in fact it usually is with another, the regulatory site, to which the name *allosteric site* is given.

Nowadays it is assumed that feedback inhibition is not restricted only to the first phase of a sequence of reactions; thus in the biosynthesis of pyrimidines not only the first phase but also the second one is susceptible to inhibition (*36*).

As a result of interaction of the metabolite with the allosteric site of an enzyme, this enzyme undergoes conformational change, which is accompanied by a decrease in affinity for the substrate (*36,41,44,45*). This change—which is reversible and is called *allosteric transition*—in the conformation of the enzyme modifies the properties of its active site and, for this very reason, the function of the enzyme.

From this explanation it is deduced that the allosteric inhibitor does not need to have any chemical resemblance to the substrate, because the allosteric site and the catalytic site are located in different portions of the enzyme (*36*). Interaction of the inhibitory drug with the allosteric site results in an alteration in the conformational state of the enzyme, which adopts a form in which its affinity, at the catalytic site, for the substrate is decreased. Hence, with the purpose of obtaining antagonists of the enzyme A, derivatives of the metabolite D can be synthesized instead of structural analogues of the metabolite A (*43*).

The new concept of feedback inhibition has been invoked to explain the mechanism of action of several drugs on nucleic acids. Aiming at the rationalization of chemotherapy, the possibility of combining this kind of inhibition with lethal synthesis was undertaken (46). The most promising fact, however, is that feedback-inhibition phenomena open the perspective of enriching the therapeutical arsenal, mainly in the sector of chemotherapeutic agents, with drugs having high specificity (43).

III. METABOLIC ANTAGONISM

There are drugs, among both pharmacodynamic and particularly chemotherapeutic agents, that owe their pharmacological action to the fact of their being structurally similar to normal cellular metabolites. For this very reason they are able to take the place of the latter in biological systems, though they may not carry out their normal functions (47,48). These altered metabolites are called *antimetabolites*.

The discovery of the antimetabolite phenomenon caused a true revolution in pharmacology (49,50), because not only did it make possible the cure of diseases that were considered incurable but also provided a new and efficient route in drug design. Nowadays the strategy of chemotherapy (51,52) consists chiefly, through studies related to comparative biochemistry (53–56), in exploring the differences of metabolism between the parasites and the hosts, with the purpose of preparing efficient antimetabolites (13).

Several authors had observed in the last century that an enzymic reaction is inhibited by the addition of compounds that are structurally similar to the substrate. However, Ehrlich, the founder of modern chemotherapy, was the first one who developed the theory of antimetabolites, at the beginning of this century, when he applied it to the search for antibacterial and antiprotozoal drugs. Nevertheless the concept of metabolic antagonism had great impulse only after Woods and Fildes (57) suggested that sulfanilamide and its derivatives act by inhibiting the utilization of *p*-aminobenzoic acid by the bacterial cell.

A. Mechanism of Action of Antimetabolites

Metabolic antagonists seem to act in two different ways: either by interfering in the synthesis of the metabolite or by preventing its utilization. The first is a case of *noncompetitive inhibition*. For instance, administration of bishydroxycoumarin to animals causes the typical syndrome of avitaminosis K_1; this deficiency is overcome by high doses of that vitamin. The second case is one of *competitive inhibition*. The classical example is that of the sulfonamides, which take the place of *p*-aminobenzoic acid in the biosynthesis of the coenzymically active form of folic acid. According to recent evidence (*58*), this form seems to be the $N^{5,10}$-formyl-5,6,7,8-tetrahydrofolic acid (*59*):

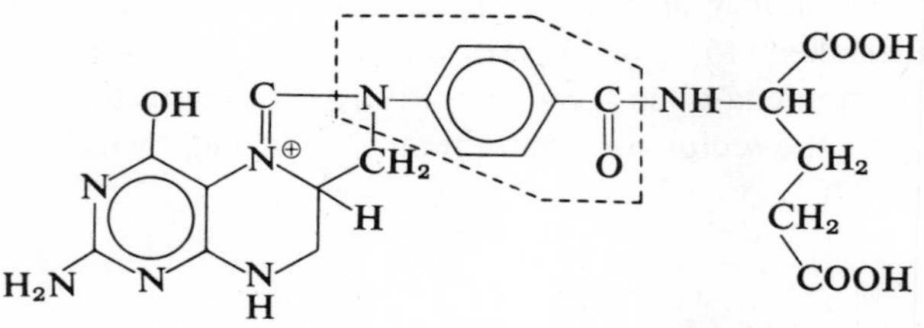

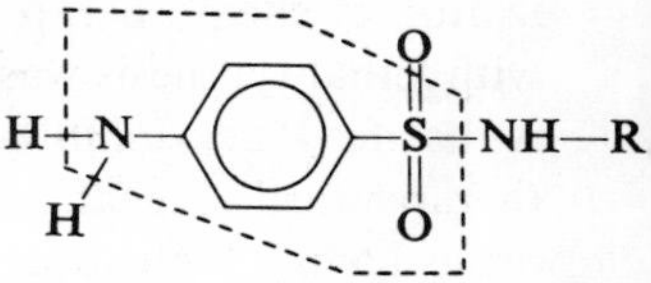

B. Examples of Antimetabolites

Many compounds have been synthesized with the aim of obtaining antimetabolites. However, only a few of them have proved to be useful, and these are being employed in therapeutics (*4,13,15,47,48,60,61*). On the other hand, many other drugs, such as the antihistaminics, a few anticoagulants, several cholinergic agents, certain adrenergic agents, some antibiotics (*26–29,62,63*), although possessing structural similarities to that of metabolites, have not resulted from the application of the antimetabolite concept, notwithstanding the fact that such an interpretation may be given (*47,64*). Neither are antimetabolites the antagonists of pharmacodynamic agents—such as nalorphine, which antagonizes morphine, and bemegride, which is an antagonist of barbiturates. Examples of antimetabolites are given below.

1. Antagonists of Amino Acids. It is known that in all organisms only 20 different amino acids are incorporated into proteins (*65*). Antagonists were prepared for several of them (*47,48*):

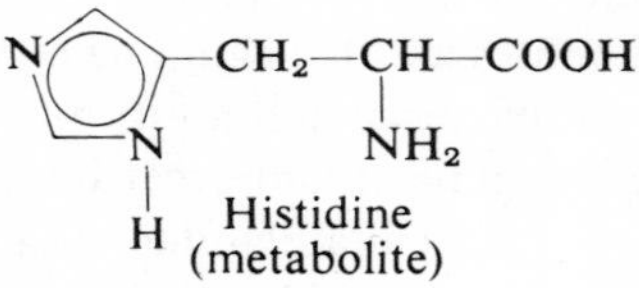

Histidine
(metabolite)

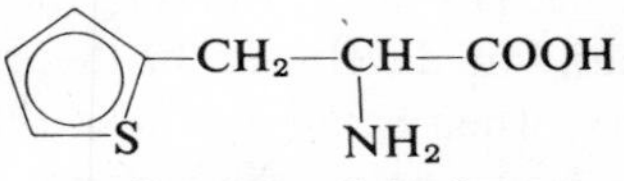

β-2-Thienylalanine
(antimetabolite)

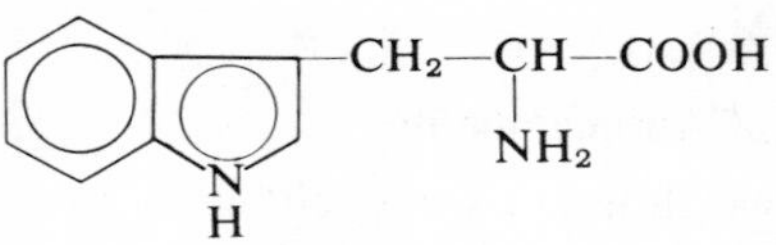

Tryptophan
(metabolite)

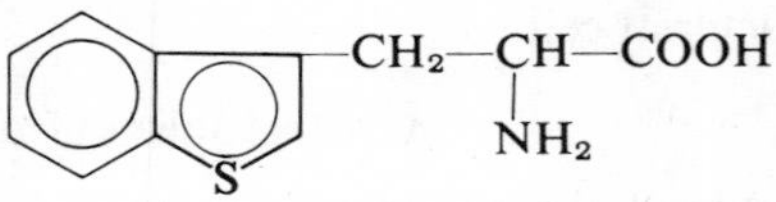

β-3-Thianaphthenylalanine
(antimetabolite)

2. Antagonists of Purines and Pyrimidines. Among many other antagonists of purines and pyrimidines are the following: 6-mercaptopurine, 6-thioguanine, 2,5-diaminopurine, 8-azaguanine, 5-fluorouracil, 6-azauracil, and

5-bromouracil. For interfering in the processes of biosynthesis related to nucleic acids, some of them and their analogs are being utilized in therapeutics, either as antiprotozoal agents, or as antiviral agents, or as cytostatic agents (*13,58,59,63,64,66–71*).

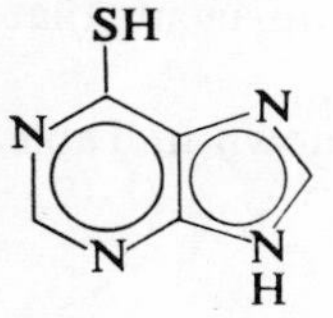

Mercaptopurine
(cytostatic)

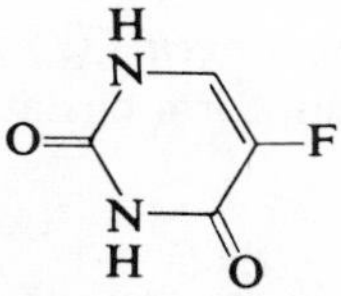

5-Fluorouracil
(cytostatic)

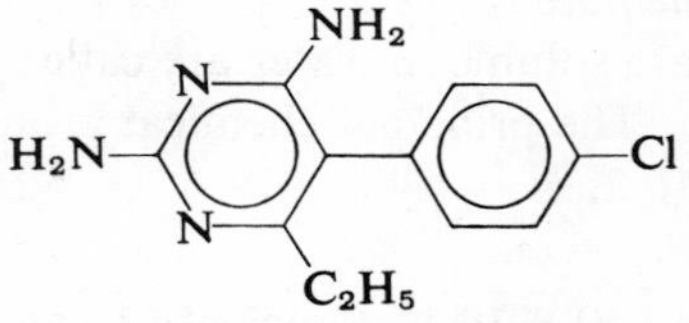

Pyrimethamine
(antimalarial)

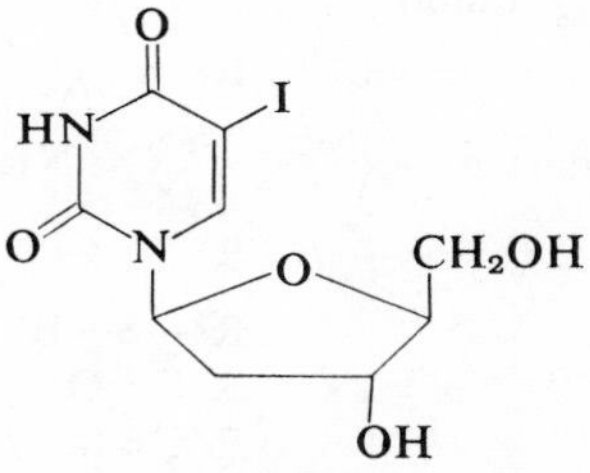

Idoxuridine
(antiviral)

3. Antagonists of Vitamins. Antagonists have been prepared for almost all vitamins (*64*). There are antagonists of thiamin, riboflavin, vitamin B_6, niacin, biotin, vitamin B_{12}, pantothenic acid, pteroylglutamic acid, choline, inositol, ascorbic acid, vitamin A, α-tocopherol, and vitamin K (*47,48*).

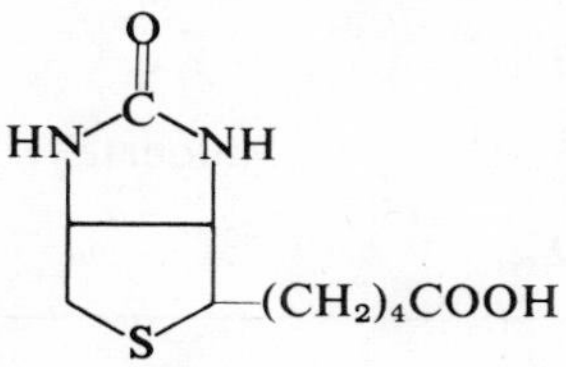

Biotin
(vitamin)

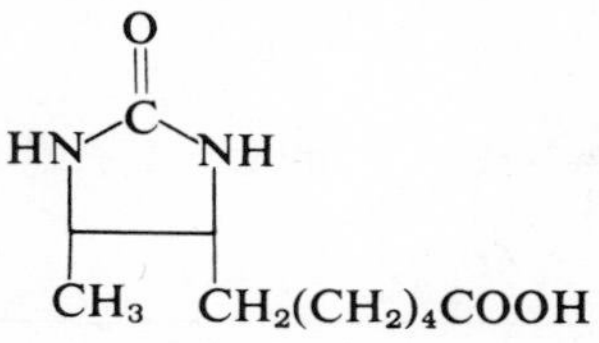

Desthiobiotin
(antivitamin)

IV. MECHANISM OF ACTION OF CHELATING AGENTS

Some substances have the property of combining with a metallic ion by donating a pair of electrons and thus forming annular compounds, or chelates, usually of five or six members (*72–74*).

Nearly all the metals can form chelates. But the main electron-donor atoms in the chelating agents are nitrogen, oxygen, and sulfur. According to the number of electron-donor groups, the ligand molecules—those that can form annular structures with a metallic ion—can be *bidentate* (two groups), *tridentate* (three groups), or *polydentate* (several groups). Chelating agents that are soluble in water are called *sequestering agents* (75,76).

The principal chemical groups that can form chelates are shown in Table 10.2.

TABLE 10.2   Principal Chelate Donor Groups (73)

Structure	Name	Structure	Name
$R—NH_2$	Primary amino		
$\begin{array}{c} R^1 \\ \diagdown \\ \quad NH \\ \diagup \\ R^2 \end{array}$	Secondary amino	$\begin{array}{c} R^1 \\ \diagdown \\ \quad C{=}NR^3 \\ \diagup \\ R^2 \end{array}$	Substituted imino
$\begin{array}{c} R^1 \\ \diagdown \\ R^2{—}N \\ \diagup \\ R^3 \end{array}$	Tertiary amino	$R^1—S—R^2$ $R^2C{=}O$ $R^2C{=}S$ $R—O^{\ominus}$ $R—S^{\ominus}$ $R—COO^{\ominus}$	Thioether Keto Thioketo Hydroxyl Thioalcohol Carboxylate
$\begin{array}{c} R^1 \\ \diagdown \\ \quad C{=}NOH \\ \diagup \\ R^2 \end{array}$	Oxime	$R—\overset{\displaystyle O}{\underset{\displaystyle OH}{\overset{\|}{P}}}—O^{\ominus}$	Phosphonate
$\begin{array}{c} R^1 \\ \diagdown \\ \quad C{=}NH \\ \diagup \\ R^2 \end{array}$	Imino	$R—\overset{\displaystyle O}{\underset{\displaystyle O}{\overset{\|}{\underset{\|}{S}}}}—O^{\ominus}$	Sulfonate

Reprinted by permission of Prentice-Hall, Inc.

Many substances present in the biological systems are chelates: insulin, hemoglobin, myoglobin, chlorophyll, vitamin B_{12}, and several enzymes. Since these have functions very vital to an organism—for instance, catalysis of oxidation-reduction reactions, oxygen transport, hydrolysis and synthesis of proteins, decarboxylation, transport of carbon dioxide (73)—the use of chelating agents as drugs (64,72,77–79) is understandable. Thus several antibacterial, tuberculostatic, antipyretic, antidiabetic, cytostatic, and fungicidal drugs are chelating agents (*78*). For instance, 8-hydroxyquinoline is utilized as a chemotherapeutic agent due to its ability to chelate iron, a metal essential to the metabolism of certain microorganisms. The same mechanism of action explains partially the tuberculostatic activity of isoniazid; another hypothesis of the mode of action of this drug is that it combines with pyridoxal (*64*).

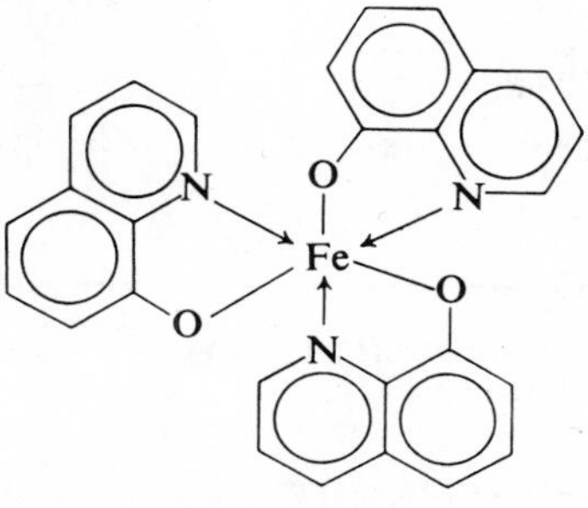

3:1-Oxine–ferric chelate
saturated (inactive)

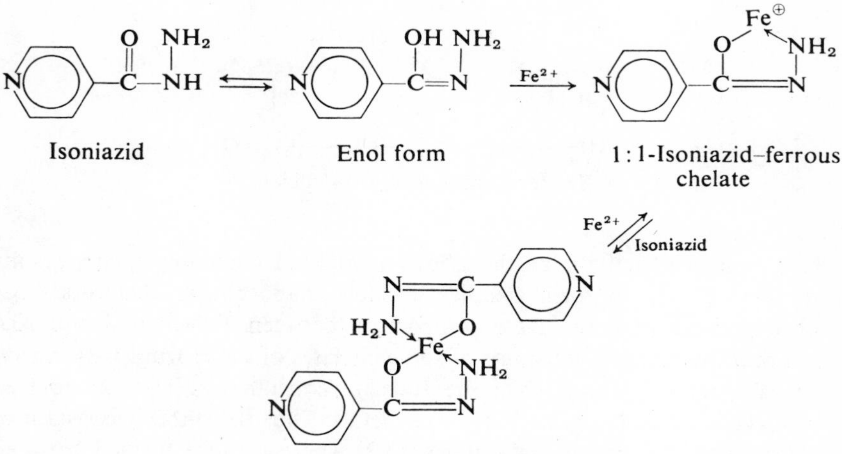

Isoniazid · Enol form · 1:1-Isoniazid–ferrous chelate

2:1-Isoniazid–ferrous chelate

Several other drugs have the property of forming chelates and owe their biological action partially or totally to this property: tetracyclines, hexachlorophene, salicylic acid, thiouracil, thiosemicarbazones, histamine, epinephrine, norepinephrine, and hydrazine (*64,72,78,80*).

Some chelating agents are used as antidotes in poisoning by metallic ions. Dimercaprol, penicillamine, desferrioxamine-B, ethylenediaminetetraacetic acid, and *trans*-1,2-diaminocyclohexanetetraacetic acid are some examples (*74*).

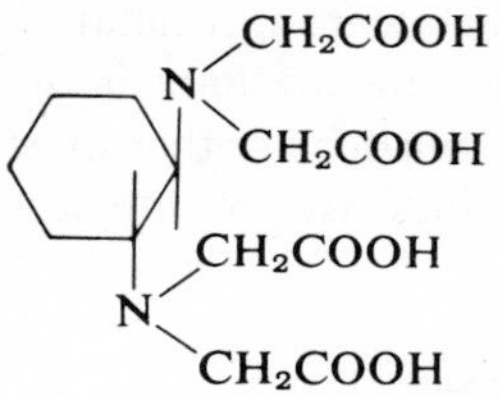

trans-1,2-Diaminocyclo-
hexanetetraacetic acid

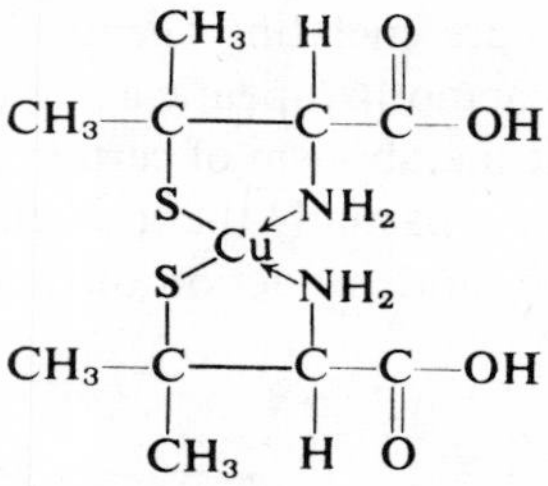

2:1-Penicillamine–copper
chelate

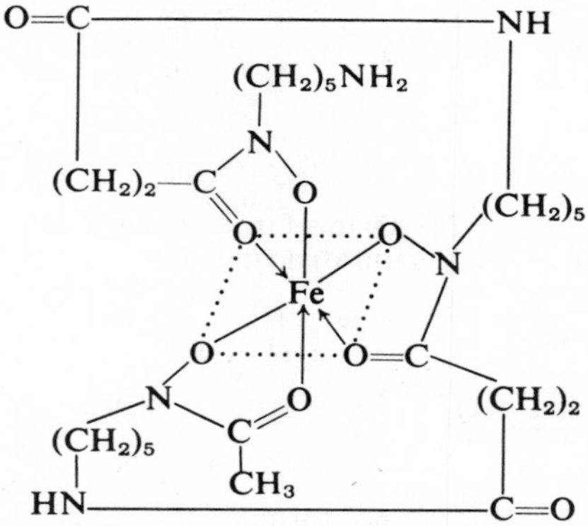

Desferrioxamine-B–iron chelate

The biological activity of the above-mentioned chelating agents results from their ability to form steadier chelates than cellular chelators (e.g., several amino acids). In fact a comparison between Tables 10.3 and 10.4 shows that the stability constants of some chelates of these drugs with heavy-metal cations are greater than the stability constants of chelates formed between cellular chelators and the same metals. Thus the stability constant of 8-hydroxyquinoline–copper chelate is 12.2, whereas those formed between copper and cellular chelators (glycine, cysteine, histidine, glutamic acid, etc.) are smaller (the greatest value being that of histidine–copper).

The main uses of chelating agents in pharmacology are threefold (*73,74*):

1. Destruction of parasitic microorganisms through chelation with essential metals—bactericidal, fungicidal, and viricidal action.
2. Inhibition of certain metals and metallic enzymes with the purpose of studying the functions of metals and of the enzymes in biological media.
3. Withdrawal of undesirable (harmful) metals from living organisms.

TABLE 10.3 Stability Constants of Substances of Therapeutic Value with Heavy-Metal Cations (78)

Ligand	log K_1 (Water, 20–30°C)					
	Cu^{2+}	Zn^{2+}	Co^{2+}	Fe^{2+}	Mn^{2+}	Fe^{3+}
8-Hydroxyquinoline	12.2	—	9.1	8.0	6.8	12.3
Salicylic acid	10.6	6.9	6.8	6.6	5.9	16.4
Gentisic acid	7.0	—	—	—	—	10.8
p-Aminosalicylic acid	—	—	—	—	—	16.1
o-Thymotic acid	9.7	—	—	—	—	15.8
Methyl salicylate	5.9	—	—	—	—	9.7
Isonicotinyl hydrazide	8.0	5.4	4.8	—	—	—
Tetracycline	7.8	4.9	5.4	5.3	4.4	9.9
Chlortetracycline	7.6	4.5	4.8	5.7	4.3	9.4
Oxytetracycline	7.2	4.6	5.1	5.6	4.3	9.6
Dimethyldithiocarbamic acid	11.4	—	—	—	—	—
2-Mercaptoethylamine	—	10.2	7.7	—	—	—

Reprinted with permission of the copyright owner.

TABLE 10.4 Stability Constants of Representative Cellular Chelators with Metal Cations (78)

Ligand	log K_1 (Water, 20–30°C)				
	Cu^{2+}	Zn^{2+}	Co^{2+}	Fe^{2+}	Mn^{2+}
Glycine	8.5	5.2	5.1	4.3	3.2
Cysteine	—	9.8	9.3	6.2	4.1
Histidine	10	6.7	7	5	< 4
Glutamic acid	—	5.4	5.1	4.6	3.3
Histamine	9.6	5.7	5.3	—	—
Glycylglycine	6.3	3.7	3.0	—	2.1
Pteroylglutamic acid	4.4	4.2	4.6	4.5	3.5
Riboflavin	7	5.6	3.9	7.1	3.4
Hypoxanthine	6.2	—	3.8	3.9	2.4
Guanosine	~6	4.6	3.2	4.3	—
Lactic acid	1.8	2.0	0.9	—	—
Oxalic acid	6	4.9	4.5	4.5	3.9

Reprinted with permission of the copyright owner.

V. ACTION OF DRUGS ON BIOLOGICAL MEMBRANES

A. Membrane Structure

The development of the electron microscope, new histochemical techniques, and biochemical analytical methods gave origin to the formulation of modern concepts on the nature of biological membranes (*81–89*). Many membrane models have been proposed (*81,84,88*). A particularly attractive one considers membranes as consisting of repeating globular lipoprotein units. Each unit is one layer thick. These units form vesicular or tubular systems (Figure 10.8).

The repeating units seem to be composed of two parts: (a) base pieces, which are subunits essential to membrane formation; (b) detachable pieces (headpieces and stalks), endowed with enzymic activity but not essential to membrane continuity. The ratio between structural and catalytic proteins seems to be 1:1. The several subunits that form one repeating unit are

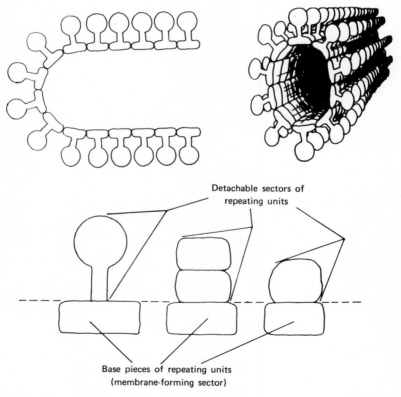

Detachable sectors of
repeating units

Base pieces of repeating units
(membrane-forming sector)

Fig. 10.8.   Schematic representation of the membrane made up by repeating units (*81*).

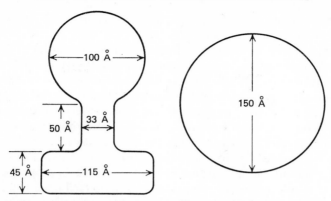

Fig. 10.9. The dimensions, in angstroms, of the elementary particle of the mitochondrial internal membrane (beef's heart) in its tripartite and spheric forms. [Adapted from (*82*).]

chemically and functionally distinct, containing different proteins, which are arranged in a characteristic manner for each subunit. Lipids constitute about 30% of the total dry weight of the membrane. Proteins attach to lipids primarily through hydrophobic interactions. This means that the hydrocarbon chains of phospholipids penetrate deeply into protein hydrophobic surfaces, while polar sectors of these phospholipid molecules impart hydrosolubility and charge to these surfaces (*82*).

Mitochondrial membranes would consist of 600 molecules of phospholipids (MW = 800) and 30 protein molecules (MW = 25,000). Considering that the base piece constitutes about 40% of the whole repeating unit, it would contain 6 catalytic protein molecules, 6 structural protein molecules, and 240 molecules of phospholipids. The dimensions of the elementary particle of the mitochondrial internal membrane are shown in Figure 10.9.

Plasma membranes present selective permeability to ions and molecules (*90–95*). This characteristic seems to reflect the tightness of fit between repeating units as well as the nature of functionality along the potential pores or channels. It is believed that metallic ions modify permeability due to the ability to alter the volume, the form, and the size of the operating units, perhaps through interaction with the anionic centers of the phospholipids— and this can induce physical transitions that essentially alter the nature of the membrane. Details on this and related subjects can be found elsewhere (*96–102*).

B. Action of Drugs on Transport Systems

Different drugs act on cellular membranes, modifying their physiological action and producing, as a consequence, pharmacological effects (*12,103*). Studies related to the various mechanisms of drug transport across membranes gave origin to a new scientific field, *transport physiology* or *transport pharmacology* (*104*).

When applied to molecular pharmacology, the mechanism of drug transport across membranes consists essentially of two phases: (a) interaction of a drug with a membrane component in order to form a complex; (b) movement of the complex from one side of the membrane to another, where the drug is liberated in the aqueous medium. In the first phase there come into play covalent, ionic, hydrogen, hydrophobic, and other bonds or interactions, discussed in Chapter 7. This interaction should be very similar to the one that is established between a drug and its receptor, as analyzed in Chapter 6. As to the second phase, various mechanisms have been propounded to explain it: simple diffusion or passive transport, facilitated diffusion, and active transport (*12,37,83,104–106*). Park (*107*) proposed nine mechanisms by which drugs and other substances can cross cell membranes: simple diffusion, solvent drag, diffusion restricted by membrane charge, diffusion restricted by a lipid barrier, facilitated diffusion (or mediated transport), exchange diffusion, active carrier transport, pinocytosis, and phagocytosis. According to Brodie (*108*), there are three ways in which substances can penetrate membranes: simple diffusion, filtration through small pores, and specialized transport systems (active transport and pinocytosis). Kruhøffer (*109*) classified these transport processes into five categories: three passive and two active. The passive ones depend only on the difference of drug concentration across the membrane, and the active ones, on the availability and utilization of cellular energy (Table 10.5). A theory on passive penetration recently presented differs from this concept for it considers that in drug action *speed* is essential and thus steady-state analyses of permeation are inadequate (*110*). The movement of chemical substances across membranes involves various thermodynamic aspects (*111*).

Pharmacological effects produced by certain drugs—such as amethopterin, local anesthetics, cardiotonic glycosides, acetylcholine—can be explained by assuming that they act on transport processes in the cellular and subcellular membrane systems, although it is not always accurate to say that the obtained effects explain their mechanism of action (*1,34*). Thus amethopterin is transported into leucocytes by facilitated diffusion (*112*). The action of acetylcholine results from the nonspecific increase it produces in membrane permeability to cations and perhaps even to anions. The increase in the periods of depolarization and polarization of myocardic membrane potential caused by quinidine is ascribed to its action on the transport of K^+ and possibly Na^+ ions. The cardiotonic glycosides mobilize the cation Ca^{2+} and transport it to the myocardium, where they cause their characteristic action: increase of systolic contraction force and decrease of cardiac rate and of conductivity.

The examples cited above refer to the action of drugs on passive transport

TABLE 10.5   Mechanisms of Passage through Cell Membranes[a] (109)

"Passive"	Simple diffusion—through continuous water phase Activated diffusion—through a nonwater phase	Rate of passage proportional to concentration difference across membrane
	Facilitated diffusion—reversible binding to membrane carrier moving by thermal agitation	
"Active" (transportation immediately dependent upon cellular energy)	Facilitated (propelled) penetration—reversible binding to membrane carrier, the movement of which is accelerated by cellular energy Unidirectional uphill transportation—transportation mechanism undefined, carrier system possibly involved	Rate of passage showing upper limit ("saturable system")

[a] Formation of vacuoles by pinocytosis may be important in some cases of cellular uptake but does not, per se, involve passage through the cell membrane.
Reprinted by permission of the Editor.

systems. Insulin, on the other hand, exerts its effect on the membrane by facilitating the diffusion of hexoses and amino acids in several tissues, for it has the ability of converting cell limitrophe lipoproteins from laminar to micellar forms, creating interstices that allow the passage of these substances (12). Copper ions act by analogous mechanisms: they facilitate the transport of various substances, such as glucose and glycerol.

Several examples can be given of substances transported by an active process: the passage of sugars (113,114), in the presence of sodium (115), across intestinal membranes; the entrance of serotonin into platelets; the incorporation of norepinephrine into the brain and heart (83,105). Ling (116,117) evaluated transport mechanisms critically and gave a mathematical treatment of membrane function. Details of transport mechanisms can be found elsewhere (118–126). With the purpose of obtaining more information on the mechanism of transport across membranes, lately such studies are being conducted on membrane models (89,127–133).

VI. MECHANISM OF ACTION OF STRUCTURALLY NONSPECIFIC DRUGS

The action of structurally nonspecific drugs, such as biological depressors (134,135), a class to which certain hypnotics, the general anesthetics, and the volatile insecticides belong, does not derive from their interaction with specific receptors, some of which were represented and discussed in Chapter 8, but results from their physicochemical properties, such as degree of ionization, solubility, surface tension, and thermodynamic activity (*64*). It seems that their action originates from the accumulation of such drugs at some point of vital importance to the cell, with consequent disorganization of a chain of metabolic processes.

In the specific case of certain hypnotics (homologs of glutarimide), analeptics (pentylenetetrazole, picrotoxin, dimefline) and related drugs, it is proposed that they act by modifying the permeability of synaptic membranes to ions, after binding nonspecifically to the outer protein layer of the membranes (*135*).

The general anesthetics were discussed extensively in Chapter 3.

In short, although it may be inaccurate to state that structurally nonspecific drugs act by a physical mechanism, it is obvious that, by behaving usually as mere foreign substances, they owe their action to the fact of being accumulated in certain body cells, due to some physical property inherent in their chemical structure (*64*).

REFERENCES

1. D. R. H. Gourley, *Progr. Drug Res.*, **7**, 11 (1964).
2. H. G. Mautner, *Pharmacol. Rev.*, **19**, 107 (1967).
3. J. F. Danielli, *Cell Physiology and Pharmacology*, Elsevier, New York, 1950.
4. J. L. Webb, *Enzyme and Metabolic Inhibitors*, 3 vols., Academic, New York, 1963–1966.
5. F. E. Hunter, Jr., and O. H. Lowry, *Pharmacol. Rev.*, **8**, 89 (1956).
6. J. J. Burns and P. A. Shore, *Ann. Rev. Pharmacol.*, **1**, 79 (1961).
7. J. A. Bain and S. E. Mayer, *Ann. Rev. Pharmacol.*, **2**, 37 (1962).
8. E. A. Zeller and J. R. Fouts, *Ann. Rev. Pharmacol.*, **3**, 9 (1963).
9. J. R. Cooper, *Ann. Rev. Pharmacol.*, **4**, 1 (1964).
10. F. Buffoni, *Pharmacol. Rev.*, **18**, 1163 (1966).
11. A. Horita and L. J. Weber, *Ann. Rep. Med. Chem.*, **3**, 252 (1968).
12. J. L. Mongar and A. V. S. de Reuck, Eds., *Enzymes and Drug Action*, Churchill, London, 1962.
13. R. M. Hochster and J. H. Quastel, Eds., *Metabolic Inhibitors—A Comprehensive Treatise*, 2 vols., Academic, New York, 1963.
14. P. A. E. Desnuelle, Ed., *Molecular Basis of Enzyme Action and Inhibition*, Pergamon, Oxford, 1963.
15. M. Dixon and E. C. Webb, *Enzymes*, 2nd ed., Academic, New York, 1964.
16. B. B. Brodie and J. R. Gillette, Eds., *Drugs and Enzymes*, Pergamon, Oxford, 1965.
17. B. G. Malmström and A. Rosenberg, *Advan. Enzymology*, **21**, 131 (1959).
18. H. Passow, A. Rothstein, and T. W. Clarkson, *Pharmacol. Rev.*, **13**, 185 (1961).

19. N. Gavrilescu and R. A. Peters, *Biochem. J.*, **25**, 2150 (1931).

20. R. A. Peters, *Biochemical Lesions and Lethal Synthesis*, Pergamon, Oxford, 1963.

21. J. Cheymol, *Actualités Pharmacol.*, **7**, 35 (1954).

22. E. A. Zeller, Ed., "Amine Oxidase Inhibitors," *Ann. N. Y. Acad. Sci.*, **80**, 551–1045 (1959).

23. T. H. Maren, *Physiol. Rev.*, **47**, 595 (1967).

24. B. A. Newton, *Ann. Rev. Microbiol.*, **19**, 209 (1965).

25. I. H. Goldberg, *Am. J. Med.*, **39**, 722 (1965).

26. W. Carter and K. S. McCarty, *Ann. Int. Med.*, **64**, 1087 (1966).

27. D. Gottlieb and P. D. Shaw, Eds., *Antibiotics I, Mechanism of Action*, Springer, New York, 1967.

28. H. J. Rogers, "The Mode of Action of Antibiotics," in E. E. Bittar, Ed., *The Biological Basis of Medicine*, Vol. II, Academic, London, 1968, pp. 421–448.

29. B. Weisblum and J. Davies, *Bacteriol. Rev.*, **32**, 493 (1968).

30. J. B. Neilands and P. K. Stumpf, *Outlines of Enzyme Chemistry*, 2nd ed., Wiley, New York, 1958.

31. H. R. Mahler and E. H. Cordes, *Biological Chemistry*, Harper and Row, New York, 1966.

32. W. P. Jencks, *Ann. Rev. Biochem.*, **32**, 639 (1963).

33. S. G. Waley, *Quart. Rev.*, **21**, 379 (1967).

34. W. C. Holland, R. L. Klein, and A. H. Briggs, *Introduction to Molecular Pharmacology*, Macmillan, New York, 1964.

35. H. Lineweaver and D. Burk, *J. Am. Chem. Soc.*, **56**, 658 (1934).

36. E. R. Stadtman, *Advan. Enzymol.*, **28**, 41 (1966).

37. J. Monod, J.-P. Changeux, and F. Jacob, *J. Mol. Biol.*, **6**, 306 (1963).

38. H. Muirhead and M. F. Perutz, *Nature*, **199**, 633 (1963).

39. J. C. Gerhart and H. K. Schachman, *Biochemistry*, **4**, 1054 (1965).

40. P. Nicholls, "Cytochrome Oxidase as an Allosteric Enzyme," in K. Okunuki, M. D. Kamen, and I. Sekuzu, Eds., *Structure and Function of Cytochromes*, University of Tokyo Press, Tokyo, 1968, pp. 76–88.

41. D. E. Koshland, Jr., *Advan. Enzymol.*, **22**, 45 (1960).

42. C. Cennamo, *J. Theoret. Biol.*, **21**, 260 (1968).

43. N. O. Kaplan and M. Friedkin, *Advan. Chemother.*, **1**, 499 (1964).

44. J. Monod, J. Wyman, and J.-P. Changeux, *J. Mol. Biol.*, **12**, 88 (1965).

45. K. Yagi, *Advan. Enzymol.*, **27**, 1 (1965).

46. K. Paigen, *Cancer Res.*, **22**, 1290 (1962).

47. G. J. Martin, *Biological Antagonism*, Blakiston, New York, 1951.

48. C. Kaiser, "Metabolite Antagonism," in A. Burger, Ed., *Medicinal Chemistry*, 2nd ed., Interscience, New York, 1960, pp. 89–132.

49. D. W. Woolley, *Advan. Enzymol.*, **6**, 129 (1946).

50. D. W. Woolley, *Progr. Drug Res.*, **2**, 613 (1960).

51. Eighth Symposium of the Society for General Microbiology, *The Strategy of Chemotherapy*, University Press, Cambridge, 1958.

52. R. Knox, "Strategy and Tactics in Antibacterial Chemotherapy," in R. J. Schnitzer and F. Hawking, Eds., *Experimental Chemotherapy*, Vol. II, Academic, New York, 1964, pp. 79–112.

53. L. G. Goodwin and R. H. Nimmo-Smith, Eds., *Drugs, Parasites and Hosts*, Little, Brown, Boston, 1962.

54. T. E. Mansour, *Advan. Pharmacol.*, **3**, 129 (1964).

55. T. von Brand, *Biochemistry of Parasites*, Academic, New York, 1966.

56. M. Florkin and B. T. Scheer, Eds., *Chemical Zoology*, 4 vols., Academic, New York, 1967–1969.

57. D. D. Woods and P. Fildes, *Chem. Ind.*, (*London*), **59**, 133 (1940).

58. R. J. Schnitzer and F. Hawking, Eds., *Experimental Chemotherapy*, 5 vols., Academic, New York, 1963–1968.

59. G. H. Hitchings and J. J. Burchall, *Advan. Enzymol.*, **27**, 417 (1965).

60. C. Mentzer, *Actualités Pharmacol.*, **7**, 173 (1954).

61. R. O. Roblin, Jr., *Ann. Rev. Biochem.*, **23**, 501 (1954).

62. E. P. Abraham, "The Antibiotics," in M. Florkin and E. H. Stotz, Eds., *Comprehensive Biochemistry*, Vol. XI, Elsevier, Amsterdam, 1963, pp. 181–224.

63. H. Busch and M. Lane, *Chemotherapy*, Year Book, Chicago, 1967.

64. A. Albert, *Selective Toxicity*, 4th ed., Methuen, London, 1968.

65. L. Fowden, D. Lewis, and H. Tristram, *Advan. Enzymol.*, **29**, 89 (1967).

66. A. Eyquem, *Antibiot. Chemother.*, (*Basel*), **5**, 165 (1958).

67. J. F. Henderson and H. G. Mandel, *Advan. Pharmacol.*, **2**, 297 (1963).

68. G. B. Elion and G. H. Hitchings, *Advan. Chemother.*, **2**, 91 (1965).

69. C. Heildelberger, *Ann. Rev. Pharmacol.*, **7**, 101 (1967).

70. G. M. Timmis and D. C. Williams, *Chemotherapy of Cancer: the Antimetabolite Approach*, Butterworths, London, 1967.

71. G. P. Warwick, *Rev. Pure Appl. Chem.*, **18**, 245 (1968).

72. M. B. Chenoweth, *Pharmacol. Rev.*, **8**, 57 (1956).

73. A. E. Martell and M. Calvin, *Chemistry of the Metal Chelates Compounds*, Prentice-Hall, New York, 1952.

74. F. P. Dwyer and D. P. Mellor, *Chelating Agents and Metal Chelates*, Academic, New York, 1964.

75. R. L. Smith, *The Sequestration of Metals*, Chapman and Hall, London, 1959.

76. S. Chaberek and A. E. Martell, *Organic Sequestering Agents*, Wiley, New York, 1959.

77. J. F. Fredrick, Ed., "Chelation Phenomena," *Ann. N.Y. Acad. Sci.*, **88**, 281–531 (1960).

78. W. O. Foye, *J. Pharm. Sci.*, **50**, 93 (1961).

79. J. Schubert, *Sci. Am.*, **214**, (5), 40 (1966).

80. M. B. Chenoweth, *Clin. Pharmacol. Therap.*, **9**, 365 (1968).

81. D. E. Green and J. F. Perdue, *Proc. Natl. Acad. Sci. U.S.*, **55**, 1295 (1966).

82. D. E. Green and R. F. Goldberger, *Molecular Insights into the Living Process*, Academic, New York, 1967.

83. L. Bolis, V. Capraro, K. R. Porter, and J. D. Robertson, Eds., *Symposium on Biophysics and Physiology of Biological Transport*, Springer, Wien, 1967.

84. D. H. Northcote, Ed., "Structure and Function of Membranes," *Brit. Med. Bull.*, **24**, 99–182 (1968).

85. R. W. Hendler, *Protein Biosynthesis and Membrane Biochemistry*, Wiley, New York, 1968.

86. E. D. Korn, *J. Gen. Physiol.*, **52**, 257s (1968).
87. L. Rothfield and A. Finkelstein, *Ann. Rev. Biochem.*, **37**, 463 (1968).
88. R. M. Dowben, Ed., *Biological Membranes*, Little, Brown, Boston, 1969.
89. W. Stoffel, *Arzneimittel-Forsch.*, **19**, 253 (1969).
90. H. Kimizuka, *J. Theoret. Biol.*, **13**, 145 (1966).
91. Physiology Society Symposium on "Ionic Permeability of Synaptic and Non-synaptic Membranes," *Federation Proc.*, **26**, 1612–1663 (1967).
92. E. Schoffeniels, *Cellular Aspects of Membrane Permeability*, Pergamon, Oxford, 1967.
93. J. S. Charnock and L. J. Opit, "Membrane Metabolism and Ion Transport," in E. E. Bittar, Ed., *The Biological Basis of Medicine*, Vol. I, Academic, London, 1968, pp. 69–103.
94. K. S. Cole, *Membranes, Ions and Impulses*, University of California Press, Berkeley, 1968.
95. P. Läuger, *Angew. Chem., Intern. Ed.*, **8**, 42 (1969).
96. J. L. Kavanau, *Structure and Function in Biological Membranes*, 2 vols., Holden-Day, San Francisco, 1965.
97. J. B. Finean, *Progr. Biophys. Mol. Biol.*, **16**, 143 (1966).
98. P. Mitchell, *Advan. Enzymol.*, **29**, 33 (1967).
99. B. D. Davis and L. Warren, Eds., *The Specificity of Cell Surfaces*, Prentice-Hall, Englewood Cliffs, N.J., 1967.
100. H. J. Rogers and H. R. Perkins, *Cell Walls and Membranes*, Spon, London, 1968.
101. E. D. Korn, "Biological Membranes," in A. Cole, Ed., *Theoretical and Experimental Biophysics*, Vol. II, Dekker, New York, 1969, pp. 1–67.
102. J. M. Diamond and E. M. Wright, *Ann. Rev. Physiol.*, **31**, 581 (1969).
103. W. R. Loewenstein, Ed., "Biological Membranes: Recent Progress," *Ann. N.Y. Acad. Sci.*, **137**, 403–1048 (1966).
104. W. Wilbrandt and T. Rosenberg, *Pharmacol. Rev.*, **13**, 109 (1961).
105. D. B. Tower, S. A. Luse, and H. Grundfest, *Properties of Membranes and Diseases of the Nervous System*, Springer, New York, 1962.
106. R. Coleman and J. B. Finean, "The Cell-Surface Membrane," in M. Florkin and E. H. Stotz, Eds., *Comprehensive Biochemistry*, Vol. XXIII, Elsevier, Amsterdam, 1968, pp. 99–126.
107. C. R. Park, "Introduction," in A. Kleinzeller and A. Kotyk, Eds., *Membrane Transport and Metabolism*, Academic, London, 1961, pp. 19–21.
108. B. B. Brodie, "Physico-Chemical Factors in Drug Absorption," in T. B. Binns, Ed., *Absorption and Distribution of Drugs*, Livingstone, Edinburgh, 1964, pp. 16–48.
109. P. Kruhøffer, *J. Pharm. Pharmacol.*, **13**, 193 (1961).
110. J. T. Penniston, L. Beckett, D. L. Bentley, and C. Hansch, *Mol. Pharmacol.*, **5**, 333 (1969).
111. A. Katchalsky, *Pure Appl. Chem.*, **16**, 229 (1968).
112. D. Kessel and T. C. Hall, *Biochem. Pharmacol.*, **16**, 2395 (1967).
113. D. H. Smyth and R. Whittam, *Brit. Med. Bull.*, **23**, 231 (1967).
114. W. F. Caspary and R. K. Crane, *Biochim. Biophys. Acta*, **163**, 395 (1968).
115. R. K. Crane, *Federation Proc.*, **24**, 1000 (1965).
116. G. N. Ling, *Ann. N.Y. Acad. Sci.*, **125**, 401 (1965).

117. G. N. Ling, *Federation Proc.*, **25**, 958 (1966).

118. E. J. Harris, *Transport and Accumulation in Biological Systems*, 2nd ed., Academic, New York, 1960.

119. A. M. Shanes, Ed., *Biophysics of Physiological and Pharmacological Actions*, American Association for the Advancement of Science, Washington, D.C., 1961.

120. A. Kleinzeller and A. Kotyk, Eds., *Membrane Transport and Metabolism*, Academic, London, 1961.

121. J. F. Hoffman, Ed., *The Cellular Functions of Membrane Transport*, Prentice-Hall, Englewood Cliffs, N.J., 1964.

122. T. B. Binns, Ed., *Absorption and Distribution of Drugs*, Livingstone, Edinburgh, 1964.

123. W. D. Stein, *The Movement of Molecules Across Cell Membranes*, Academic, New York, 1967.

124. E. Heinz, *Ann. Rev. Physiol.*, **29**, 21 (1967).

125. L. Gross, *J. Theoret. Biol.*, **15**, 298 (1967).

126. A. Rothstein, *Ann. Rev. Physiol.*, **30**, 15 (1968).

127. P. Mueller, D. O. Rudin, H. Ti Tien, and W. C. Wescott, "Formation and Properties of Bimolecular Lipid Membranes," in J. F. Danielli, K. G. A. Pankhurst, and A. C. Riddiford, Eds., *Recent Progress in Surface Science*, Vol. I, Academic, New York, 1964, pp. 379–393.

128. C. Huang, L. Wheeldon, and T. E. Thompson, *J. Mol. Biol.*, **8**, 148 (1964).

129. T. E. Andreoli, M. Tieffenberg, and D. C. Tosteson, *J. Gen. Physiol.*, **50**, 2527 (1967).

130. L. Bolis and B. A. Pethica, Eds., *Membrane Models and the Formation of Biological Membranes*, North-Holland, Amsterdam, 1968.

131. P. Mueller, and D. O. Rudin, *J. Theoret. Biol.*, **18**, 222 (1968).

132. L. Finkelstein and A. Cass, *J. Gen. Physiol.*, **52**, 145s (1968).

133. A. D. Bangham, *Progr. Biophys. Mol. Biol.*, **18**, 29 (1968).

134. W. S. Root and F. G. Hofmann, Eds., *Physiological Pharmacology*, Vol. I, Academic, New York, 1963.

135. A. Shulman, G. M. Laycock, and A. S. Buchanan, "A Molecular Basis for the Action of Certain Drugs in the Central Nervous System," in E. J. Ariëns, Ed., *Physico-Chemical Aspects of Drug Action*, Pergamon, Oxford, 1968, pp. 355–375.

SUBJECT INDEX